Health Communication
Research Measures

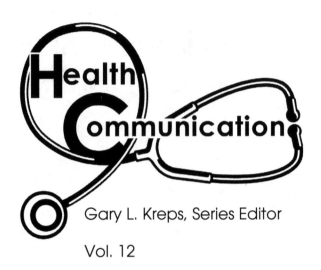

Gary L. Kreps, Series Editor

Vol. 12

The Health Communication series is part of
the Peter Lang Media and Communication list.
Every volume is peer reviewed and meets
the highest quality standards for content and production.

PETER LANG
New York • Bern • Frankfurt • Berlin
Brussels • Vienna • Oxford • Warsaw

Health Communication Research Measures

Edited by DO KYUN KIM and JAMES W. DEARING

PETER LANG
New York • Bern • Frankfurt • Berlin
Brussels • Vienna • Oxford • Warsaw

Library of Congress Cataloging-in-Publication Data
Health communication research measures /
edited by Do Kyun Kim, James W. Dearing.
P. ;cm. — (Health communication; vol. 12)
[DNLM: 1. Health Communication. 2. Research. WA 590]
I. Kim, Do Kyun, editor. II. Dearing, James W., editor.
III. Series: Health communication (New York, N.Y.); v. 12.
R118   610.1'4—dc23   2015023828
ISBN 978-1-4331-2903-2 (hardcover)
ISBN 978-1-4331-2902-5 (paperback)
ISBN 978-1-4539-1682-7 (e-book)
ISSN 2153-1277

Bibliographic information published by **Die Deutsche Nationalbibliothek**.
Die Deutsche Nationalbibliothek lists this publication in the "Deutsche
Nationalbibliografie"; detailed bibliographic data are available
on the Internet at http://dnb.d-nb.de/.

Cover image: ©iStock.com/stevecoleimages

© 2016 Do Kyun Kim and James W. Dearing
Peter Lang Publishing, Inc., New York
29 Broadway, 18th floor, New York, NY 10006
www.peterlang.com

Printed in the United States of America

Contents

Introduction

Social science theorists have long envisioned how social scientists could organize so that the knowledge borne from our work might contribute to the improvement of both science and society (Campbell, 1971; Cronbach, 1982). Such aspiration requires that researchers understand what their forefathers did before them and with what results so that we may incrementally improve (Merton, 1965). In the health promotion field, progress in this direction has occurred, for example, through the production of consensus statements about standards of evidence (Flay et al., 2005).

Alas, the challenge of learning incrementally and cumulatively from others' work is daunting. Not only are we limited in terms of how much each of us can know (Simon, 1955), but the expansion of scientific knowledge continues unabated. We publish our results in more journals than ever before and increasingly cite others' work that appears in new and far flung journals (Acharya et al., 2014). If modern society can be thought of as an information processor, then it is at present an increasingly decentralized one.

Researchers and policy makers who attend to issues of research measurement have attempted to coalesce what we know. For certain measures, compendiums exist of their validity, reliability, long and short forms, and adaptations to suit particular applications or topics, along with examples for how to use them and interpret results (Kiresuk, Smith, & Cardillo, 1994) Online resources such as the Measurement Instrument Database for the Social Sciences do not as of yet cover much of relevance to the scholar of health communication. Other online resources such as the Grid-Enabled Measures portal sponsored by the U.S. National Cancer Institute list many measures (834 as of April 2015) but very few concern communication.

The present book is a modest effort to better share what is known about health communication research measures in a format that is accessible and will be used. Ours is not a comprehensive collection. Other measures could well be included. Nor is this an especially broad perspective since we focus on quantitative measures that are suited to survey research. Yet we submit that the measures included here are centrally important to the study of health communication whether one's academic home is public health, health services research, or communication science. These measures do well by the standards of scale development (DeVellis, 2003) though for most of these topics what you have in your hands is a living literature that will continue to evolve. What the chapters herein represent are up-to-date reports about key social science constructs and ways of measuring them, whether your interest is in patient-provider dyadic communication, uncertainty management, self-efficacy, disclosure, social norms, social support, risk perception, health care team performance, message design and effects, health and numerical literacy, communication satisfaction, social influence and persuasion, stigma, health campaigns, reactance, or other topics. We thank the chapter authors for summarizing their own work and that of others in brief, informative, and illustrative accounts. They have done a terrific job.

Do Kyun Kim
Lafayette, Louisiana

James W. Dearing
East Lansing, Michigan

Acharya, A., Verstak, A., Suzuki, H., Henderson, S., Iakhiaev, M., Lin, C., & Shetty, N. (2014). Rise of the rest: The growing impact of non-elite journals. Nonpublished paper. October 9. Google Inc.

Campbell, D. T. (1971). Methods for the experimenting society. Paper presented at the meeting of the American Psychological Association. Washington DC.

Cronbach, L.J. (1982). *Designing evaluations of educational and social programs.* San Francisco: Jossey-Bass.

DeVellis, R. F. (2003). *Scale development: Theory and applications.* Second edition. Thousand Oaks, CA: Sage.

Flay, B. R., Biglan, A., Boruch, R. F., Gonzalez Castro, F., Gottfredson, D., Kellam, S., Moscicki, E. K., Schinke, S., Valentine, J. C., & Ji, P. (2005). Standards of evidence: Criteria for efficacy, effectiveness and dissemination. *Prevention Science, 6,* 151–175.

Kiresuk, T. J., Smith, A., & Cardillo, J. E. (1994). *Goal attainment scaling: Applications, theory, and measurement.* Hillsdale, NJ: Lawrence Erlbaum.

Merton, R. K. (1965). *On the shoulders of giants.* New York: Free Press.

Simon, H. A. (1955). A behavioral model of rational choice. *Journal of Economics, 69,* 99–118.

1. *Communication Competence*

JOHN BANAS,
University of Oklahoma
& DANIEL R. BERNARD,
California State University, Fresno

In his book *Blink*, Gladwell (2005) informs readers that the best predictor of malpractice lawsuits is not, in fact, the degree to which a doctor erred in performing her or his duties but rather the quality of the doctor-patient interaction as perceived by the patient. This example is typical of Gladwell's writing in several ways: it distills a great deal of research into a pithy and memorable factoid, it presents an empirical reality that is counterintuitive to readers, and it elevates a research area to new importance.

As counterintuitive as the above example might be for many, scholars of health communication have long recognized the importance of knowledge and skill regarding effective and appropriate communication, which taken together form the construct of communication competence. Indeed, health and interpersonal communication researchers have long championed the importance of communication competence for mental, physical, and emotional health outcomes. In their *Handbook of Interpersonal Competence Research*, Spitzberg and Cupach (1989) reviewed research that found people who lack communicative competence to be at increased risk for a variety of negative health outcomes, including: anxiety, depression, hypertension, loneliness, premature mortality, therapeutic outcomes, low self-esteem, and suicide.

Researchers have examined health and communication competence in a variety of ways. Scholars have looked at the predictors of competence, the outcomes of communication competence, as well as how competence is interdependent with other variables in health processes. Examples of research include how communication competence influences health outcomes (such as stress and burnout among health care workers), or how perceptions of competence affect health care encounters (such as how patient and physician competence shape primary care medical interviews).

Kreps' (1988) Relational Health Communication Competence Model (RHCCM) demonstrates how communication competence can be a central construct in health communication research. The RHCCM is a theoretical framework that explicitly recognizes the centrality of communication competence for understanding interdependent communication roles in health care. It is through communication competence that people can accomplish instrumental tasks, such as convincing people to perform actions or providing corrective feedback after a poor performance, while also maintaining interpersonal relationships. The RHCCM predicts that high levels of communication competence lead to "therapeutic communication, social support, satisfaction, information exchange, and cooperation," whereas poor communication competence leads to "pathological communication, lack of social support, dissatisfaction, information barriers, and lack of cooperation" (Kreps, 1988, p. 354).

The field of communication has a longstanding interest in competence, leading to several separate definitions and measures of the construct. Although the current page limit makes discussing all of the definitions impossible, the present chapter presents three scales, Wiemann's (1977) communicative competence scale, Spitzberg's (2007) Conversational Skill Rating Scale (CSRS), and Guerrero's (1994) Communication Competence Scale. These three scales have been used in contemporary health communication studies, and they offer different approaches to the measurement of perceived communication competence.

Measuring Communication Competence

Attempting to consolidate the cognitive and behavioral perspectives (which produced overlapping and occasionally contradictory definitions) regarding communication competence into one multi-dimensional scale, Wiemann (1977) explained communicative competence as other-oriented communication that is also successful in accomplishing the goals of the speaker. Specifically he described it as "the ability of an interactant to choose among available communication behaviors in order that he (she) may accomplish his (her) own interpersonal goals during an encounter while maintaining the face and line of his (her) fellow interactants within the constraints of the situation" (p. 198). This description underscores the self-presentation theoretical underpinnings of Wiemann's scale.

Communicative competence is conceptualized as a plurality of communication behaviors that include empathy, affiliation, behavioral flexibility, relaxation, and interaction management (Wiemann, 1977; Wiemann &

Backlund, 1980). *Interaction management* was originally labeled "general competence" and describes the smooth synchronization of turn-taking among interactants. *Empathy* describes concern for others' feelings and the ability to understand others. *Affiliation* describes general likeability and listening skill. *Behavioral flexibility* is a measure of rigidity and a person's ability to adapt to changing situations. *Relaxation* is how comfortable a person is with communication and interacting with new people.

Wiemann (1977) tested 57 Likert-type items and eventually retained 36 (see Table 1). The scale can be used for both self-report or for evaluating others. As a whole, the reliabilities of the scale are quite good, with recent studies reporting Cronbach's alphas ranging from .87 (Wright, Rosenberg, Egbert, Ploeger, Bernard, & King, 2013) to .97 (McKinley & Perino, 2013). Wright, Banas, Bessarabova, and Bernard (2010) reported reliabilities for each of the subscales, revealing adequate reliabilities: interaction management (Cronbach's α = .70), affiliation (Cronbach's α = .68), empathy (Cronbach's α = .74), social relaxation (Cronbach's α = .72), and behavioral flexibility (Cronbach's α = .69).

Although Wiemann (1977) and Wiemann and Backlund (1980) explicated five clear dimensions about communication competence, the factor structure of the scale was problematic from the start. Indeed, Wiemann's initial investigation only revealed four dimensions, and many of the items loaded on factors that were inconsistent with theoretical predictions. Despite these problems with fitting the theorized factor structure with the original data, a more recent study by Wright, Banas et al. (2010) found support for the theorized five-factor measurement model. It should be noted that Wright, Banas et al. only used 27 of the 36 items as 9 items were dropped to improve the reliability and fit of the structural equation model that was tested in their study (the 27 items are marked with an asterisk below). The factor loadings were quite good, ranging from .59 to .85.

Table 1. Communicative Competence Scale (CCS; Wiemann, 1977).

Interaction Management (Originally General Competence)
1. I find it easy to get along with others.*
2. I am "rewarding" to talk to.*
3. I can deal with others effectively.*
4. I do not mind meeting strangers.*
5. I generally say the right thing at the right time.*
6. I interrupt others too much. (R)
7. I am easy to talk to.

Interaction Management (Originally General Competence)

8. My conversation behavior is not "smooth." (R)

9. I am an effective conversationalist.

10. I don't follow the conversation very well. (R)

11. I pay attention to the conversation.

Affiliation

1. I am a good listener.*

2. My personal relations are cold and distant.* (R)

3. I like to be close and personal with people.*

4. I am supportive of others.*

5. I am a likeable person.*

6. People can go to me with their problems.*

7. I am interested in what others have to say.

Empathy

1. I ignore other people's feelings.* (R)

2. I generally know how others feel.*

3. I let others know I understand them.*

4. I understand other people.*

5. I listen to what people say to me.*

6. I can easily put myself in another person's shoes.*

7. I won't argue with someone just to prove I am right.

8. I usually do not make unusual demands on my friends.

Social Relaxation

1. I am relaxed and comfortable when speaking.*

2. I am generally relaxed when conversing with a new acquaintance.*

3. I enjoy social gatherings where I can meet new people.*

4. I am not afraid to speak with people in authority.*

5. I like to use my voice and body expressively.*

Behavioral Flexibility

1. I can adapt to changing situations.*

2. I treat people as individuals.*

Behavioral Flexibility

3. I generally know what type of behavior is appropriate in any given situation.*

4. I am flexible.*

5. I am sensitive to others' needs of the moment.*

(Items with (R) are reverse coded.)

In a recent study of communication competence, social support, and depression of college students comparing Facebook and face-to-face support networks, Wright et al. (2013) used Wiemann's (1977) CSS but treated it as a unidimensional scale instead of a multi-dimensional one labeled interpersonal competence. The reliability was good (α = .85).

In addition to Wiemann's scale, Spitzberg (2007) developed the Conversational Skills Rating Scale (CSRS). Spitzberg and colleagues have been researching communication competence for a great deal of time. Although the CSRS has primarily been associated with pedagogical purposes, Spitzberg notes that it was designed for a wide range of research applications. One of the features that distinguish the scale is the focus on conversational skills: "CSRS was developed to provide a subjectively based, yet relatively specific, assessment of the skills component of conversational interaction" (2007, p. 4).

The CSRS has been widely studied, including research related to health communication. An early application of the scale was used to examine the connection between interpersonal competence and loneliness over time (Spitzberg & Hurt, 1987b). More recently, Spitzberg and Cupach (2002) outlined several psychological and physiological health contexts related to interpersonal competence. Specifically, Spitzberg and Cupach suggested that lacking interpersonal competence may exacerbate existing health conditions because these individuals are likely unable to marshal social resources for support.

The CSRS (Table 2) is comprised of 25 molecular items and 5 molar items. The molecular items measure specific conversational behaviors that comprise conversational competence and molar items measure general perceptions of competence. The CSRS is subdivided into four clusters: *attentiveness* (i.e., other-orientation), *composure* (i.e., calmness, confidence), *expressiveness* (e.g., facial and vocal), and *coordination* (i.e., controlling the flow of the conversation, or interaction management). The 25 molecular items are measured on a 5-point, Likert-type scale (1 = Inadequate, 2 = Fair 3 = Adequate, 4 = Good, 5 = Excellent). The 5 molar items are measured on a seven-point, semantic-differential scale. The order of the items have been re-sequenced since the scale was first posited (Spitzberg and Hurt, 1987a) so that behaviors considered immediately apparent are listed first and more subtle items are listed later (Spitzberg, 2007). The CSRS can be used to measure self, other, and third person assessment of competence. Although the factor structure has varied some across different contexts, Spitzberg (2007) argues that, "in terms of validity, it has generally produced validity coefficients in the expected direction and of reasonable magnitude" (p. 18). Internal consistency has consistently been over .80, and is usually in the high .80s to low .90s.

Table 2. Conversational Skills Rating Scale (CSRS; Spitzberg, 2007).

(CSRS Molecular items)
1. Speaking rate (neither too slow nor too fast)
2. Speaking fluency (pauses, silences, "uh", etc.)
3. Vocal confidence (neither too tense/nervous nor overly confident sounding)
4. Articulation (clarity of pronunciation and linguistic expression)
5. Vocal variety (neither overly monotone nor dramatic voice)
6. Volume (neither too loud nor too soft)
7. Posture (neither too closed/formal nor too open/informal)
8. Lean toward partner (neither too forward nor too far back)
9. Shaking or nervous twitches (aren't noticeable or distracting)
10. Unmotivated movements (tapping feet, fingers, hair-twirling, etc.)
11. Facial expressiveness (neither blank nor exaggerated)
12. Nodding of head in response to partner statements
13. Use of gestures to emphasize what is being said
14. Use of humor and/or stories
15. Smiling and/or laughing
16. Use of eye contact
17. Asking of questions
18. Speaking about partner (involvement of partner as a topic of conversation)
19. Speaking about self (neither too much nor too little)
20. Encouragements or agreements (encouragement of partner to talk)
21. Personal opinion expression (neither too passive nor too aggressive)

(CSRS Molecular items)
22. Initiation of new topics
23. Maintenance of topic and follow-up comments
24. Interruption of partner speaking turns
25. Use of time speaking relative to partner

Attentiveness = 8,12,18,19,20,21
Composure = 2,3,6,7,9,10
Expressiveness = 4,5,11,13,14,15,16
Coordination = 1,17,22,23,24,25

(CSRS Molar items: semantic differential)
1. Poor Conversationalist/Good Conversationalist
2. Socially Unskilled/Socially Skilled
3. Incompetent Communicator/Competent Communicator
4. Inappropriate Communicator/Appropriate Communicator
5. Ineffective Communicator/Effective Communicator

Similar to the molar items of Spitzberg's CSRS, Guerrero's (1994) Communication Competence Scale uses items that "were chosen to represent broad, global perceptions of communication competence and to tap social skill, effectiveness, and appropriateness" (p. 139). Whereas the molar items of the CSRS balance the 25 molecular items with very global assessment, Guerrero's scale attempts to capture global perceptions of all communication competence in 6 items. The scale development is quite different from the previous two scales described as Guerrero's simply borrowed items from previous scales and created a new measure. As such, there are no formal tests of validity; however, she found the measure to be reliable (Alpha reliability of .74). The scale has been successfully utilized in health communication research, as Schrodt (2006) successfully adapted her scale in his study of communication competence and health in stepchildren. He found stepfamily types "predict meaningful differences in stepchildren's perceptions of communication competence for stepfamily members, but the results also revealed a small, but meaningful and consistent trend in stepchildren's mental health" (p. 327). Alpha coefficients for the scale were .70 for self-reports, .86 for mothers, .82 for fathers, and .86 for stepparents.

Table 3. Guerrero's (1994) Communication Competence Scale.

1.	I am (my partner is) a good communicator
2.	I am (my partner is) a good listener
3.	I do *not* (my partner does *not*) solve problems effectively (R)
4.	My (my partner's) communication is usually appropriate to the situation at hand
5.	I have (my partner has) a wide variety of social skills
6.	It is hard for me (my partner) to communication (her/his) feeling clearly (R)

(Items with (R) are reverse coded.)

Use of Existing Measures and Future Studies

This chapter reviewed three scales commonly used in contemporary health communication scholarship. The first two scales, Wiemann's (1977) communicative competence scale (CCS) and Spitzberg's (2007) Conversational Skills Rating Scale (CSRS), are multi-dimensional, whereas Guerrero's (1994) communication competence scale is a brief six items designed to measure competence in a global and unidimensional manner. All three scales are easily adapted to measure self- versus other-reports.

Our goal for this chapter was to present health researchers with several options for measuring communication competence. Those interested in a rigorously tested scale that measures specific behavioral manifestations of conversational competence may prefer Spitzberg's CSRS. Those informed by Kreps' theoretical model of communication competence may benefit from Wiemann's approach. Last, those worried about respondent fatigue or interested in a global unidimensional construct of communication competence may prefer Guerrero's scale.

Finally, although there is widespread recognition about the importance of communication competence, there has not been a recent attempt to systematically examine the various measures of competence. One fruitful approach in this direction would be to simultaneously compare existing scales to be able to ascertain their explanatory and/or predictive power, factor structure, and adequacy of fit. Furthermore, comparing existing scales (and potentially modifying and/or combining scale items) would answer the question about whether context-based competence measures (e.g., computer-mediated communication competence) outperform more general competence measures that could easily be adapted to fit particular contexts.

Recommended Readings

McKinley, C. J., & Perino, C. (2013). Examining communication competence as a contributing factor in health care workers' job satisfaction and tendency to report errors. *Journal of Communication in Healthcare, 6,* 158–165.

McManus, T. G., & Donovan, S. (2012). Communication competence and feeling caught: Explaining perceived ambiguity in divorce-related communication. *Communication Quarterly, 60,* 255–277.

Morreale, S., Staley, C., Stavrositu, C., & Krakowiak, M. (2015). First-year college students' attitudes toward communication technologies and their perceptions of communication competence in the 21st century. *Communication Education, 64,* 107–131.

Robbins, S. A., & Merrill, A. F. (2014). Understanding posttransgressional relationship closeness: The roles of perceived severity, rumination, and communication competence. *Communication Research Reports, 31,* 23–32.

References

Gladwell, M. (2005). *Blink: The power of thinking without thinking.* New York: Little, Brown, and Co.

Guerrero, L. K. (1994). "I'm so mad I could scream:" The effects of anger expression on relational satisfaction and communication competence. *Southern Journal of Communication, 59*(2), 125–141. doi: 10.1080/10417949409372931.

Kreps, G. L. (1988). Relational communication in health care. *Southern Speech Communication Journal, 53,* 344–359. doi: 10.1080/10417948809372736.

McKinley, C. J., & Perino, C. (2013). Examining communication competence as a contributing factor in health care workers' job satisfaction and tendency to report errors. *Journal of Communication in Healthcare, 6,* 158–165. doi: 10.1179/1753807613Y.0000000039.

Schrodt, P. (2006). A typological examination of communication competence and mental health in stepchildren. *Communication Monographs, 73,* 309–333. doi: 10.1080/03637750600873728.

Spitzberg, B. H. (2007). CSRS, the Conversational Skills Rating Scale: An instructional assessment of interpersonal competence. In *Conversational Skills Rating Scale: An Instructional Assessment of Interpersonal Competence* (pp. i–53). National Communication Association.

Spitzberg, B. H., & Cupach, W. R. (1989). *Handbook of Interpersonal Competence.* New York: Springer-Verlag.

Spitzberg, B. H., & Cupach, W. R. (2002). Interpersonal skills. In M. L. Knapp & J. R. Daly (Eds.), *Handbook of interpersonal communication* (3rd ed., pp. 564–611). Newbury Park, CA: Sage.

Spitzberg, B. H., & Hurt, H. T. (1987a). The measurement of interpersonal skills in instructional contexts. *Communication Education, 36,* 28–45.

Spitzberg, B. H., & Hurt, H. T. (1987b). The relationship of interpersonal competence and skills to reported loneliness across time. *Journal of Social Behavior and Personality, 2* (No. 2, Part 2), 157–172.

Wiemann, J. M. (1977). Explication and test of a model of communicative competence. *Human Communication Research, 3*(3), 195–213. doi: 10.1111/j.1468-2958.1977. tb00518.x.

Wiemann, J. M., & Backlund, P. (1980). Current theory and research in communicative competence. *Review of Educational Research, 50*(1), 185–199. doi: 10.3102/00346543050001185.

Wright, K., Banas, J. A, Bessarabova, E., & Bernard, D. R. (2010). Healthcare worker burnout: An initial analysis of a structural equation model. *Health Communication, 25*,1–8. doi: 10.1080/10410231003775206.

Wright, K., Rosenberg, J., Egbert, N., Ploeger, N. A., Bernard, D. R., & King, S. (2013). Communication competence, social support, and depression among college students: A model of facebook and face-to-face support network influence. *Journal of Health Communication, 18,* 41–57. doi: 10.1080/10810730.2012.688250.

2. Disclosure

KATHRYN GREENE,
Rutgers University
& AMANDA CARPENTER,
Rutgers University

Disclosure is an expanding area of health communication research. Sharing information is important for how patients experience and manage illness. Research examines disclosure to providers, in personal relationships (e.g., partners or family), and in social networks (e.g., friends or coworkers). Several studies have developed scales to measure disclosure as a communication process including focus on patterns of sharing along with timing and message choices.

Disclosure is defined as "an interaction between at least two individuals where one intends to deliberately divulge something personal to another" (Greene, Derlega, & Mathews, 2006, p. 411). In health, disclosure often focuses on sharing a diagnosis or an event (e.g., surgery or pregnancy). Disclosure has been associated with several important outcomes for both individuals and relationships. First, people who disclose have greater access to social support and resources. Next, people who disclose may find better ways of coping with stressful life events with increased access to resources such as support groups. Third, people who disclose report closer relationships with increased trust and openness. Fourth, there is an opportunity for catharsis and reduced anxiety from holding in information (Greene, Carpenter, Catona, & Magsamen-Conrad, 2013). Finally, disclosure can lead to more effective health care if patient disclosure results in health care providers who are aware of all relevant health information.

Health communication scholars studying disclosure have focused on information management, topic avoidance, privacy, and secrets. Some of this research includes patient-provider communication (including why patients withhold certain information from their physician), and other studies focus on disclosure within interpersonal relationships (for example, choosing not to disclose an illness in a newly developing or established romantic relationship).

This chapter focuses on one measure that considers factors such as breadth, depth, and frequency of disclosure rather than considering disclosure as a single unidimensional event. Past research has focused on disclosure of a diagnosis (e.g., cancer or HIV) or single feature (e.g., adoption or sexual orientation) but often missed how patients or partners/providers share their experience of an illness and how information sharing ebbs and flows through both illness and relationship trajectories.

Disclosure measurement has lacked consistency, in part due to the range of foci and several theories, frameworks, and models that attempt to explain the complex disclosure process. Research examines predictors of disclosure including uncertainty, communication efficacy, relationships with the disclosure target, anticipated response, and assessment of the information. Yet, disclosure is often measured by intent to share some piece of information to some target person (e.g., "I am likely to tell this person [my mother] about my diabetes diagnosis"), but this is not the same as a measure that assesses if the information is known: "This person (my partner) knows about my diabetes diagnosis." In the remainder of the chapter we outline several existing measures of disclosure and offer suggestions for future research.

Measuring Disclosure

One available measure of health disclosure was developed to address the multidimensional nature of the construct and has been used with patient samples including cardiology, cancer, and nonvisible health issues. It has also been developed (and used) in dyadic studies and targeting patients with partners/spouses and patients without partners but focusing on "others" (a family member or friend).

Checton and Greene (2012) initially elaborated on theorizing by Omarzu (2000) to develop a scale measuring patterns of disclosure about a health condition. They asked 203 cardiology patients about ongoing disclosure to a spouse/partner about their health condition. The authors developed scales related to breadth, depth, and frequency of disclosure. All items were measured on 5-point Likert-type scales with a higher score equal to more of the disclosure feature. Breadth addressed the range of topics disclosed, measured by 4 items with acceptable reliability ($\alpha = 0.82$, $M = 3.69$, $SD = .92$). Confirmatory factor analysis (CFA) indicated that items loaded onto this latent construct, χ^2 (26) = 46.48, $p < 0.01$, CFI = 0.97, RMSEA = 0.07. Depth focused on the degree of disclosure intimacy, with 4 items and acceptable reliability ($\alpha = 0.75$, $M = 3.82$, $SD = .82$). CFA yielded good fit, depth χ^2 (26) = 48.43, $p < 0.01$, CFI = 0.97, RMSEA = 0.07. Frequency tapped how often participants disclosed, with 4 items measuring this variable (α = 0.84, M = 3.09, SD = .86). CFA indicated all items loaded onto the latent construct, χ^2 (26) = 33.43, p = 0.15, CFI = 0.99, RMSEA = 0.04. The three disclosure aspects were strongly correlated (range r = .46 – .72).

A number of studies assessed validity through examining correlations between breadth, depth, frequency and other variables. In Checton and Greene (2012) the 3 disclosure variables were correlated with communication efficacy, relational quality, and support such that the higher the breadth, depth, and frequency of disclosure, the higher communication efficacy, higher perceived partner support, and better perceived relational quality. For association with assessment of the information, breadth and depth were directly related yet frequency was inversely related to symptom uncertainty. Thus, symptoms can dampen some aspects of disclosure while simultaneously increasing others.

In an extension of the 2012 study, Checton and Greene (2014b) examined 253 cardiology patients who reported/did not report that they "shared everything" with their partners. Additional questions focused on sharing specific health related information. Sharing specific physical symptoms was correlated with disclosure depth and frequency but not breadth, and sharing psychological/emotional symptoms was correlated with all three disclosure features. Patients who reported "sharing everything" reported greater breadth, depth, and frequency of sharing with their partner, however, on specific health disclosure items patients who reported "sharing everything" with their partner were not higher in disclosing physical and psychological/emotional health information. Thus, these findings caution researchers against using a broad "share everything" item if assessing disclosure with partners.

Another extension of the 2012 study (Checton & Greene, 2014a) compared 273 cardiology patients who reported sharing with either a partner/spouse or an "other" (family member or friend for patients without a spouse). Patients reported higher disclosure breadth, depth, and frequency to partners compared to others. Additionally, cardiology patients reported higher physical and psychological/emotional disclosure and more "heart healthy talk" to spouses than to others.

In a separate study, similar breadth and depth measures were used as indicators of open cancer-related communication (Venetis, Magsamen-Conrad, Checton, & Greene, 2014). This is a dyadic study of 95 couples (N = 190) where one partner had a cancer diagnosis. They present additional CFAs confirming the disclosure factor structures. In paired t-tests, partners reported greater perceptions of disclosure breadth and depth than the patients. Reported breadth and depth were strongly correlated, and both were inversely correlated with topic avoidance for both patients and partners. Finally, the partner's caregiver burden was correlated with the partners' disclosure breadth and depth but not the patients'.

The items for three patterns of disclosure about a health condition to a spouse are presented in Table 1. The scale includes parallel items adapted for patients without a spouse (targeting an "other" such as a family member or a friend) as well as versions of the measure for the partner or the other for use in dyadic studies.

Table 1. Checton and Greene's (2012) Patterns of Disclosure about a Health Condition.

Please indicate your agreement with each of the following statements:

(Breadth)

1. I discuss a wide variety of issues related to my health condition.
2. There are some issues about my health condition that I do not talk about. (R)
3. There are some areas related to my health condition that I avoid discussing. (R)
4. I am hesitant to share small health concerns.

(Depth)

1. I have heart-to-heart talks with my spouse about my health condition.
2. My spouse and I only talk about superficial issues related to my health condition. (R)
3. I hold back from sharing intimate issues about my health condition with my spouse. (R)
4. I share my innermost fears about my health condition with my spouse.

(Frequency)

1. We often talk about my health condition.
2. I rarely talk about my health condition. (R)
3. My spouse and I have frequent conversations about my health condition.
4. How often do you talk with your spouse about your health condition?

*(R) indicates reverse-scored

Other Related Measures

There are other disclosure related measures that may be useful for health communication research. Greene et al. (2012) developed measurement for components of the health disclosure decision-making model (DD-MM). The disclosure decision-making model (Greene, 2009) suggests that 3 components (assessment of information with 5 facets, assessment of the receiver with 2 components, and disclosure efficacy), affect the decision to disclose or not disclose health information. Greene et al. (2012) sampled participants with nonvisible illnesses including sexually transmitted infections, eating disorders, diabetes, and mental health issues. Patients reported about their disclosure experiences with one person who knew their diagnosis and another with whom they had not yet shared the diagnosis. For the purposes of this chapter, we focus on additional measures of disclosure efficacy and anticipated response to disclosure.

Disclosure efficacy. A number of researchers of health disclosure include a construct related to efficacy, either communication or disclosure efficacy. Disclosure efficacy is described as the perceived ability to disclose personal information to another person. Greene et al. (2012) measured disclosure efficacy using 2 items in a sample of 183 patients with a nonvisible health condition ($M = 3.63$, $SD = .94$). A sample item was, "I have trouble finding the right words when I share my health information" (R) with responses ranging from 1 (strongly disagree) to 7 (strongly agree). Efficacy was negatively correlated with perceptions of the information in terms of stigma, prognosis, and relevance but not significantly associated with relational quality.

Checton and Greene (2012) used four 5-point Likert type items ($\alpha = 0.84$, $M = 4.56$, $SD = .59$) to measure efficacy in a sample of 203 cardiology patients. A sample item included "I am confident that I can share information about my health condition with my spouse when I want to." Efficacy was directly related to breadth, depth, and frequency of disclosure to spouse. In a related use of this measure, Checton and Greene (2014a) reported no difference in cardiology patients' and partners' ratings of efficacy.

Checton, Greene, Magsamen-Conrad, and Venetis (2012) used five 5-point Likert type items to measure communication efficacy (patient $\alpha = 0.81$, $M = 4.40$, $SD = .58$; partner $\alpha = 0.86$, $M = 4.26$, $SD = .63$) in a sample of 308 dyads ($N = 616$) where one person had a chronic health condition. Results indicated a single factor for patients (eigenvalue = 2.93, 59% variance, loadings above .70) and partners (eigenvalue = 3.26, 66% variance, loadings above .80). Patient and partner perceptions of the patient's communication efficacy were moderately correlated ($r = .27$). Thus, there is only moderate agreement between spouses on patients' efficacy. Additionally, communication efficacy was correlated with uncertainty, but efficacy was correlated with health care management for partners but not patients.

Magsamen-Conrad, Checton, Venetis, and Greene (2015) measured communication efficacy using six 5-point Likert type items with a sample of 95 couples ($N = 190$) where one had been diagnosed with cancer. Factor analysis indicated a single factor for patients (eigenvalue = 4.18, 70% variance, all items loading above .73) and partners (eigenvalue = 3.25, 65% variance, all items loading above .72). Communication efficacy was strongly correlated with cancer management for both patient and partner, but efficacy was also inversely correlated with prognosis uncertainty. Finally, patients reported higher efficacy than partners.

For researchers interested in using an efficacy measure related to disclosure, note that the above scales use both five and seven-point responses and additionally range from 2 to 6 items. Finally, Greene et al. (2013) developed a brief HIV disclosure intervention targeting increases in disclosure efficacy, but they use semi-structured interviews that may not be as useful for measurement. The intervention is beneficial for practice and prevention, however, using interviews in data collection introduces some challenges. On the benefit side, semi-structured or unstructured interviews can provide greater depth of response when participants generate content instead of reacting to provided stimulus items. In contrast, researchers must weigh these benefits with the labor costs of interviews, generally smaller sample sizes, and inability to compare some responses precisely.

Anticipated response. Beyond efficacy, a number of researchers are including anticipated response as a predictor of health disclosure. Anticipated response is described as expectations of how the disclosure recipient would react upon learning the health information. In the Greene et al. (2012) study of patients with nonvisible illnesses, anticipated reaction was comprised of 2 latent variables, anticipated response and anticipated outcome measured in response to "If I shared my health diagnosis with this person." Anticipated response was measured with 4 items, $\chi^2 (8) = 6.51$, $p = 0.58$, CFI = 0.99, RMSEA = 0.01, $\alpha = 0.80$. A sample item was, "This person would offer emotional support." Anticipated outcome was defined as expectations of positive relational outcomes and was measured with 3 items, $\chi^2 (13) = 29.50$, $p = 0.01$, CFI = 0.97, RMSEA = 0.08, $\alpha = 0.74$. A sample item included, "I am concerned about how this person will feel about me after hearing the health information."

Anticipated response and anticipated outcome were positively associated, such that expectations of a supportive response were related to expectations of positive relationship outcomes. Anticipated outcome and disclosure efficacy were also related, such that expectations of positive relationship outcomes related to higher perceived ability to disclose information. Finally, anticipated response was correlated with prognosis and closeness as well as disclosure depth.

Privacy rules. Another measure developed by Venetis et al. (2012) in three studies operationalizes prior restraint phrases, which are privacy rules about information. Perception of ownership, explicit privacy rules, and implicit privacy rules were scales developed for the study based on communication privacy management theory (CPM, Petronio, 2002). CPM postulates that people "own" and create boundaries around information. To protect private information, people use rules to indicate what information should not be shared further. Items were developed in Study 1 and used Likert-type scales ranging from 1 (strongly disagree) to 5 (strongly agree). Perception of ownership items asked participants if they "owned" the health information and if others had a right to share this health information ($\alpha = 0.67$, $M = 4.16$, $SD = 0.78$). 6 explicit privacy rule items loaded onto one latent construct, χ^2 (9) = 25.99, $p = 0.01$, CFI = 0.98, RMSEA = 0.07, $\alpha = 0.90$, $M = 2.68$, $SD = 1.09$. These items asked if participants told recipients not to share their information, clarity in issuing privacy rules, and timing related to explicit rules. Implicit privacy rules measured if the discloser perceived that the recipient knew not to share the information without being specifically told ($\alpha = 0.57$, $M = 3.88$, $SD = 0.57$). In the dyadic Study 2, an additional measure beyond anticipated further revealing included was actual further revealing, asking disclosure recipients if they shared the information with others.

Ownership was positively related to both implicit and explicit privacy rules such that the higher the perception of ownership, the more participants specifically asked recipients not to share their information and the more certain participants felt that recipients would not share their information even if they did not specifically ask them. Explicit and implicit privacy rules were not related, but both were related to information valence. Ownership and anticipated revealing were positively correlated, such that the higher perception of ownership, the higher expectation that the disclosure recipient would reveal the information. Ownership and actual further revealing were negatively correlated, such that the higher perception of ownership, the less likely recipients were to share information. In terms of effectiveness of either type of privacy rules, neither implicit nor explicit privacy rules fully protected information from further sharing (see pilot study and Study 2). That is, even when we share information with others using "please don't tell anyone" types of qualifications and phrases, some others still choose to share further. Thus, people should continue to carefully evaluate decisions to share and how to balance those risks and benefits, even with close others.

Table 2. Venetis et al. (2012) Privacy Rules.

(Perception of Ownership)
1. I feel that I "own" my health information.
2. Others do not have the right to share my health information.

(Explicit Privacy Rules)
1. I asked this person not to share the health information with anyone else.
2. We never discussed if s/he could share the health information with others. (R)
3. I was clear about who this person could tell/not tell the health information.
4. Before I shared the health information with this person, I asked him/her not to share the information with anyone.
5. After I shared the health information with this person, I asked him/her not to share the information with anyone.
6. I never asked this person to keep the health information to him/herself. (R)

(Implicit Privacy Rules)
1. Although I did not ask this person not to, s/he knows not to tell others.
2. I know that s/he won't share my health information even if I didn't ask him/her to keep the information to him/herself.

Reasons for/against disclosure. Other health disclosure measures developed in the HIV/AIDS literature include the reasons for and against disclosure, based on an integrative model of HIV-disclosure decision-making (Derlega, Winstead, Greene, Serovich, & Elwood, 2004). The model includes the social environment, relational and individual factors, and the interplay between these levels to affect reasons why people would or would not disclose their HIV status. HIV-positive patients completed surveys focused on reasons for and for not disclosing. Reasons for disclosure included 24 items highlighting five reasons for disclosing including catharsis, duty to inform/educate, desire to test reactions, a close/support relationship, and similarity. Reliabilities (α) ranged from 0.60 to 0.90. Reasons for nondisclosure contained 23 items and highlighted six reasons for not disclosing including privacy, self-blame/self-concept difficulties (note association with stigma and identity), communication difficulties, fear of rejection, protecting the other, and superficial relationship. Reliabilities (α) ranged from 0.75 to 0.91.

Disclosure personality measures. Two additional measures treat disclosure as an individual difference rather than focusing on message features or other communication components. These measures focus on how individuals manage information based on personal tendencies different from previously reviewed scales emphasizing changes in disclosure patterns related to the health information or a diagnosis.

Larson and Chastain's (1990) self-concealment scale considered the construct separate from disclosure. Sample items include "If I shared all my secrets with my friends, they'd like me less" and "My secrets are too embarrassing to share with others." Items are measured on a 5-point Likert-type scale (1 = strongly disagree, 5 = strongly agree). The scale consists of 10 items with good reliability ($\alpha = 0.83$) in samples of human service workers, participants at a professional training conference, and psychology graduate students.

Kahn and Hessling's (2001) disclosure distress measure taps concealment versus disclosure of distress. The index includes 12 items measured on a 5-point Likert-type scale. Instructions ask participants to indicate the extent to which they agree or disagree with each item. Sample items include "I usually seek out someone to talk to when I am in a bad mood" and "I try to find people to talk with about my problems." The survey was validated through several studies with undergraduate students, and reliabilities (α) ranged from 0.92 to 0.95.

Use of Existing Measures and Future Studies

This chapter reviewed measures that have been used in health disclosure studies, focusing on one measure that assesses breadth, depth, and frequency of sharing health information. Many studies create new scales, yet most of the scales presented in this chapter can be adapted for certain illnesses and diseases. Several of the existing scales can be easily modified to apply in the health communication context instead of creating unique scales for each new context. Some of the measures can be adapted for similar illnesses and diseases, for example, measures for HIV/AIDS can easily be applied to other stigmatized health conditions such as mental illness. We encourage use of similar or adapted measures to allow for comparison of findings across samples and context.

Continuing to use these scales with various populations and in different health contexts can improve both theory and psychometrics. One important consideration in measuring disclosure is distinguishing it from privacy, secrets, concealment, and other information management concepts. This is vital for improving validity. Future studies should distinguish disclosure from other similar concepts to continue to contribute to the growing literature on information management and health communication.

Recommended Readings

Checton, M. G., & Greene, K. (2014). Elderly patients' heart-related conditions: Disclosing health information differs by target. *Psychology, Health, & Medicine, 20,* 594–604.

Checton, M. G., & Greene, K. (2014). "I tell my partner everything...(or not)": Patients' perceptions of sharing health-related information with their partner. *Journal of Family Nursing, 20,* 164–184.

Checton, M. G., Magsamen-Conrad, K., Venetis, M. K., & Greene, K. (2015). A dyadic approach: Applying a developmental-conceptual model to couples coping with chronic illness. *Health Education and Behavior, 42,* 257–267.

Greene, K., Derlega, V. J., & Mathews, A. (2006). Self-disclosure in personal relationships. In A. Vangelisti & D. Perlman (Eds.), *Cambridge handbook of personal relationships* (pp. 409–427). Cambridge, England: Cambridge University Press.

Magsamen-Conrad, K., Checton, M. G., Venetis, M. K., & Greene, K. (2014). Communication efficacy and couples' cancer management: Applying a dyadic appraisal model. *Communication Monographs.* Advanced online publication, *82,* 179–200.

Venetis, M. K., Greene, K., Checton, M. G., & Magsamen-Conrad, K. (2015). Decision-making in cancer-related topic avoidance. *Journal of Health Communication, 20,* 303–313.

Venetis, M. K., Magsamen-Conrad, K., Checton, M., & Greene, K. (2014). Cancer communication and partner burden: An exploratory study. *Journal of Communication, 64,* 82–102.

References

Checton, M. G., & Greene, K. (2012). Beyond initial disclosure: The role of prognosis and symptom uncertainty in patterns of disclosure in relationships. *Health Communication, 27,* 145–157.

Checton, M. G., & Greene, K. (2014a). Elderly patients' heart-related conditions: Disclosing health information differs by target. *Psychology, Health, & Medicine.* Advanced online publication.

Checton, M. G., & Greene, K. (2014b). "I tell my partner everything...(or not)": Patients' perceptions of sharing health-related information with their partner. *Journal of Family Nursing, 20,* 164–184.

Checton, M. G., Greene, K., Magsamen-Conrad, K., & Venetis, M. K. (2012). Patients' and partners' perspectives of chronic illness and its management. *Families, Systems, & Health, 30*, 114–129.

Derlega, V. J., Winstead, B. A., Greene, K., Serovich, J., & Elwood, W. N. (2004). Reasons for HIV disclosure/nondisclosure in close relationships: Testing a model of HIV-disclosure decision-making. *Journal of Social and Clinical Psychology, 23*, 747–767.

Greene, K. (2009). An integrated model of health-disclosure decision-making. In T. D. Afifi & W. A. Afifi (Eds.), *Uncertainty and information regulation: Theories and applications* (pp. 226–253). New York: Routledge.

Greene, K., Carpenter, A., Catona, D., & Magsamen-Conrad, K. (2013). The Brief Disclosure Intervention (BDI): Facilitating African Americans' disclosure of HIV. *Journal of Communication, 63*, 138–158.

Greene, K., Derlega, V. J., & Mathews, A. (2006). Self-disclosure in personal relationships. In A. L. Vangelisti and D. Perlman (Eds.), *The Cambridge handbook of personal relationships* (pp. 409–427). New York: Cambridge University Press.

Greene, K., Magsamen-Conrad, K., Venetis, M. K., Checton, M. G., Bagdasarov, Z., & Banerjee, S. C. (2012). Assessing health diagnosis disclosure decisions in relationships: Testing the disclosure decision-making model. *Health Communication, 27*, 356–368.

Kahn, J. H., & Hessling, R. M. (2001). Measuring the tendency to conceal versus disclose psychological distress. *Journal of Social and Clinical Psychology, 20*, 41–65.

Larson, D. G., & Chastain, R. L. (1990). Self-concealment: Conceptualization, measurement, and health implications. *Journal of Social and Clinical Psychology, 9*, 439–455.

Magsamen-Conrad, K., Checton, M. G., Venetis, M. K., & Greene, K. (2014). Communication efficacy and couples' cancer management: Applying a dyadic appraisal model. *Communication Monographs*. Advanced online publication.

Omarzu, J. (2000). A disclosure decision model: Determining how and when individuals will self-disclose. *Personality and Social Psychology Review, 4*, 174–185.

Petronio, S. (2002). *Boundaries of privacy: Dialectics of disclosure*. Albany: State University of New York Press.

Venetis, M. K., Greene, K., Magsamen-Conrad, K., Banerjee, S. C., Checton, M., & Bagdasarov, Z. (2012). "You can't tell anyone but…": Exploring the use of privacy rules and revealing behaviors. *Communication Monographs, 79*, 344–365.

Venetis, M. K., Magsamen-Conrad, K., Checton, M., & Greene, K. (2014). Cancer communication and partner burden: An exploratory study. *Journal of Communication, 64*, 82–102.

3. *Health Belief Model*

HYE-JIN PAEK,
Hanyang University, South Korea

Which factors affect people's health-related outcomes? This has long been an important question in health communication and associated research fields. In particular, one line of research has documented that people's perceptions of risks about a health problem are significant determinants of health-related attitudes and behaviors. The important roles of such risk perceptions have been highlighted in several health research theories, for example the Health Belief Model, Motivation Protection Theory, and the Extended Parallel Process Model. Among these theories, the Health Belief Model (HBM) was the first to use key risk perception variables as antecedents to health-related behaviors.

The Health Belief Model (HBM) was developed in the 1950s to discover reasons that could explain the lack of popularity of an x-ray screening program provided by the U.S. Public Health Service. HBM was developed based on the value-expectancy framework, which highlights people's behavior as a function of the subjective value of an outcome and their expectation that taking a specific action will achieve that outcome (Janz, Champion, & Strecher, 2002). If this premise is applied more specifically to the health domain, it can be assumed that people desire to avoid an illness, and that they will expect that taking a certain healthy action would prevent them from becoming ill.

Originally, the HBM comprised five key constructs: four risk perception concepts and the concept of cues to action. The four risk perceptions include perceived susceptibility, perceived severity, perceived benefit, and perceived barrier. Perceived susceptibility refers to people's subjective beliefs about their likelihood of contracting a disease. It includes estimates of vulnerability, belief in the diagnosis, and susceptibility to illness in general (Janz & Becker, 1984). Perceived severity refers to people's levels of perceived seriousness about the disease. It includes evaluations of health consequences such as death, disability, and pain, as well as social consequences such as detriments to work, family life, and social relations.

Together, these two risk perceptions lead to a perceived threat, which in turn motivates action. But the perceived threat won't be sufficient to trigger the recommended action unless perceived benefits outweigh its perceived barriers (Rosenstock, 1974). Perceived benefits refer to people's subjective beliefs that the risk can be managed or reduced by actions recommended for health. Perceived barriers refer to people's beliefs that negative aspects of a recommended health behavior—such as physical (e.g., pain, side effects) and psychological (e.g., difficulty, inconvenience, time) factors—may prevent them from following the behavior. These two perception variables are categorized as risk perceptions together with the perceived susceptibility and severity variables, or health beliefs.

These antecedents can be stimulated by cues to action aimed at health-related outcomes. Cues to action include both internal and external cues to activate readiness to action and facilitate a series of decision-making processes related to health (Janz et al., 2002; Mattson, 1999). Internal cues to action aid the development of people's perceptions of their physical health status or symptoms. These symptoms can be personally experienced or observed from close friends and family. External cues include media cues represented by media campaigns, and interpersonal communications with friends, family, doctors, and health professionals about the target disease and/or preventive behaviors. The last addition to HBM is self-efficacy, or one's confidence in successfully performing a recommended health behavior. This concept was a late addition to HBM, and it was added to overcome the model's weak explanatory power. But because the role of self-efficacy is more pronounced in other theoretical models such as Theory of Planned Behavior and Social Cognitive Theory, the concept is not highlighted much in HBM literature.

While HBM introduced important risk perception and health belief variables to predict health behaviors, studies testing HBM show some mixed results. The first systematic review of HBM research revealed that perceived barriers, benefits, and susceptibility were significant predictors of behavior, whereas severity was not (Janz & Becker, 1984). This same study also concluded that HBM may be better suited for preventive health behaviors such as tuberculosis (TB) screening and vaccinations, but not much for lifestyle-related health such as diet and jogging. Another meta-analytic study (Harrison, Mullen, & Green, 1992) pointed out that each of the HBM constructs was significantly related to behavior or behavioral intention, although their explanatory power is small. The most recent meta-analysis of HBM studies with a more rigorous statistical method found that the four risk perceptions were generally significant predictors of health-related outcomes; however, the results were inconsistent (Carpenter, 2010). Among the four risk perceptions, perceived severity had a relatively weak relationship with likelihood of adopting the target behavior. In the studies that examined prevention, susceptibility was at most a weak predictor of behavior.

Despite some of the mixed evidence supporting it, HBM has been applied to various health topics such as nutrition, exercise, smoking, TB, immunization, cancer, and HIV/AIDS (Paek, Shin, & Lee, 2014). A series of attempts have been made to establish an HBM scale, particularly in cancer research.

Measuring Health Beliefs

HBM variables are measured based on underlying conceptual definitions and propositions. Depending on which health problem is being studied, these measures will have different referents in item wording. For example, in TB studies, the variables can be measured as follows (Paek et al., 2014): for perceived susceptibility, "there is a high possibility that I may contract TB"; for perceived severity, "TB is more severe than other diseases," "TB is a very serious illness," "TB is a very painful disease," and "If I get TB, my life will be ruined"; for perceived benefit, "TB screening will protect my family," "I believe TB screening will protect me," and "TB screening may reduce the anxiety of contracting the disease"; for perceived barrier, "I don't have enough time for TB screening" and "The TB screening fee is a burden for me."

More systematic efforts have been made to establish and apply the HBM scale in cancer-related research. Victoria Champion pioneered such efforts and other cancer researchers have replicated her scale and/or modified it to fit the different cancer contexts. For scale development, the following procedures were taken: (1) focus group and expert interviews to check existing scales' content validity, (2) survey to measure people's responses to the selected HBM question items, (3) exploratory and confirmatory factor analysis using the survey results to check construct validity (discriminant/ convergent validity), (4) internal and test-retest reliability analysis to secure the measurement's reliability and stability, and (5) predictive validity by examining mean differences of each variable depending on stages of behavioral action.

Revising her own HBM scale from breast cancer and mammography studies, Champion (1999) came up with 19 items using a 5-point Likert scale

(1 = strongly disagree to 5 = strongly agree): 3 susceptibility items, 5 benefit items, and 11 barrier items. The items are as follows:

Perceived susceptibility
1. It is likely that I will get breast cancer.
2. My chances of getting breast cancer in the next few years are great.
3. I feel I will get breast cancer sometime during my life.

Perceived benefits
1. If I get a mammogram and nothing is found, I do not worry as much about breast cancer.
2. Having a mammogram will help me find breast lumps early.
3. If I find a lump through a mammogram, my treatment for breast cancer may not be as bad.
4. Having a mammogram is the best way for me to find a very small lump.
5. Having a mammogram will decrease my chances of dying from breast cancer.

Perceived barriers
1. I am afraid to have a mammogram because I might find out something is wrong.
2. I am afraid to have a mammogram because I don't understand what will be done.
3. I don't know how to go about getting a mammogram.
4. Having a mammogram is too embarrassing.
5. Having a mammogram takes too much time.
6. Having a mammogram is too painful.
7. People doing mammograms are rude to women.
8. Having a mammogram exposes me to unnecessary radiation.
9. I cannot remember to schedule a mammogram.
10. I have other problems more important than getting a mammogram.
11. I am too old to need a routine mammogram.

It should be noted that Champion's HBM scale does not include perceived severity items because, presumably, people perceive cancer to be a serious health problem without much variation. In other health contexts, though, people's perceived severity may vary. This scale has been applied in many countries to breast cancer studies that use HBM. Applying the scale and modifying it to fit cervical cancer and Pap smear contexts in Turkey, Guvenc and his associates (2011) took a similar procedure to come up with the following HBM scale:

Perceived susceptibility
1. It is likely that I will get cervical cancer in the future.
2. My chances of getting cervical cancer in the next few years are high.
3. I feel I will get cervical cancer some time during my life.

Perceived severity
1. The thought of cervical cancer scares me.
2. When I think about cervical cancer, my heart beats faster.
3. I am afraid to think about cervical cancer.
4. Problems I would experience with cervical cancer would last a long time.
5. Cervical cancer would threaten a relationship with my boyfriend, husband, or partner.
6. If I had cervical cancer my whole life would change.
7. If I developed cervical cancer, I would not live longer than 5 years.

Perceived benefits
1. Having regular Pap smear tests will help to find changes to the cervix, before they turn into cancer.
2. If cervical cancer was found at a regular Pap smear test its treatment would not be so bad.
3. I think that having a regular Pap smear test is the best way for cervical cancer to be diagnosed early.
4. Having regular Pap smear tests will decrease my chances of dying from cervical cancer.

Perceived barriers
1. I am afraid to have a Pap smear test for fear of a bad result.
2. I am afraid to have a Pap smear test because I don't know what will happen.
3. I don't know where to go for a Pap smear test.
4. I would be ashamed to lie on a gynecologic examination table and show my private parts to have a Pap smear test.
5. Having a Pap smear test takes too much time.
6. Having a Pap smear test is too painful.
7. Health professionals doing a Pap smear test are rude to women.
8. I neglect or cannot remember to have a Pap smear test regularly.
9. I have other problems more important than having a Pap smear test in my life.
10. I am too old to have a Pap smear test regularly.
11. There is no health center close to my house to have a Pap smear test.
12. If there is cervical cancer development in my destiny, having a Pap smear test cannot prevent it.

13. I prefer a female doctor to conduct a Pap smear test.

14. I will never have a Pap smear test if I have to pay for it.

It should be noted that Guvenc et al. (2011) also tested the health motivation construct together with the four HBM variables and found one factor structure totaling nine items that include the perceived benefit items and some of the health motivation items. The perceived benefit items presented above include only the items specific to the health context of inquiry (i.e., Pap smear test). Researchers who wish to use HBM and measure perceived benefits should be aware that the perceived benefit measures could possibly overlap with other relevant constructs, such as health motivation, health orientation, and attitudes toward health. Because the HBM scale used by Guvenc et al. (2011) was translated into Turkish and then back into English, item wording may not be as idiomatic as the original phrasings used in English-speaking countries. Nevertheless, it demonstrates the validity and applicability of the HBM scale in other countries.

In addition to cancer contexts, Hoffman (1996) developed a 25-item HBM scale in HIV/AIDS contexts, which was applied in the study by Winfield and Whaley (2002). The scale included 5 perceived susceptibility items (e.g., "I don't think I will ever be exposed to the virus that causes HIV and AIDS"—reverse coded), three perceived severity items (e.g., "Becoming HIV infected is the worst thing that could happen to me"), 6 perceived benefit items (e.g., "Condoms can provide effective protection against AIDS and HIV disease"), 6 perceived barrier items (e.g., "I would find it difficult to do the things I need to do to protect myself from HIV/AIDS"), and 5 self-efficacy items (e.g., "I can convince my partner to practice safer sex") (p. 335). The 5-point Likert scale response options were used with 1 = strongly disagree to 5 = strongly agree.

Use of Existing Measures and Future Studies

HBM has been one of the most commonly used theoretical models to predict health-related behaviors. Although the relationships among the key concepts still need further explication, the concepts themselves are frequently used as determinants of health-related outcomes—particularly the concepts of perceived susceptibility, perceived severity, perceived barriers, and perceived benefits. In health communication, implications are provided to develop messages that highlight these risk perceptions and health beliefs depending on which factors were found to be most strongly related to the specific health-related outcomes of inquiry.

A few caveats should be noted with respect to using the HBM scales for major risk perceptions to predict an array of health behaviors.

First, depending on which health problems and recommended health behaviors are at issue, the role of the four major risk perceptions in predicting the health behavior may vary. As discussed above, meta-analytic studies show differential roles of the risk perception and health belief variables in different health-related outcomes.

Second, perceived benefits and barriers comprise multiple dimensions (e.g., physical, social, psychological, environmental) and therefore require several question-items for measurement. Studies have generally shown that these multiple dimensions comprise one factor to measure the respective perception variables. However, that may not always be the case across health contexts and situations. It is also possible that these dimensions play a differential role in predicting health-related outcomes. For this reason, researchers should measure multiple dimensions of perceived benefit of and barriers to recommended health behaviors and then perform factor analysis to ensure the factor structure.

For a related third point, perceived barriers and benefits need to be measured with a number of questions that are specific to the health problem under study. But in evaluation research, it may not be feasible to include a lengthy list of questions to measure just one variable. Accordingly, researchers may need to make strategic decisions to shorten the list of questions they ask. To determine the most important pool of question items, they may need to perform focus group and/or expert interviews.

Fourth, while the four risk perception variables are the core content of HBM, the concept of cues to action has been under-explicated, and that of self-efficacy has been underemphasized. For a test of the HBM scale including both self-efficacy and cues to action, see Winfield and Whaley (2002).

Lastly, all the variables would need to be modified to fit each relevant health issue.

Recommended Readings

Chew, F., Palmer, S., Slonska, Z., & Subbiah, K. (2002). Enhancing health knowledge, health beliefs, and health behavior in Poland through a health promoting television program series. *Journal of Health Communication*, 7(3), 179–196. http://doi.org/10.1080/10810730290088076

Gozum, S. & Aydin, I. (2004). Validation evidence for Turkish adaptation of Champion's health belief model scale. *Cancer Nursing*, 27, 491–498.

Kasmaei, P., Shokravi, F. A., Hidarnia, A., Hajizadeh, E., Atrkar-Roushan, Z., Shirazi, K. K., & Montazeri, A. (2014). Brushing behavior among young adolescents: does perceived severity matter. *BMC Public Health, 14*(1), 8. http://doi.org/10.1186/1471-2458-14-8

Rodriguez-Reimann, D. I., Nicassio, P., Reimann, J. O. F., Gallegos, P. I., & Olmedo, E. L. (2004). Acculturation and health beliefs of Mexican Americans regarding tuberculosis prevention. *Journal of Immigrant Health, 6*(2), 51–62.

Taymoori, P., & Berry, T. (2009). The validity and reliability of Champion's Health Belief Model Scale for breast cancer screening behaviors among Iranian women. *Cancer Nursing, 32*(6), 465–472. http://doi.org/10.1097/NCC.0b013e3181aaf124

References

Becker, M. H. (1974). The health belief model and personal health behavior. *Health Education Monographs, 2*, 324–508.

Carpenter, C. J. (2010). A meta-analysis of the effectiveness of health belief model variables in prediction behavior. *Health Communication, 25*(8), 661–669.

Champion V. L. (1999). Revised susceptibility, benefits, and barriers scale for mammography screening. *Research in Nursing & Health, 22*, 341–348.

Guvenc, G., Akyuz, A., & Açikel, C. H. (2011). Health Belief Model Scale for cervical cancer and Pap smear test: Psychometric testing. *Journal of Advanced Nursing, 67*, 428–437.

Harrison, J. A., Mullen, P. D., & Green, L. W. (1992). A meta-analysis of studies of the health belief model with adults. *Health Education Research, 7*(1), 107–116.

Hoffman, M. (1996). *Development of the health belief model for AIDS questionnaire.* Unpublished manuscript, University of Maryland at College Park.

Janz, N. K., & Becker, M. H. (1984). The health belief model: A decade later. *Health Education Quarterly, 11*, 1–47.

Janz, N. K., Champion, V. L., & Strecher, V. J. (2002). The health belief model. In K. Glanz, B. K. Rimer, & F. M. Lewis (Eds.), *Health behavior and health education: Theory, research, and practice* (3rd ed., pp. 45–66). San Francisco: Jossey-Bass.

Mattson, M. (1999). Toward a reconceptualization of communication cues to action in the health belief model: HIV test counseling. *Communication Monographs, 66*, 240–265.

Paek, H.-J., Shin, K., & Lee, B. K. (August, 2014). Exploring cues to action in health belief model: A test case of tuberculosis screening in South Korea. Paper presented at the annual conference of the Association for Education in Journalism and Mass Communication Convention. Montreal, Canada.

Rosenstock, I. M. (1974). Historical origin of the health belief model. In M. H. Becker (Eds.), *The health belief model and personal health behavior* (pp. 1–8). Thorofare, NJ: Charles B. Slack, Inc.

Winfield, E. B., & Whaley, A. L. (2002). A comprehensive test of the health belief model in the prediction of condom use among African American college students. *Journal of Black Psychology, 28*, 330–346.

4. Communication Campaign Evaluation

CHRISTOPHER E. BEAUDOIN,
Texas A&M University
& MICHAEL T. STEPHENSON,
Texas A&M University

Communication campaign evaluations are based in the tenets of social science, including being systematic, objective, and replicable. They can consider assorted consequences—intended and unintended, immediate and long-term—and can encompass different types of assessment, whether formative, process, or outcome (Valente, 2002). They can determine how to best improve a campaign, if staff are carrying out activities in a specified manner, and if a communication campaign is successful, as well as why it is or why it is not. Researchers have used different approaches to evaluating communication campaigns in different contexts (see Hornik [2002] for an excellent overview). In terms of outcome assessment, an evaluation can determine whether a communication campaign causes a significant change in an intended outcome, including behaviors such as healthy diet, physical activity, condom use, or cigarette smoking. For example, an evaluation can empirically assess whether the Truth campaign is effective in causing a decrease in teen cigarette smoking (Sly, Heald, & Ray, 2001). This national campaign, with funding from the American Legacy Foundation, targeted youth with an industry manipulation strategy that portrayed tobacco industry executives as being predatory, manipulative, and greedy. Its evaluations were varied, including a quasi-experimental design with four cross-sectional surveys and two intermediate tracking surveys. The current chapter, with a focus primarily on outcome evaluation, aims to articulate how researchers can best evaluate theory-based communication campaigns, including issues related to study design, data collection, intervention specification, and measurement.

Causation is central to determining if a communication campaign is successful in influencing its intended outcomes (Shadish, Cook, & Campbell, 2002). There are four criteria for determining causation. First, the outcome variable must change over time (e.g., a decrease in cigarette smoking from time 1 to time 2). Second, the communication campaign must precede such over-time change in the outcome variable (e.g., the campaign begins before the aforementioned decrease in cigarette smoking). Third, respondents' exposure to the communication campaign must be correlated with the intended increase or decrease in the outcome (e.g., the more a person is exposed to an anti-smoking campaign, the more he/she experiences a decrease in cigarette smoking). Fourth, the determination of such over-time change and correlation must be non-spurious. In other words, there must be evidence that the results are genuine and not confounded by alternative processes (e.g., changes in cigarette sales taxation). Thus, a campaign evaluator has the formidable task of ensuring that a campaign is an antecedent of an intended outcome, determining that the intended outcome varies over time and according to respondents' exposure to the campaign, and diminishing concerns for alternative explanations for such over-time change and correlation.

Measuring the Effectiveness of Communication Campaigns

Study Design and Data Collection

The determination of time order, of course, necessitates data collection from at least two points in time. For instance, evaluators often collect measurements of an outcome variable before a communication campaign (i.e., pre-campaign) and after the communication campaign (i.e., post-campaign). Such an approach can permit proper time-order and test for the postulated change in the outcome variable. Longitudinal data collection can involve panel or cross-sectional samples of respondents. A panel sample consists of data from interviews of individual respondents at more than one time. (Thus, each respondent is interviewed more than once.) In contrast, a cross-sectional sample consists of data from the interview of individual respondents at just one point in time. Thus, consistent with the example in the previous paragraph, evaluators can use a panel sample to measure cigarette smoking before and after a communication campaign, with survey interviews of the exact same individuals at both points in time—pre-campaign and post-campaign (see Figure 1, Design Type 1). With self-reported responses from identical individuals in the panel data set, the evaluator can test whether there is significant change in the outcome variable from pre-campaign to post-campaign. Taking a different approach, evaluators can use cross-sectional samples to make longitudinal measurements. They can collect data from one cross-sectional sample before the communication campaign—and then collect data from a completely different cross-sectional sample after the communication campaign (see Figure 1, Design Type 2). With self-reports on cigarette smoking prevalence from both distinct cross-sectional samples, the evaluators can test whether there is significant change in the outcome variable from pre-campaign to post-campaign.

Figure 1. Evaluation Design for Communication Campaigns.

Design Type	Pre-Campaign	Campaign	Post-Campaign
1. Panel	O_1	X	O_2
2. Longitudinal Cross-Sectional	O_1	X	
		X	O_2
3. Panel with Post-Cross-Sectional	O_1	X	O_2
		X	O_2
4. Treatment/Control	O_1	X	O_2
	O_1		O_2

O=Observation; X=Intervention

There are pros and cons to using panel or cross-sectional samples. The primary strength of panel data is that an evaluator can demonstrate over-time change in an outcome, as well as in antecedent variables, with data *from the exact same sample of individuals.* This characteristic of panel data permits it—unlike cross-sectional data—to make inferences of causation. A con of panel data, however, involves attrition. While an evaluator may have a large representative sample at pre-campaign, attrition will decrease the size of the sample—sometimes, substantially—and often can change the demographic makeup of the resulting panel sample. Thus, even if a researcher began with a representative sample at pre-campaign, the post-campaign sample may not well represent the population. It may be that certain types of individuals are more likely than others to withdraw from the panel sample between pre-campaign and post-campaign, with such a problem exacerbated by the length of time between panel surveys. For instance, in the evaluation of school-based interventions across the high school years, there is commonly higher attrition among lower performing students, who, also, tend to be more likely to smoke cigarettes and use illicit drugs. (To compensate for minor or moderate discrepancies between the resulting panel sample and the population, researchers can weight their statistical analyses.) Unlike panel samples, cross-sectional longitudinal samples can be administered in a manner that tends to make them less prone to sampling bias, thus, resulting in longitudinal samples that are more consistent with population parameters. In particular, researchers can seek a representative sample at pre-campaign and another, distinct representative sample at post-campaign. (To address any differences between the O_1 and O_2 cross-sectional data sets—normally, minor in nature—researchers can weight data.) Another con of a panel sample is the threat of testing bias. In particular, if researchers ask a respondent about his/her cigarette smoking pre-campaign, there is the possibility that the interview itself will cause a change in how the person subsequently consumes cigarettes and reports on such consumption at post-campaign. In using different cross-sectional samples, an evaluator can eliminate this threat to validity. Furthermore, in a more complex research design, an evaluator can add a post-intervention cross-sectional sample to a traditional panel sample, thus, moving from Design Type 1 to Design Type 3 (see Figure 1). In this manner, previous evaluations (Beaudoin, 2007) have mitigated concerns for testing bias by demonstrating that the outcome variable does not significantly differ between the panel sample at O_2 and the cross-sectional sample at O_2.

Notably, however, to yield accurate findings in some communication campaign contexts, it may be helpful to have even greater survey refinement than pre-post designs. For example, a media campaign in Kentucky used a cohort survey design with monthly assessments to track marijuana use among adolescents, beginning at age 12 and progressing to age 16 (Palmgreen, Donohew, Lorch, Hoyle, & Stephenson, 2001). This monthly survey approach helped the researchers account for the normal upward trend in marijuana initiation and use across these early teen years. By conducting monthly survey interviews in both the treatment and control conditions, the researchers documented over-time increases in marijuana use in both conditions, but a relative decrease in the treatment condition.

Study Design and Intervention Specification

Along with selecting a suitable sampling approach, an evaluator must also specify the intervention. Critical in specifying the intervention and control conditions in evaluations of communication campaigns, there are three types of assignment: individual, group, and self-selective (Valente, 2001). Individual assignment refers to how a researcher can determine (via random assignment) which specific individuals are exposed to a communication campaign and which specific individuals are not exposed. Per random assignment in a laboratory experiment, researchers can determine which half of a sample will see a communication campaign (i.e., the treatment group) and which half of the sample will not see the communication campaign (i.e., the control group) (see Figure 1, Design Type 4). The gold standard for determining causation, laboratory experiments, permit a researcher to determine time order, test for correlation, and, by manipulating only the independent variable and keeping all else constant in the treatment and control groups, eliminate most concerns regarding alternative explanations. Simply put, a researcher can isolate the effects of a message (e.g., a communication campaign ad) on a dependent variable (e.g., behavioral intention). Despite its strength in determining causation, an individual level of assignment is not possible for most types of communication campaigns given their message dissemination patterns and their broad and dispersed audiences in which a researcher cannot implement random assignment and, thus, cannot ensure which individuals will be exposed—or not exposed—to a communication campaign. Individual assignment, however, can be used in some distinct scenarios, including in randomized controlled trials. For example, in a new media campaign, researchers could randomly assign individuals to treatment and control groups and conduct pre- and post-interviews, with only the treatment group receiving email or text messages with preventive health recommendations in between the two interviews. Then, the researchers could test whether individuals in the treatment group who received the email or text recommendations develop stronger preventive behaviors than their counterparts in the control group. For example, one study employed a randomized controlled trial to assess the effects of health promotion via email and phone text messages in the context of youth sexual health (Lim et al., 2012). The treatment group, which received messages across the 12-month intervention, developed higher levels of knowledge about sexually transmitted infections (STI) than the control group. In addition, as compared to their control group counterparts, women in the treatment group were more likely to have an STI test and discuss sexual health with a clinician.

As noted earlier, such study designs and related random assignment at the individual level are not possible when disseminating messages to mass audiences (e.g., traditional television advertisements). In cases where individual assignment is not possible, some of the tenets of a laboratory experiment can be used in natural settings with the implementation of group level of assignment. Group assignment refers to how the researcher can determine which specific groups (e.g., communities or schools) are exposed to a communication campaign and which specific groups are not exposed. Such evaluations, often called community trials, permit manipulating the presence of a communication campaign in a treatment community, while having it absent in a comparative control community (see Figure 1, Design Type 4). In such scenarios, measurement is of the presence of a campaign in a community, not of whether specific individuals in the community are actually exposed to the campaign. For example, in a media campaign on adolescent marijuana use in Kentucky, the intervention was assigned by county, with one county receiving the televised media campaign (i.e., the treatment group) and another county receiving no intervention at all (i.e., the control group) (Palmgreen et al., 2001). This evaluation plan was possible because the two counties were well matched in terms of demographic and cultural variables.

Commonly, however, communication campaigns have not been evaluated with individual assignment (for reasons noted earlier) or group assignment, for various reasons including the following two formidable challenges: 1) matching equivalent treatment and control communities before the advent of a communication campaign; and 2) making sure that experimental messages do not spread from a treatment community to contaminate a control community. (In the first regard, for example, imagine the difficulty of trying to find a control city for New Orleans following Hurricane Katrina or, for that matter, at any other time.) Thus, in evaluations of communication campaigns, researchers often rely on self-selection assignment, which refers to how subjects in a study determine for themselves whether they will expose themselves to a communication campaign (e.g., an individual decides if he/she will—or will not—watch a specific health campaign advertisement on television). This permits campaign evaluation without using an equivalent control group and necessitates that researchers measure respondents' campaign exposure as a means to creating "pseudo-exposed" groups and "pseudo-unexposed" groups. In particular, respondents who self-report exposure to a campaign become the pseudo-exposed group, whereas respondents who self-report non-exposure to the campaign become the pseudo-unexposed group. In such cases, the measurement of campaign exposure is essential to specify the intervention.

Measuring Communication Campaign Exposure

When self-selection assignment is used, it is necessary to measure respondents' campaign exposure. In particular, if a person reports that he/she was exposed to a campaign, it would be expected that he/she would be more likely to achieve an intended campaign outcome than a counterpart who reported not being exposed to the campaign. In addition, survey measurement of respondents' campaign exposure can be useful when assignment is at the group level. In such instances, an evaluator would expect the following: 1) respondents in a treatment community would be more likely to adopt an intended campaign outcome than respondents in a control community; and 2) in the treatment community, respondents who report being exposed to the campaign would be more likely to adopt an intended campaign outcome than respondents who report not being exposed to the campaign. (Thus, per Design Type 4 in Figure 1, we could measure campaign exposure among individuals in the treatment group.)

Different survey techniques have been implemented to measure campaign exposure, which refers to the level to which a person is aware of or can recall a communication campaign or specific communication campaign ad. These approaches vary between unaided and aided, unconfirmed and confirmed, and campaign exposure and ad exposure. The difference between unconfirmed and confirmed involves whether respondents are simply asked to indicate if they saw or heard a campaign or campaign ad (i.e., unconfirmed awareness)—or whether, via open-ended questioning, they can subsequently provide details about the campaign or campaign ad (i.e., confirmed recall). Thus, confirmation is requisite to the measurement of recall, but not awareness. The distinction between unaided and aided refers to how much detail is provided to a respondent to describe a specific campaign or campaign advertisement.

Some evaluations have relied on measures of unconfirmed awareness, which can be unaided or aided. For example, in measuring aided ad awareness, Stephenson and colleagues (2002) provided respondents with a four-sentence description of four different campaign ads and then asked about their certainty of having seen each ad, with responses scaled from 1 (very certain I did not see it) to 4 (very certain I saw it). In another measurement of aided ad awareness, Hornik and colleagues (2008) played a short clip of an ad for respondents and then asked the following close-ended question:

- "Have you ever seen or heard this ad?"

Then, respondents who answered "yes" were asked the following close-ended question:

- "In recent months, how many times have you seen or heard this ad?"

This latter two-item approach permits measurement, first, of aided ad awareness in a dichotomous manner (yes/no) and, second, of aided ad awareness on a ratio scale.

Evaluations can also use aided and unaided ad recall, unconfirmed and confirmed, pertinent to campaign ads or the campaign itself. Using one such approach, Sly, Heald, and Ray (2001) measured awareness of four Truth campaign ads, beginning with the following aided prompt:

- "Have you recently seen an anti-smoking advertisement that showed 'cue'?" (Inserted for 'cue' was a description of one of four specific Truth campaign advertisements.)

Responses were dichotomous (yes/no), with respondents who answered "yes" being coded as aware of an ad. To measure aided confirmed recall, two additional items were used. First, without any additional cues provided, respondents were asked to describe the ad that they had reported being aware of. Second, without any additional cues provided, respondents were asked to describe the main message or theme of the ad that they had reported being aware of. Via these two open-ended questions, respondents who could well describe the ad or its main message or theme were coded as having confirmed ad recall. Furthermore, Sly, Heald, and Ray (2001) measured unaided awareness and unaided confirmed recall of the Truth campaign itself. To measure unaided campaign awareness, respondents were asked if they were aware of any anti-tobacco or anti-smoking campaign taking place in Florida. Those who answered "yes" were coded as being campaign aware. Next, respondents who were coded as aware were asked, via open-ended questioning, to provide a major theme of the campaign. If they did so correctly in regards to the Truth campaign, they were then coded for having confirmed campaign recall.

More recently, a hybrid approach was used by Agha and Beaudoin (2012) in their evaluation of the Touch condom campaign in Pakistan. The family planning campaign had one television ad, which, in running about 3.5 minutes long, was part public service announcement and part entertainment education. Unaided and aided techniques were used to measure recall of the campaign ad. To begin, respondents were asked the following unaided question:

- "During the last 3 months, have you seen any advertisements on television about contraceptive methods or reproductive health services?"

Two subsequent steps were then taken to measure unaided confirmed ad recall. In a first unaided approach, respondents who answered "yes" to the previous question were then asked the following open-ended question:

- "What did you see in the advertisements?"

Respondents were coded as having confirmed ad recall if their responses were consistent with at least one of the following 12 main elements of the Touch condom advertisement: 1) a group of students playing basketball in college; 2) one of the students playing guitar while the other students sit together and enjoy the music; 3) a newly admitted female student coming in front of those students who are enjoying music and asking about a classroom; 4) the guitarist focusing his eyes on the newly present woman; 5) a professor giving a lecture in a class with the woman and the man who was playing the guitar; 6) the guitarist and the new female student sitting in the library and chatting with each other and, after that, both talking on cell phones; 7) parents of the guitarist meeting with parents of the female student at her home to talk about marriage; 8) after marriage, the couple enjoying their honeymoon in a frozen icy country scene; 9) the husband sitting outside a clinic or maternity ward where their baby is born; 10) the husband going to a supermarket to buy Touch condoms; 11) a Greenstar cup shown in the kitchen; and 12) the couple and their parents sitting with the new baby and drinking tea. This first unaided approach, thus, results in confirming respondents' initial unaided ad awareness. In a second aided approach, respondents who said "no" to the initial unaided ad awareness question were then asked (constituting aided ad awareness) the following question specific to contraceptive methods or reproductive health services:

- "Did you see an advertisement in the last 3 months in which a young couple met, got married and had a happy married life?"

Respondents who answered "yes" were coded as having aided ad awareness and then asked to complete six jingles from the campaign ad. If respondents could properly complete at least one jingle, they were coded for having aided confirmed ad recall. For their final statistical analyses, Agha and Beaudoin (2012) then grouped respondents coded as "unaided confirmed ad recall" and "aided confirmed ad recall" to make up an overall group who had confirmed campaign ad recall.

Critical to such measurement of campaign exposure is validity (see Niederdeppe [2014] for review). Validity is the degree to which an empirical measurement fits the actual meaning of the concept it is intended to represent. In being exclusively dependent on self-report, measures of ad awareness (Hornik et al., 2008), of course, are prone to response bias, as well as problems respondents may have in remembering if they actually saw or heard a specific campaign ad. In contrast, two-question measurement of confirmed ad recall (Agha & Beaudoin, 2012; Sly et al., 2001) requires respondents to come up with details of a campaign ad on their own, which mitigates problems with response bias, but not with memory. In such cases of confirmed ad recall, it is also possible that respondents did not actually see or hear an advertisement firsthand and, instead, heard about it via interpersonal communication. Certainly, we expect measures of unconfirmed ad awareness to result in higher assessments of exposure than measures of confirmed ad recall (Niederdeppe, 2014).

Use of Existing Measures and Future Studies

Researchers are recommended to take the most rigorous approach possible in their evaluations of communication campaigns. There are pros and cons to each approach when it comes to study design, data collection, and intervention specification. There are also pros and cons to each type of exposure measurement, whether unaided or aided, unconfirmed or confirmed, and campaign-specific or ad-specific. Most campaigns derive merit from measuring respondents' campaign exposure. Such is essential to measuring campaigns in which self-selection assignment is used, but can also be advantageous when group assignment is implemented.

Additional Resources

CDC, Building Our Understanding: Key Concepts of Evaluation: http://www.cdc.gov/ nccdphp/dch/programs/healthycommunitiesprogram/tools/pdf/eval_planning. pdf

CDC, Research & Evaluation, Gateway to Health Communication & Social Marketing Practice: http://www.cdc.gov/healthcommunication/research/

Additional Readings

Niederdeppe, J. (2014). Conceptual, empirical, and practical issues in developing valid measures of public communication campaign exposure. *Communication Methods and Measures, 8*(2), 138–161.

Shadish, W. R., Cook, T. D., & Campbell, D. T. (2002). *Experimental and quasi-experimental designs for generalized causal inference.* Boston: Houghton Mifflin Co.

Valente, T. W. (2001). Evaluating communication campaigns. In R. E. Rice & C. K. Atkin (Eds.), *Public communication campaigns* (3rd ed., pp. 105–124). Thousand Oaks, CA: Sage.

Valente, T. W. (2002). *Evaluating health promotion programs.* Oxford: Oxford University Press.

References

Agha, S., & Beaudoin, C. E. (2012). Assessing a thematic condom advertising campaign on condom use in urban Pakistan. *Journal of Health Communication, 17*(5), 601–623.

Beaudoin, C. E. (2007). Mass media use, neighborliness, and social support: Assessing causal links with panel data. *Communication Research, 34*(6), 637–664. doi: 10.1177/0093650207307902.

Hornik, R. C. (Ed.). (2002). *Public health communication: Evidence for behavior change.* New York: Lawrence Erlbaum.

Hornik, R. C., Jacobsohn, L., Orwin, R., Piesse, A., & Kalton, G. (2008). Effects of the national youth anti-drug media campaign on youths. *American Journal of Public Health, 98*(12), 2229–2236.

Lim, M. S., Hocking, J. S., Aitken, C. K., Fairley, C. K., Jordan, L., Lewis, J. A., & Hellard, M. E. (2012). Impact of text and email messaging on the sexual health of young people: a randomised controlled trial. *Journal of Epidemiology and Community Health, 66*(1), 69–74.

Niederdeppe, J. (2014). Conceptual, empirical, and practical issues in developing valid measures of public communication campaign exposure. *Communication Methods and Measures, 8*(2), 138–161.

Palmgreen, P., Donohew, L., Lorch, E. P., Hoyle, R. H., & Stephenson, M. T. (2001) Television campaigns and adolescent marijuana use: Tests of a sensation seeking targeting. *American Journal of Public Health, 91,* 292–296.

Shadish, W. R., Cook, T. D., & Campbell, D. T. (2002). *Experimental and quasi-experimental designs for generalized causal inference.* Boston. Houghton Mifflin Co.

Sly, D. F., Heald, G. R., & Ray, S. (2001). The Florida "truth" anti-tobacco media evaluation: Design, first year results, and implications for planning future state media evaluations. *Tobacco Control, 10,* 9–15.

Stephenson, M. T., Morgan, S. E., Lorch, E. P., Palmgreen, P., Donohew, L., & Hoyle, R. H. (2002). Predictors of exposure form an antimarijuana media campaign: Outcome research assessing sensation seeking targeting. *Health Communication, 14*(1), 23–43.

Valente, T. W. (2001). Evaluating communication campaigns. In R. E. Rice & C. K. Atkin (Eds.), *Public communication campaigns* (3rd ed., pp. 105–124). Thousand Oaks, CA: Sage.

Valente, T. W. (2002). *Evaluating health promotion programs.* Oxford: Oxford University Press.

5. *Health Information Seeking*

Z. JANET YANG,
State University of New York at Buffalo
& SUSAN LAVALLEY,
State University of New York at Buffalo

In the last two decades, there has been a steady stream of research on information seeking in mass communication as well as in interpersonal communication, information and library science, health psychology and behavior, and beyond (Case, 2002; Lambert & Loiselle, 2007). In the area of health communication, for instance, researchers have proposed several models of information seeking, including the Health Information Model (Longo, 2005), the Theory of Motivated Information Management (Afifi & Weiner, 2004), the Comprehensive Model of Information Seeking (Johnson & Meischke, 1993), the Health Information Acquisition Model (Freimuth, Stein, & Kean, 1989) and the Risk Information Seeking and Processing Model (Griffin, Dunwoody, & Neuwirth, 1999).

These models are developed based on evidence from both qualitative and quantitative research. Although the specific mechanisms that account for health information seeking vary from model to model, most of them identify a perceived *need* for information as a key motive that drives health information seeking behaviors. This need for information, from an evaluative perspective, depicts the specific utility that health information serves to enable individuals to better manage their health outcomes.

Health information seeking is a purposive act that is initiated by a perceived need for health information (Johnson & Case, 2012). Given the breadth of this definition, measurement of health information seeking varies greatly from study to study. While most studies focus on the sources of health information, existing measurement strategies have also included the frequency, content, and evaluations of health information seeking. Below, we review scale development associated with each of these measurement strategies. In particular, we primarily focus on empirical studies published since 2010 as an earlier study has systematically reviewed methods and measures commonly used to study active health information seeking in the literature from 1978 to 2010 (Anker, Reinhart, & Feeley, 2011).

Measuring Health Information Seeking

A large number of studies on health information seeking adopt questions from the National Cancer Institute's Health Information National Trends Survey (HINTS) (Manganello & Clayman, 2011; K. M. Oh, Kreps, Jun, Chong, & Ramsey, 2012; Peretti-Watel et al., 2014; Tian & Robinson, 2013). Across different data collection years, two questions are consistently used to measure health information seeking: 1) Have you ever searched for health or medical information (yes/no)? 2) The most recent time you looked for information about health or medical topics, where did you go first? (Internet, books/magazines/ news, health provider, friends/family, other). Following this approach, research applying Channel Complementarity Theory (Ruppel & Rains, 2012) subsequently asks participants if they have looked anywhere else for such information and, if so, to identify the next source they used. This procedure is repeated until respondents indicate that they have not used any more sources.

Some studies go into greater detail while exploring information sources (Yang et al., 2011), incorporating both local news sources and online support groups, in addition to the sources included in the HINTS database (Table 1). Additional sources may also include one or more doctors, another type of health care provider such as nurses, family or friends who are in the medical field, family or friends who are not in the medical field, other cancer patients or survivors, co-workers, support groups, pamphlets or books, television, radio, public library, resource center at a hospital or clinic, and cancer information or support organizations (Blance-Hartigan, Blake, & Viswanath, 2014).

Table 1. Sample scale for health information sources (Yang et al., 2011).

On a scale of 0 to 10, where 0 is "none" and 10 is "a lot," how much attention would you pay to information about [health topic] from…?	
Interpersonal sources	Family members
	Friends and coworkers
Traditional media	Local newspapers
	Local radio or television stations
New media	Health-related websites
	Internet support groups

Other research specifies the type of health matters inquired about through various online and offline sources. For example, information seekers may inquire about actual medical issues such as a specific disease or medical problem; prescription or over-the-counter drugs; specific doctor or hospital; depression, anxiety, stress, or mental health issues (treatment health information). They may also seek information about broader, more mundane health issues such as diet, nutrition, vitamins or nutritional supplements, and exercise or fitness (lifestyle health information) (Dobransky & Hargittai, 2012). Findings from this study suggest that women are considerably more likely to turn to traditional sources (e.g., medical professional, friends or family) for treatment health information than are men.

Frequency

Besides sources of information, frequency of search is also widely used to measure health information seeking. Again, HINTS data are often adapted to assess the frequency of online and offline information seeking. For example, to assess online health information seeking, participants are usually asked, "How often did you use the Internet to look for health or medical information for yourself [for someone else]?" Response options include "at least once a week," "at least once a month (but less than once a week)," "less than once a month, but at least six times a year," "less than six times a year," and "never." (Neumark, Lopez-Quintero, Feldman, Hirsch Allen, & Shtarkshall, 2013).

   Other research relies on self-reported time spent online (hours/minutes per week) seeking information regarding treatments, medications, parenting, diet, exercise, illness or disease, medical or dental insurance benefits, and medical or health care equipment. Respondents were asked "about how much time" they spent "during a typical week" obtaining health information online (Weaver III, Thompson, Weaver, & Hopkins, 2009). Then, within each content area, responses were totaled to reflect online health information seeking per week, in minutes.

   Some studies supplement frequency measures with perceived quality of various sources of health information. For instance, one study that specifically examines seniors' use of the Internet for health information asked participants to rate frequency of use (Table 2) and perceived quality of various sources (McMillan & Macias, 2008). In addition, respondents were asked to indicate how much they agreed that words like "sincere" and "dependable" applied to online health information using a 5-point Likert scale (α = .88). Similarly, other studies have asked users to assess the quality of health websites, including whether the website is believable, trustworthy, accurate, complete, and biased (reverse-coded) (α = .87) (Rains & Karmikel, 2009).

Table 2. Sample scale for health information seeking frequency (McMillan & Macias, 2008).

How often do you use the following sources of health information (5-point scale)?
Search engines (e.g., Google.com)
General commercial health sites (e.g., WebMD)
Commercial portal sites (e.g., Yahoo.com)
Sites by media companies
Sites by educational institutions
Sponsored commercial health sites
Sites by governmental agencies
Sites by nonprofit groups
Sites by hospitals, clinics, etc.

Content

Research on health information seeking tends to be topic-specific. In particular, cancer-related information seeking has generated great research interest. For instance, research that measures the content of cancer-related information seeking has included these topics—side effects of treatment; treatment or treatment options; likelihood of surviving; type of cancer; what to expect when dealing with cancer; diet/nutrition; staying healthy or health in general; non-traditional medicine, or alternative or complementary medicine; how to cope with stress, fear, depression or anxiety; doctors; facilities where you could get treatment; financial assistance or help with money; work or employment issues (Galarce et al., 2011).

For cancer-related information seeking, a comparison is often drawn between nonclinical sources and medical professional sources. Lewis et al. (2012) developed a measure containing three questions related to cancer patients' information seeking (Table 3).

Table 3. Sample scale for clinical and non-clinical sources of cancer-related information (Lewis et al., 2012).

Questions	Check all that apply for each question:	
1. Think back to the first few months after you were diagnosed with your cancer. In making decisions about what treatments to choose, did you actively look for information about treatments from any sources?	Non-clinical sources	Friends or family members Other cancer patients Television or radio Books or brochures Newspapers or magazines Support groups (face-to-face and online) Telephone hotlines
2. What sources did you use when you were actively looking for any information related to your cancer?		
3. Where have you actively looked for information about quality of life issues (i.e. physical problems, how to reduce cancer recurrence)?		
	Clinical sources	Treating doctors Other doctors Other health care professionals

Sexual health information seeking represents another key topic of research. Specifics topics examined include unwanted pregnancy, abortion, HIV/AIDS, and other STIs (Chang, 2014). Respondents were asked "during the past three months, how often did you discuss each of these issues with your best friends?" Each question was measured on a 5-point scale with 1 representing "never" and 5 "very often" ($\alpha = .78$). To examine generic online health information seeking, researchers have also inquired about other topics such as "a specific disease or medical problem," "environmental health hazards," and "doctors or other health professionals" (H. J. Oh, Lauckner, Boehmer, Fewins-Bliss, & Li, 2013).

Evaluation

Individuals' evaluations of their seeking experience represent another strategy to assess health information seeking. Some studies focus on individuals' frustration and confusion that are caused by health information seeking (Arora et al., 2008). For instance, using HINTS questions, frustration is evaluated through four questions: 1) You wanted more information but did not know where to find it; 2) It took a lot of effort to get the information you needed; 3) You did not have the time to get all the information you needed; 4) You felt frustrated during your search for the information. Confusion is assessed with two questions: 1) You were concerned about the quality of the information; 2) The information you found was too hard to understand ($\alpha = .82$).

Other studies focus on the role of patient satisfaction in cancer-related information seeking, centering on patients' reliance on the Internet as compared to other information sources. For instance, on a 4-point scale ranging from "very" through "somewhat" and "not at all" to "don't use," cancer patients were asked to evaluate the Internet and other sources' comprehensiveness, accuracy, credibility, relevance, convenience of use, and whether the information provided is easy to understand and helps them make a decision. Sources evaluated include Internet ($\alpha = .81$), online support groups ($\alpha = .85$), cancer specialist ($\alpha = .83$), other health care provider ($\alpha = .89$), television ($\alpha = .85$), radio ($\alpha = .87$), magazines and newspapers ($\alpha = .81$), and brochures from clinics ($\alpha = .83$). Patients also rate the extent to which they use the Internet to supplement and verify information from their cancer specialist, for an explanation of their illness, for decisions about treatments and medications, for information on side effects, and to check the credentials of their oncologist, hospital, or clinic ($\alpha = .79$) (Tustin, 2010).

Concerning patients with newly diagnosed prostate cancer, researchers have used descriptive paragraphs to depict five different health information seeking behavior profiles: intense (having a keen interest in detailed cancer information), complementary (process of getting "good enough" cancer information), fortuitous (search for cancer information mainly from others with a diagnosis of cancer), minimal (a limited interest for cancer information), and guarded (avoidance of some cancer information) (Lambert, Loiselle, & Macdonald, 2009a, 2009b). Applying these profiles, past research has asked patients to select the pattern that best describes how they wish to receive information to help them make a treatment decision (Davison & Breckon, 2012).

Similar to this approach, past research has also employed Likert-type scales to assess individuals' information seeking activities that are not related to specific sources. Typical items include: 1) When the topic of [specific health topic] comes up, I'm likely to tune it out; 2) I am likely to search for information about [specific health topic]; 3) I look for information about [specific health topic] to understand it better ($\alpha = .70$) (Yang, 2012).

Behavior versus Intention

Lastly, the measurement strategies reviewed above mostly rely on individuals' reflections of their past information seeking behaviors. In contrast, several studies have attempted to track actual health information seeking. For instance, focusing on breast cancer patients, a research team from the University of Wisconsin's Comprehensive Health Enhancement Support System (CHESS), a well established and widely studied interactive website, developed a web browser to automatically collect information about users at the individual keystroke level as patients utilized the system. This allows the research team to create a log file with each user's code name, date, time spent, and URL of every web page requested from the CHESS web server database. For each CHESS information service and topic sought out, the total time spent browsing each type of information indicates cancer patients' information-seeking activities (Kim, Shah, Namkoong, McTavish, & Gustafson, 2013).

To measure public information seeking behaviors related to cervical cancer, cervical screening, and HPV vaccination, researchers have relied on Google Insights for Search, a database of all Google searches that can be analyzed by week of access and country of user. This tool does not provide absolute numbers of searches but a relative figure based on changes in search activity for the time period under study (Metcalfe, Price, & Powell, 2011).

On the opposite spectrum, several studies have examined health information seeking as individuals' intentions to seek health information in the near future (Hovick, Kahlor, & Liang, 2014; Kahlor, 2010; Rains, 2008). Table 4 shows sample items for health information-seeking intentions that achieve good reliability ($\alpha = .97$).

Table 4. Sample scale for health information-seeking intentions (Hovick et al., 2014).

Please indicate whether you agree with the following items (1 = strongly disagree, 7 = strongly agree)

---

1. I plan to seek information about my cancer risks in the near future.
2. I will try and seek information about my cancer risks in the near future.
3. I intend to find more information about my cancer risks soon.
4. I intend to look for information about my cancer risks in the near future.
5. I will look for information related to my cancer risks in the near future.

Use of Existing Measures and Future Studies

This chapter reviewed scales that have been used in empirical research to assess health information seeking. As Anker et al. (2011) showed, a majority of studies prior to 2010 measured general health information seeking (i.e., whether the participant engaged in a search for health information) through cross-sectional study designs. A large proportion of those studies used open-ended questions to assess health information seeking content or dichotomous measures to assess desire for health information. Other studies used Likert-type scales to assess frequency of source/channel use or dichotomous measures to assess information sources/channels utilized. Focusing on certain aspects of information seeking, some studies used Likert-type scales to assess information or source credibility, barriers to health information seeking/self-efficacy, intentions to seek health information, and reasons for seeking information.

Looking at studies published since 2010, these trends largely remain the same. However, recent research has also utilized more creative strategies such as using descriptive scenarios to describe different information seeking styles and incorporating technology to track actual health information seeking behavior. In addition, a large proportion of empirical studies focus on online information seeking. Health information seeking activities involve dynamic processes that are largely context-specific (i.e. they can change based on prognosis of diseases, and upon the cognitive versus affective states of the information seeker). Thus, in addition to measuring health information seeking as an outcome variable, researchers should pay more attention to the processes and mechanisms that account for health information seeking. That is, health information seeking research should employ more diverse measurement topics such as barriers to health information seeking, self-efficacy, and motivations for health information seeking.

Recommended Readings

Afifi, W., & Weiner, J. (2004). Toward a theory of motivated information management. *Communication Theory, 14*, 167–190.

Brashers, D. E. (2001). Communication and uncertainty management. *Journal of Communication, 51*(3), 477–497.

Case, D. O. (2002). *Looking for information: A survey of research on information seeking, needs and behavior.* San Diego, CA: Academic Press.

Johnson, J. D., & Case, D. O. (2012). *Health Information Seeking.* New York: Peter Lang.

Niederdeppe, J., Hornik, R. C., Kelly, B. J., Frosch, D. L., Romantan, A., Stevens, R. S., & Schwartz, J. S. (2007). Examining the dimensions of cancer-related information seeking and scanning behavior. *Health Communication, 22*(2), 153–167.

References

Afifi, W., & Weiner, J. (2004). Toward a theory of motivated information management. *Communication Theory, 14*, 167–190.

Anker, A. E., Reinhart, A. M., & Feeley, T. H. (2011). Health information seeking: A review of measures and methods. *Patient Education and Counseling, 82*, 346–354.

Arora, N., Hesse, B., Rimer, B., Viswanath, K., Clayman, M., & Croyle, R. (2008). Frustrated and confused: The American public rates its cancer-related information-seeking experiences. *Journal of General Internal Medicine, 23*(3), 223–228. doi: 10.1007/s11606-007-0406-y.

Blance-Hartigan, D., Blake, K. D., & Viswanath, K. (2014). Cancer survivors' use of numerous information sources for cancer-related information: Does more matter? *Journal of Cancer Education, 29*, 488–496.

Case, D. O. (2002). *Looking for information: A survey of research on information seeking, needs and behavior.* San Diego, CA: Academic Press.

Chang, L. (2014). College students' search for sexual health information from their best friends: An application of the theory of motivated information management. *Asian Journal of Social Psychology, 17*(3), 196–205. doi: 10.1111/ajsp.12063.

Davison, B. J., & Breckon, E. N. (2012). Impact of health information-seeking behavior and personal factors on preferred role in treatment decision-making in men with newly diagnosed prostate cancer. *Cancer Nursing, 35*(6), 411–418.

Dobransky, K., & Hargittai, E. (2012). Inquiring minds acquiring wellness: uses of online and offline sources for health information. *Health Communication, 27*(4), 331 343. doi: 10.1080/10410236.2011.585451.

Freimuth, V. S, Stein, J. A., & Kean, T. J. (1989). *Searching for health information: The Cancer Information Service model.* Philadelphia: University of Pennsylvania Press.

Galarce, E. M., Ramanadhan, S., Weeks, J., Schneider, E. C., Gray, S. W., & Viswanath, K. (2011). Class, race, ethnicity and information needs in post-treatment cancer patients. *Patient Education and Counseling, 85*(3), 432–439. http://dx.doi.org/10.1016/j.pec.2011.01.030

Griffin, R. J., Dunwoody, S., & Neuwirth, K. (1999). Proposed model of the relationship of risk information seeking and processing to the development of preventive behaviors. *Environmental Research, 80*(2), S230-S245.

Hovick, S. R., Kahlor, L., & Liang, M. (2014). Personal cancer knowledge and information seeking through PRISM: The planed risk information seeking model. *Journal of Health Communication, 19*, 511–527.

Johnson, J. D., & Case, D. O. (2012). *Health Information Seeking*. New York: Peter Lang.

Johnson, J. D., & Meischke, H. (1993). A comprehensive model of cancer-related information seeking applied to magazines. *Human Communication Research, 19*, 343–367.

Kahlor, L. (2010). PRISM: A planned risk information seeking model. *Health Communication, 25*, 345–356.

Kim, S. C., Shah, D. V., Namkoong, K., McTavish, F. M., & Gustafson, D. H. (2013). Predictors of online health information seeking among women with breast cancer: the role of social support perception and emotional well-being. *Journal of Computer-Mediated Communication, 18*(2), 98–118. doi: 10.1111/jcc4.12002.

Lambert, S. D., & Loiselle, C. G. (2007). Health information seeking behavior. *Qualitative Health Research, 17*, 1006–1019.

Lambert, S. D., Loiselle, C. G., & Macdonald, M. E. (2009a). An in-depth exploration of information-seeking behavior among individuals with cancer: Part 2: Understanding differential patterns of active information seeking. *Cancer Nursing, 32*(1), 26–36.

Lambert, S. D., Loiselle, C. G., & Macdonald, M. E. (2009b). An in-depth exploration of information-seeking behavior among individuals with cancer: Part 1: Understanding differential patterns of active information seeking. *Cancer Nursing, 32*(1), 11–23.

Lewis, N., Martinez, L. S., Freres, D. R., Schwartz, J. S., Armstrong, K., Gray, S. W.,... Hornik, R. C. (2012). Seeking cancer-related information from media and family/friends increases fruit and vegetable consumption among cancer patients. *Health Communication, 27*(4), 380–388. doi: 10.1080/10410236.2011.586990.

Longo, D. R. (2005). Understanding health information, communication and information seeking of patients and consumers: A comprehensive and integrative model. *Health Expectations, 8*, 189–194.

Manganello, J. A., & Clayman, M. L. (2011). The association of understanding of medical statistics with health information seeking and health provider interaction in a national sample of young adults. *Journal of Health Communication, 16*, 163–176. doi: 10.1080/10810730.2011.604704.

McMillan, S. J., & Macias, W. (2008). Strengthening the safety net for online seniors: factors influencing differences in health information seeking among older Internet users. *Journal of Health Communication, 13*(8), 778–792. doi: 10.1080/10810730802487448.

Metcalfe, D., Price, C., & Powell, J. (2011). Media coverage and public reaction to a celebrity cancer diagnosis. *Journal of Public Health, 33*(1), 80–85. doi: 10.1093/pubmed/fdq052.

Neumark, Y., Lopez-Quintero, C., Feldman, B. S., Hirsch Allen, A. J., & Shtarkshall, R. (2013). Online health information seeking among Jewish and Arab adolescents in Israel: Results from a national school survey. *Journal of Health Communication, 18*(9), 1097–1115. doi: 10.1080/10810730.2013.778360.

Oh, H. J., Lauckner, C., Boehmer, J., Fewins-Bliss, R., & Li, K. (2013). Facebooking for health: An examination into the solicitation and effects of health-related social support on social networking sites. *Computers in Human Behavior, 29*(5), 2072–2080. http://dx.doi.org/10.1016/j.chb.2013.04.017

Oh, K. M., Kreps, G. L., Jun, J., Chong, E., & Ramsey, L. (2012). Examining the health information–seeking behaviors of Korean Americans. *Journal of Health Communication, 17*(7), 779–801. doi: 10.1080/10810730.2011.650830.

Peretti-Watel, P., Seror, V., Verger, P., Guignard, R., Legleye, S., & Beck, F. (2014). Smokers' risk perception, socioeconomic status and source of information on cancer. *Addictive Behaviors, 39*(9), 1304–1310. http://dx.doi.org/10.1016/j.addbeh.2014.04.016

Rains, S. A. (2008). Seeking health information in the information age: The role of Internet self-efficacy. *Western Journal of Communication, 72*, 1–18.

Rains, S. A., & Karmikel, C. D. (2009). Health information-seeking and perceptions of website credibility: Examining web-use orientation, message characteristics, and structural features of websites. *Computers in Human Behavior, 25*, 544–553.

Ruppel, E. K., & Rains, S. A. (2012). Information sources and the health information-seeking process: an application and extension of channel complementarity theory. *Communication Monographs, 79*(3), 385–405. doi: 10.1080/03637751.2012.697627.

Tian, Y., & Robinson, J. D. (2013). Media complementarity and health information seeking in Puerto Rico. *Journal of Health Communication, 19*(6), 710–720. doi: 10.1080/10810730.2013.821558.

Tustin, N. (2010). The role of patient satisfaction in online health information seeking. *Journal of Health Communication, 15*(1), 3–17. doi: 10.1080/10810730903465491.

Weaver III, J. B., Thompson, N. J., Weaver, S., & Hopkins, G. L. (2009). Healthcare non-adherence decisions and Internet health information. *Computers in Human Behavior, 25*, 1373–1380.

Yang, Z. J. (2012). Too scared or too capable? Why do college students stay away from the H1N1 flu vaccine? *Risk Analysis, 32*, 1703–1716. doi: 10.1111/j.1539-6924.2012.01799.x.

Yang, Z. J., McComas, K. A., Gay, G., Leonard, J. P., Dannenberg, A. J., & Dillon, H. (2011). Information seeking related to clinical trial enrollment. *Communication Research, 38*, 856–882.

6. Health Literacy Assessment

SHOOU-YIH DANIEL LEE,
University of Michigan
& TZU-I TSAI,
National Yang-Ming University, Taiwan

Health literacy is a requisite ability and skill for health promotion and self-care. Systematic research and effective interventions are impossible without accurate measurement. Thus, a global interest in health literacy has led to numerous efforts in developing health literacy instruments in different languages and countries.

A popular approach to health literacy instrument development is translation of existing instruments—such as Rapid Estimate of Adult Literacy in Medicine (REALM), Test of Functional Health Literacy in Adults (TOFHLA) and its short form TOFHL-S, and Newest Vital Sign (NVS)—that were developed in the United States (e.g.,Connor, Mantwill, & Schulz, 2013; Han, Kim, Kim, & Kim, 2011; Jović-Vraneš, Bjegović-Mikanović, Marinković, & Vuković, 2013). A related approach is modification of existing instruments—e.g., changing the spelling, converting numerical units to ensure format-concordance with the target population, using passages that are specific to the new context of application (Ko, Lee, Toh, Tang, & Tan, 2012; Rowlands et al., 2013).

Translation and modification of existing instruments are time and cost-efficient. However, they may fail to account for cultural differences—as well as structural, financial, and operational differences in health care delivery systems—that may influence individual abilities to comprehend and utilize health information, communicate with health care providers, and access appropriate health services (Beaton, Bombardier, Guillemin, & Ferraz, 2000). Take English-language instruments as an example. British English and American English differ significantly in phonology, vocabulary, spelling, and grammar (Crystal, 2004). The language differences aside, English-speaking countries, such as the UK, the USA, Canada, Australia, and New Zealand, do not share the same customs, attitudes, values, and worldviews. Significantly, the structural, financial, and operational differences in their health care delivery systems are likely to limit the application of a health literacy instrument across those countries.

Attempts to develop a new health literacy instrument are rare, likely because they are costly, time consuming, and not conducive to cross-cultural comparisons. Nevertheless, new instrument development maximizes the likelihood of linguistic and cultural appropriateness. The purpose of this chapter is to describe a methodology that was employed to develop a new and theoretically sound instrument for measuring health literacy in Mandarin Chinese in Taiwan. The methodology is generic and has wide application for instrument development in other languages and countries.

Measuring Health Literacy: Developing the Mandarin Health Literacy Scale (MHLS) [1]

Development of MHLS Items

To ensure that the MHLS was theoretically sound, we first invested in constructing a conceptual framework (Figure 1) based on a thorough review of the literature, in-depth interviews of health consumers, and discussions with an expert panel. The framework specified (1) four capabilities that an individual needed to adequately deal with personal health issues (obtaining information, understanding information, processing information, and decision-making); (2) six major types of health information and services that an individual encountered in a health care system (health promotion and maintenance, health signs and medical symptoms, diagnosis, treatment/medication, treatment/surgery, and treatment/self-care); and (3) three domains of literacy skills: prose (the ability to read and understand text), document (the ability to locate and use information in a document), and numeracy (the ability to apply arithmetic operations and use numerical information).

This framework guided the development of a draft instrument through a 3-step process that included (1) item pool development, (2) item selection, and (3) evaluation of readability.

Figure 1. The MHLS Framework.

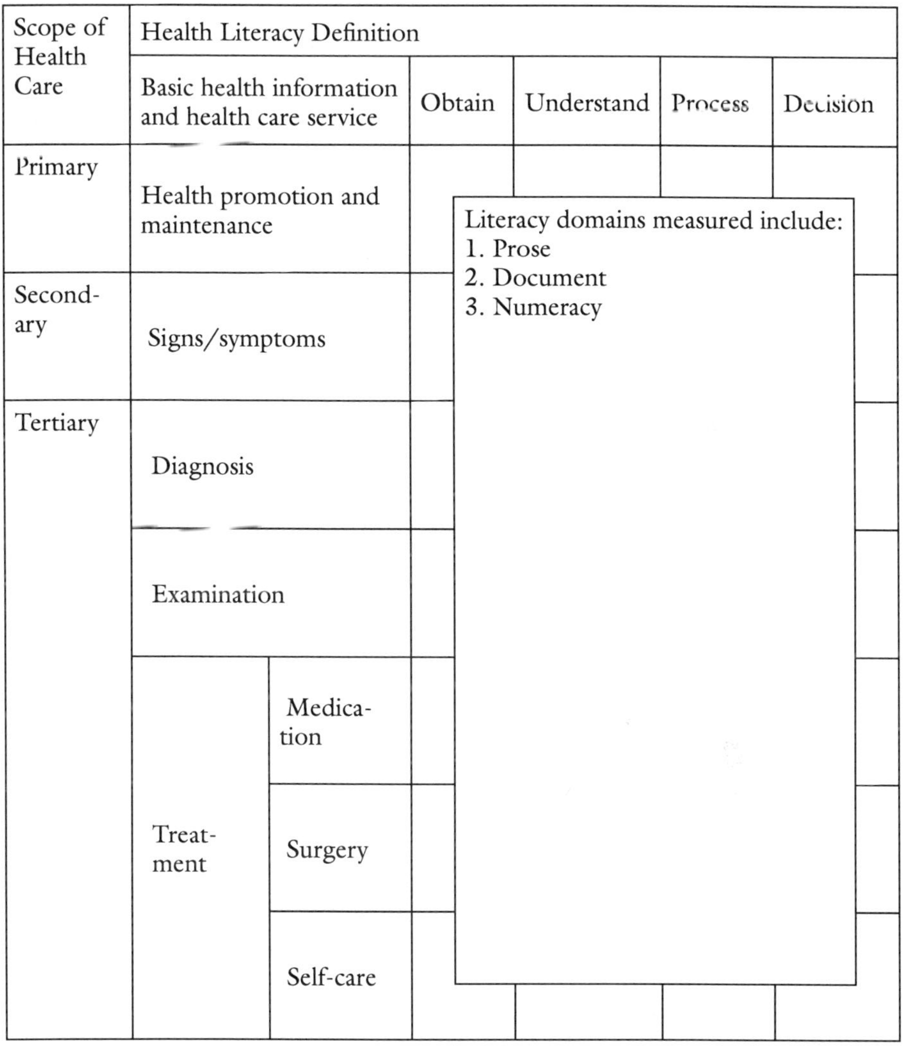

Scope of Health Care	Health Literacy Definition				
	Basic health information and health care service	Obtain	Understand	Process	Decision
Primary	Health promotion and maintenance				
Second-ary	Signs/symptoms	Literacy domains measured include: 1. Prose 2. Document 3. Numeracy			
Tertiary	Diagnosis				
	Examination				
	Treat-ment — Medica-tion				
	Treat-ment — Surgery				
	Self-care				

Source: Tsai, T. I., Lee, S. Y., Tsai, Y. W., & Kuo, K. N. (2011). Methodology and validation of health literacy scale development in Taiwan. *Journal of Health Communication, 16*(1), 50 61.

Item pool development. A group of health care experts, including physicians and health behavior and communication specialists, used the framework as a guide and followed the template of existing instrument (primarily TOFHLA) to construct a pool of 183 test items, grouped in four sections that reflected real-life literacy abilities. The first section assessed reading and comprehension abilities. The tasks involved reading five short, health-related passages regarding cardiovascular diseases, asthma, degenerative arthritis, cold and influenza, and tuberculosis and then locating, selecting, or integrating text or quantitative information to answer questions specific to each of the passages. The second section included Cloze-type questions that simulated the dialogue between a patient and a physician in an ambulatory setting regarding the symptoms, diagnosis, and treatment of seven common diseases (cough, fever, cellulitis, chest muscle pain, insomnia, urinary tract infection, and tuberculosis). The third section used six prescription labels with variation in dosage, path, and schedule to assess abilities to comprehend both text and numeric information and to correctly follow the directions. The final section incorporated two appointment slips, three examination instructions, two billing statements, and two consent forms to assess abilities to comprehend text information, read a map, tell the time, identify the date, understand billing information, and follow clinical instructions in order to navigate the health care system.

Item selection. A Delphi panel of 23 experts, including physicians, nurses, pharmacists, health educators, health care administrators, and health services researchers, participated in three rounds of evaluation and discussion to select test items. In the first round, the panel rated the *appropriateness* and *clarity* of each item on a 5-point Likert scale and provided suggestions for revision if necessary. The research team collected and summarized ratings, incorporated the suggestions in revising test items, and sent the revision back to the panel. The second round involved the panel weighing the *importance* (very, somewhat, and not at all) and *difficulty* (very difficult, somewhat difficult, and easy) of each item and sending the results, along with comments, to the research team for summarization. The final round, a round-table discussion, was held among the panel to review the results from the first two rounds of evaluation and to form consensus on a final set of items to be included in the health literacy scale. The panel eliminated inappropriate and redundant items (items assessing the same ability and showing a similar difficulty level) as well as items that less than two-thirds of the panel considered to be important. The final set included 63 items, which were equally distributed across four sections: health materials (15 items), outpatient dialogue (16 items), prescription labels (17 items), and health-related written documents (15 items). Nineteen of those items assessed numeracy skills and 44 assessed comprehension abilities.

Evaluation of readability. We recruited 18 4th to 9th-grade teachers at urban, suburban, and rural schools to review and rephrase the 63 test items, because there was no established standard to assess readability in Mandarin Chinese (a problem not uncommon in other languages) and because the reading level of an average Taiwanese was between grades 5 to 8. We also conducted a cognitive, "think aloud" interview with 67 4th to 9th-grade students to help us revise the items. The revised instrument was then administered to 518 students in grades 4 to 9 to ensure appropriate readability. Results of these evaluations led us to reword and rephrase some of the items to improve the readability of the scale. No item was deleted at this stage.

MHLS Validation

To validate the scale, we field-tested it with a random sample of 323 Taiwanese adults (age 18 and over). The field-test questionnaire included the 63 MHLS items as well as questions regarding the subject's socio-demographic information, general health status, health knowledge, reading habits, and receipt of assistance with written health materials. The MHLS items were self-administered and the remainder of the questionnaire was administered in-person by trained interviewers.

Using the field-test data, we employed item response theory (IRT) and item total correlation to calibrate the MHLS scale (Embretson & Reise, 2000). We eliminated 13 items that had either low item-total correlations or appeared to provide redundant information in terms of discrimination and difficulty. Of the 50 retained items, 33 concerned text reading and 17 were assessments of numeracy.

Finally, we assessed the convergent validity, predictive validity, internal reliability, and split-half reliability of the remaining 50 items. Convergent validity was assessed by correlating a subject's score on the 50 items to his/her years of formal schooling. Predictive validity was evaluated by correlating a subject's score to his/her health status, health knowledge, self-reported reading habits, and self-reported reading assistance. Internal reliability was examined using the Cronbach's alpha. Split-half reliability was determined by randomly splitting the 50 items into two equal parts and correlating the scores on both halves.

Psychometric Qualities and Research Use of MHLS

The total score of the remaining 50 items on MHLS was significantly correlated with years of formal education ($r = 0.72$, $p<0.001$), indicating high convergent validity. The score was also significantly related to reading habit ($r = 0.34$, $p<0.001$), health knowledge ($r = 0.55$, $p<0.001$), and receipt of assistance with reading written health materials ($r = -0.52$, $p<0.001$), suggesting good predictive validity. The MHLS also displayed high internal reliability (Cronbach's alpha = 0.97) and split-half reliability ($r = 0.90$, $p<0.001$).

By examining the scatter plot of the MHLS score and years of formal schooling as well as the distributions and 95% confidence intervals of the score for different educational attainment groupings (≤6 years, 7–12 years, 13–16 years, and ≥17 years), we classified health literacy into three levels: inadequate (0–30), marginal (31–42), and adequate (43–50). In our study sample, 15.4% had inadequate health literacy, 17.1% had marginal health literacy, and 67.6% had adequate health literacy. The proportion of individuals with inadequate health literacy increased with age, ranging from 4.0% in the 18–30 group to 45.9% in the ≥60 group. There was no significant gender difference in terms of inadequate health literacy.

We have used the MHLS in several studies (Lee, Tsai, & Tsai, 2013; Lee, Tsai, Tsai, & Kuo, 2010, 2011, 2012; Tsai, Lee, & Chang, 2014; Tsai, Lee, & Tsai, 2013). Results indicate that individuals with lower health literacy have poorer physical and psychological health status; were less likely to seek health information; more likely to interpret medication label incorrectly; had more problems communicating with health care providers; and were less likely to participate in health decision-making and practice health promoting behaviors. We have shown that health literacy is directly and indirectly related to health promotion behaviors via socio-cognitive factors such as self-efficacy and health locus of control.

Use of the MHLS Measure and Future Studies

We should note several caveats in the methodology described above. First, the methods we employed were meant to develop an instrument that assessed general health literacy. They may be adapted to assess health literacy in relation to specific diseases or health problems (e.g., diabetes, mental health) and populations (e.g., adolescents, older adults). Second, we did not evaluate individuals' abilities to communicate with health care providers and to critically appraise the accuracy of health information (Heijmans, Waverijn, Rademakers, van der Vaart, & Rijken, 2015). Development of communicative and critical health literacy would require a different methodology. Third, the instrument we developed was primarily for research use. Modifying or shortening it for screening purposes would require further work.

A major lesson we learned is the importance of a sound conceptual framework in guiding the scale development. The framework made explicit how we conceptualized health literacy. Without that, we may not have been able to effectively work with expert panels in reaching a common understanding of health literacy and developing and selecting test items that reflected the key dimensions of the concept. An explicit framework could also facilitate our revision and improvement of the instrument to account for continuing evolution of the health literacy concept.

Our scale development benefited from the collaboration with a heterogeneous panel of experts with diverse backgrounds in medicine, nursing, pharmacy, adult education, health behavior and health education, health communication, and health services research. The diversity of expert panels provided a check-and-balance, helping to uncover "blind spots" of the research team in the scale development process. The struggle to forge a common understanding among panelists of health literacy also increased our appreciation that health literacy is multidimensional, composed of not one but several skills, and that the skills an individual needs to make personal health decisions and seek proper care are specific to the structure of a country's health care delivery system.

This contextual understanding of health literacy points to the inadequacy of cross-cultural adaption of existing instruments. We offer instead a generic methodology for developing health literacy instruments that are culturally appropriate and country specific.

Note

1. The description in this section is adapted from an article published in the *Journal of Health Communication* (T. I. Tsai, Lee, Tsai, & Kuo, 2011)

Recommended Readings

Haun, J. N., Valerio, M. A., McCormack, L. A., Sørensen, K., & Paasche-Orlow, M. K. (2014). Health literacy measurement: An inventory and descriptive summary of 51 instruments. *Journal of Health Communication, 19,* 302–333.

McCormack, L., Bann, C., Squiers, L., Berkman, N. D., Squire, C., Schillinger, D., Ohene-Frempong, J., & Hibbard, J. (2010). Measuring health literacy: A pilot study of a new skills-based instrument. *Journal of Health Communication, 10,* 51–71.

McCormack, L., Haun, J., Sørensen, K., & Valerio, M. (2013). Recommendations for advancing health literacy measurement. *Journal of Health Communication, 18,* 9–14.

Tsai, T.-I., Lee, S.-Y., Tsai, Y.-W., & Kuo, K. N. (2011). Methodology and validation of health literacy scale development in Taiwan. *Journal of Health Communication, 16,* 50–61.

References

Beaton, D. E., Bombardier, C., Guillemin, F., & Ferraz, M. (2000). Guidelines for the process of cross-cultural adaptation of self-report measures. *Spine, 25,* 3186–3191.

Connor, M., Mantwill, S., & Schulz, P. (2013). Functional health literacy in Switzerland–validation of a German, Italian, and French health literacy test. *Patient Education and Counseling, 90*(1), 12–17.

Crystal, D. (2004). *The Cambridge encyclopedia of the English language* (2nd ed.). Cambridge: Cambridge University Press.

Embretson, S. E., & Reise, S. P. (2000). *Item response theory for psychologists*. Mahwah, NJ: Erlbaum.

Han, H. R., Kim, J., Kim, M. T., & Kim, K. B. (2011). Measuring health literacy among immigrants with a phonetic primary language: A case of Korean American women. *Journal of Immigrant and Minority Health, 13*(2), 253–259.

Heijmans, M., Waverijn, G., Rademakers, J., van der Vaart, R., & Rijken, M. (2015). Functional, communicative and critical health literacy of chronic disease patients and their importance for self-management. *Patient Education and Counseling, 98*(1), 41–48.

Jović-Vraneš, A., Bjegović-Mikanović, V., Marinković, J., & Vuković, D. (2013). Evaluation of a health literacy screening tool in primary care patients: Evidence from Serbia. *Health Promotion International, 29*(4), 601–607.

Ko, Y., Lee, J., Toh, M., Tang, W., & Tan, A. (2012). Development and validation of a general health literacy test in Singapore. *Health Promotion International, 27*(1), 45–51.

Lee, S.-Y. D., Tsai, T.-I., & Tsai, Y.-W. (2013). Accuracy in self-reported health literacy screening: A difference between men and women. *BMJ Open, 3*(11), e002928.

Lee, S.-Y. D., Tsai, T.-I., Tsai, Y.-W., & Kuo, K. N. (2010). Health literacy, health status, and healthcare utilization of Taiwanese adults: Results from a national survey. *BMC Public Health, 10*, 614.

Lee, S.-Y. D., Tsai, T.-I., Tsai, Y.-W., & Kuo, K. N. (2011). Health literacy and women's health-related behaviors in Taiwan. *Health Education & Behavior, 39*(2), 210–218.

Lee, S.-Y. D., Tsai, T.-I., Tsai, Y.-W., & Kuo, K. N. (2012). Development and validation of the short-form Mandarin Health Literacy Scale. *Taiwan Journal of Public Health, 31*(2), 184–194.

Rowlands, G., Khazaezadeh, N., Oteng-Ntim, E., Seed, P., Barr, S., & Weiss, B. (2013). Development and validation of a measure of health literacy in the UK: The newest vital sign. *BMC Public Health, 13*(1), 116.

Tsai, T.-I., Lee, S.-Y. D., & Chang, L.-Y. (2014). Misunderstanding of medication labels: Results of national survey in Taiwan. *Taiwan Journal of Public Health, 33*(3), 238–250.

Tsai, T.-I., Lee, S.-Y. D., & Tsai, Y.-W. (2012). *Health literacy, health behaviors, and health status*. Health and Medicine in South Asia. Academic Sinica. Taipei, Taiwan.

Tsai, T.-I., Lee, S.-Y. D., & Tsai, Y.-W. (2013). Explaining selected health behaviors in a national sample of Taiwanese adults. *Health Promotion International*. doi:10.1093/heapro/dat085.

Tsai, T. I., Lee, S. Y., Tsai, Y. W., & Kuo, K. N. (2011). Methodology and validation of health literacy scale development in Taiwan. *Journal of Health Communication, 16*(1), 50–61.

7. Media Literacy

BRUCE E. PINKLETON,
Washington State University
& ERICA WEINTRAUB AUSTIN,
Washington State University

Researchers have documented the potentially harmful contributions of media message exposure to negative outcomes in a variety of contexts including alcohol abuse (e.g., Anderson, de Bruijn, Angus, Gordon, & Hastings, 2009; Hoffman, Pinkleton, Austin, & Reyes-Velazquez, 2014), tobacco use (e.g., Davis, Gilpin, Loken, Viswanath, & Wakefield, 2008; Pinkleton, Austin, Cohen, Miller, & Fitzgerald, 2007), and sexual decision-making (e.g., Chandra, Martino, Collins, Elliott, Berry, Kanouse, & Miu, 2008; Hestroni, 2007; Pinkleton, Austin, Chen, & Cohen, 2012, 2013). Media also can have beneficial effects to the extent that users can make distinctions effectively between beneficial or truthful information versus unhealthy or deceptive information. As a result, many experts are looking for viable strategies to help reduce negative media influence and to enhance the potential for positive media influence on message receivers' decision-making and behavior.

In general, scholars define media literacy broadly in terms of an individual's ability to access, analyze, evaluate, and communicate messages using a wide range of communication tools and forms (Aufderheide, 1993). Media literacy primarily focuses on activating individuals' logic-based information processing in an effort to help counteract the impact of messages by helping increase individuals' skepticism toward media messages and strengthening their critical thinking (e.g., Austin, Pinkleton, Hust, & Cohen, 2005; Hobbs & Frost, 2003; Pinkleton et al., 2007). Consistent with this perspective, the intent of media literacy education is to help people—often adolescents—develop the tools necessary to analyze the veracity of media messages and use them effectively in decision-making. Austin (2014) writes that media-literate individuals possess capabilities that develop with maturation, such as the cognitive sophistication to control attentional processes, relevant competencies resulting from vicarious and/or personally experienced learning, and the skills necessary to apply competencies as appropriate. Scholars have completed a number of reviews concerning media literacy and related topics (e.g., Bergsma & Carney, 2008; Hobbs, 2011; Jeong, Cho, & Hwang, 2012; Potter, 2010).

The impact of media literacy training should be most evident through assessments of individuals' beliefs related to decision-making processes, because media literacy holds that increased understanding of media messages should alter their influence. Evaluations of media literacy programs typically are based on theoretical concepts from social cognitive theory (Bandura, 1986), expectancy theory (Goldman, Brown, & Christiansen, 1987) and theories of heuristic and systematic message processing (e.g., Chen & Chaiken, 1999). These concepts are reflected in constructs associated with the Message Interpretation Process (MIP) Model—consistent with the Integrative Model of Behavioral Prediction (Fishbein & Capella, 2006)—because it treats decision-making as a process of message evaluation and understanding rather than as a simple response to message stimuli (Austin et al., 2005).

The results of a meta-analysis concerning media literacy programs conducted by Jeong and colleagues (2012) indicate that media literacy interventions typically produce effects on outcomes they classify as either media relevant or behavior relevant. Media-relevant outcomes include knowledge of media, understanding of persuasive intent of advertising, skepticism toward media messages, and the like. Behavior-relevant outcomes include normative perceptions of the behavior of social-reference groups, attitudes toward performing specific behaviors, and self-efficacy to perform these behaviors such as refusing tobacco or choosing to delay sex. As a result of their research, Jeong and colleagues (2012) indicate media literacy programs generally are effective as interventions producing desired effects on most media- and behavior-relevant outcomes; the authors suggest that such curricula have the potential to reduce potentially harmful message effects (Jeong et al., 2012).

The following measures have appeared in a variety of publications and conference papers about research with adolescents and young adults, for topics ranging from substance use to sexual health and public affairs, with acceptable-to-high reliability coefficients. This is not a comprehensive list of evaluative indexes but rather a sample of indexes that have proven useful in past media literacy evaluations. In most instances, item response scales are 7-point, modified Likert scales with strongly disagree and strongly agree (or other applicable response descriptors) as anchors.

Measuring Media Literacy: Constructs and Measures

Knowledge Questions Example

The questions in this example are based on sexual health but similar questions can address any media literacy-relevant topic. In an experiment, these questions can serve as a manipulation check to ensure the participants who received media literacy training benefitted in terms of knowledge gain, and no alpha is necessary.

- About what percentage of teens report that they have had sexual intercourse?
  10%   20%   50%   80%   Don't know
- Most teens who have had sex wish they had waited.
- A vaccine is available to prevent the HPV sexually transmitted infection.
- Some sexually transmitted diseases can be treated but not cured.
- Not having sex is the only 100% guaranteed way to avoid sexually transmitted diseases.
- Condoms are 100% effective at preventing pregnancy.
- Most birth control methods also prevent sexually transmitted diseases.

Perceived Realism

Participants indicate the extent to which media portrayals seem true to life by answering questions concerning perceived realism. Examples of alphas for perceived realism have included .76 and .80, potentially depending on variables such as participants' age.

- Advertising [might be TV, movies, music] about [relevant descriptor] is a realistic source of information for what makes people popular.
- Advertising [might be TV, movies, music] about [relevant descriptor] is a realistic source of information for what makes people successful.
- Advertising [might be TV, movies, music] concerning [relevant descriptor] is a realistic source of information for how people who [engage in relevant behavior] act.

Perceived Similarity

Participants indicate the extent to which people they see in advertising or other media messages mirror people they know in their own lives. Correlations for two-index items measuring similarity have been significant; the alpha for a scale similar to the following scale was .80.

- People in [relevant descriptor] ads are like people I know.
- People in [relevant descriptor] ads are like people in my community.
- People in [relevant descriptor] ads are like people in my family.
- People in [relevant descriptor] ads are like people in my school.

Wishful Identification

Measures of wishful identification assess the extent to which participants desire to emulate people they see in the media. Examples of alphas for wishful identification have included .64 and .76.

- I wish I could be like people in [relevant descriptor] ads.
- I wish I could look like people in [relevant descriptor] ads.
- I wish I could do what people in [relevant to descriptor] ads do.
- I wish I could have as much fun as people in [relevant descriptor] ads have.

Perceived Media Influence

Measures of perceived media influence assess participants' understanding of the extent to which media influence adolescents' sexual or other behavior. Alphas typically have ranged from .70 to .82.

- Media messages change the way kids in my school think about [relevant descriptor].
- Media messages change the way teens think about [relevant descriptor].
- [Relevant descriptor] behaviors shown on TV [or adapt to other media platforms] change the way teens my age behave.

Perceived Media Myths

Participants indicate their knowledge of fallacies concerning mediated portrayals of a topic and its consequences by answering the following questions. Alphas typically have ranged from .71 to .84.

- People on TV make it seem okay (or appropriate) for teens to engage in [dangerous/unhealthy behavior].
- People on TV make is seem as if most teens are [engaging in dangerous/unhealthy behavior].
- Shows on television make it seem like popular people [engage in dangerous/unhealthy behavior].

The following questions concerning perceived media myths are reverse worded.

- Characters on TV make it seem as if few teens choose not to [engage in dangerous/unhealthy behavior].
- Characters on TV make it seem like [specific negative consequences] rarely happen [when teens engage in relevant dangerous/unhealthy behavior].

Perceived (Tactic-based) Desirability

Participants indicate the extent to which they find media portrayals of a topic enticing when completing items concerning tactic-based desirability. For example, the following items measured perceived, tactic-based desirability of advertising in an evaluation of a media literacy program concerning adolescent sexual health. Alphas for desirability typically have ranged from .78 to .88.

- When people in ads act sexy, it makes the products more interesting to me.
- I like ads that show people flirting.
- Ads that show people acting sexy get my attention.
- My favorite ads include people flirting.

Perceived (Social-comparison-based) Desirability

Indexes of perceived social-comparison-based desirability concern participants' reference-group members. In these instances, desirability measures address the extent to which participants are attracted by attributes of reference group members in media messages. These measures of desirability assess participants' responses to ads or other media messages based on the extent to which they contain actors that appear to be popular or unpopular, happy or sad, attractive or unattractive, successful or unsuccessful, and appear to have many friends or few friends.

As an additional note, in some instances measures of desirability have produced what appear to be boomerang effects because participants' ratings of message desirability remain steady or increase as a result of media literacy training. Further analyses have confirmed that these are in fact beneficial interactions resulting from a media-literacy intervention. That is, media literacy can diminish the influence of desirable but unrealistic media messages without reducing adolescents' appreciation for media messages (Austin, Pinkleton, & Chen, 2015; see also Austin, Pinkleton, & Funabiki, 2007).

Critical Thinking

Critical thinking concerning media is reflected in message receivers' competencies to assess media message content. Measures of critical thinking assess the extent to which individuals analyze media messages in a discriminating manner based on their possession of relevant capabilities, competencies, and skills (Austin, 2014).

Critical thinking about message content. The following three-item scale produced an alpha of .76 (Austin, Pinkleton, Radanielina Hita, Ran, 2015).

- I look for more information before I believe something I see in advertising [or other relevant media messages].
- I think about the truthfulness of advertisements [or other relevant media messages] before I accept them as true.
- It is important to think twice about what advertising messages [or other relevant media messages] say.

Critical thinking about message sources. The following three-item scale produced an alpha of .88 (Austin et al., 2015).

- I think about why someone created a message I see on TV.
- I think about how someone created a message I see on TV.
- I think about what the creator of a television message wants me to think.

Combined critical thinking index. Items similar to the following items might serve as part of a combined critical thinking scale or might serve in separate critical thinking scales concerning message content or message sources.

- I think about how someone created a message I see.
- I think about what the creator of a message wants me to think.
- I think about why someone created a message I see.
- It is important to think twice about what messages say.
- I look for more information before I believe something I see in messages.
- I think about things I see before I accept them as believable.

Expectancies Index

Participants indicate their beliefs concerning engaging in applicable or relevant behaviors by answering questions concerning expectancies. The following two scales, created for adolescent participants, address efficacy for different topics (the first for alcohol consumption and the second for engaging in sex). Alphas for expectancies typically have ranged from .67 to .84, depending on variables such as participants' age and the complexity of the referent topic.

Expectancies for alcohol consumption

- Drinking alcohol makes you feel happy.
- Beer is a good reward after a hard day.
- Drinking alcohol makes a party more fun.
- You will find alcohol at a good party.
- Drinking alcohol is a good way to relax.

Expectancies for sexual behavior

- Having sex shows a person is an adult.
- Being sexually active makes a person cool.
- Having sex makes a person popular.
- Being sexually active helps people fit in with others they want to have as friends.

Efficacy Index

Participants indicate their sense of their ability to control choices or outcomes concerning an issue by answering questions addressing efficacy. The following measures of efficacy, for example, concern sexual decision-making. Alphas for efficacy typically have ranged from .62 to .77, depending on variables such as participants' age and complexity of the referent topic.

- It's realistic for me to choose not to be sexually active.
- I can choose to resist pressure to engage in sexual behavior.
- If my friends participate in sexual behavior I probably will too (reverse worded).
- If my friends don't participate in sexual behavior I probably won't either.

Curriculum Evaluation Index

Media literacy typically involves a lesson or series of lessons that participants can evaluate. When it is appropriate or useful, participants can evaluate the media literacy curriculum by answering questions similar to these (alpha .87).

- The [media literacy topic] lessons will be useful for me.
- The [media literacy topic] lessons were interesting.

- The [media literacy topic] lessons have taught me things I did not know before.
- The [media literacy topic] lessons made me think.
- The [media literacy topic] presenters seemed to understand my concern.
- Before the [media literacy topic] program, I had never thought about what my life would be like if [negative health issue being targeted happened].
- The [media literacy topic] presenters knew what they were talking about.

Sometimes media literacy curriculum is taught by peer presenters. In these cases, the curriculum evaluation can include the following questions.

- Having presenters my age helps me understand the lessons better.
- I thought it was a good idea to have teens presenting the [media literacy topic] lessons.

Use of Existing Measures and Future Studies

Health promotion experts continue to seek and evaluate potential best practices as they work to reduce the influence of harmful media messages and increase the influence of positive media messages on message receivers' decision-making and behavior. The scales discussed in this chapter have proven useful identifying and understanding evidence-based outcomes resulting from media literacy training in a variety of contexts. One of the benefits of using these scales is that they enable researchers to examine variables as part of decision-making processes rather than simply examining decision-making outcomes. Research on information processing and message interpretation indicates that the skills and motivations with which individuals approach media messages play a more-important role in their decision-making than simple exposure (Austin et al., 2006). Audience members make sense of messages according to their own personal experience, ability, and need, and these often have logical and affective components (Austin, 2014; Pinkleton et al., 2013). Accordingly, some constructs have their basis in logic-oriented interpretations. Perceived similarity of a portrayal, for example, reflects how closely a portrayal reflects personal experience (Pinkleton, Austin, Van de Vord, 2010). The model also accounts for more affective aspects of interpretations, usually through measurement of the construct of perceived desirability.

As a result, the successful evaluation of media literacy programming requires a clear understanding of the needs of the individuals receiving a curriculum and also the specific, intended outcomes of the curriculum. When evaluating a media literacy program created for young people, for example, it is important to ensure that participants can easily read and understand each item. In addition, participants must have the opportunity to receive unbiased help from a trained adult when necessary and also have enough time to complete the entire questionnaire without feeling rushed or distressed. In addition, given the relatively large reading and comprehension differences existing among young people, it is important to have simple distractor tasks available for those who complete the questionnaire early so they do not disturb other participants who still are working to complete a questionnaire. To prepare a successful evaluation instrument requires careful pretesting and fine-tuning—typically more than once—and also time spent listening to those familiar with the environments in which testing will take place. This may mean numerous planning and evaluation meetings with teachers, for example, to ensure evaluation instruments are well written and clear and also that testing procedures are clearly understood to avoid biasing participants' responses. Ultimately, evaluating media literacy programs can be a complicated endeavor. To fail to carefully consider and plan the entirety of the evaluation process is to risk an incomplete or misleading evaluation outcome.

In terms of future research, it will be important for scholars to continue working to both understand message receivers' decision-making processes and to test and refine media construct measurement and evaluations of media literacy. One of the biggest limitations of previous media literacy evaluations has been the cross-sectional nature of evaluation data, which makes it impossible to draw conclusions about causality. In addition, evaluation findings typically are limited to single samples (e.g., college students or adolescents in a single state or region). Because decision-making models typically hypothesize that media message interpretations contribute to decisions over time, it is important for researchers to replicate and extend evaluation studies in a longitudinal design.

Ultimately, it is important for researchers to understand how young people and other potentially vulnerable message receivers process and interpret marketing and other media messages. Researchers and public health professionals need to continue their work developing effective educational programs and prevention campaigns resulting in message receivers' understanding and development of critical thinking skills. Media literacy evaluation measures help in this process by providing experts with evidence-based evaluation tools and an ability to help identify and evaluate best practices concerning media literacy.

Recommended Readings

Austin, E. W., Pinkleton, B. E., Austin, B. W., & Van de Vord, R. (2012). The relationships of information efficacy and media literacy skills to knowledge and self-efficacy for health-related decision-making. *Journal of American College Health, 60,* 548–554.

Austin, E. W., Pinkleton, B. E., Hust, S. J. T., & Cohen, M. (2005). Evaluation of an American Legacy Foundation/Washington State Department of Health media literacy pilot study. *Health Communication, 18,* 75–95.

Pinkleton, B. E., Austin, E. W., Chen, Y., & Cohen, M. (2012). The role of media literacy in shaping adolescents' understanding of and responses to sexual portrayals in mass media. *Journal of Health Communication, 17,* 460–476.

Pinkleton, B. E., Austin, E. W., Chen, Y., & Cohen, M. (2013). Assessing effects of a media literacy-based intervention on U.S. adolescents' responses to and interpretations of sexual media messages. *Journal of Children and Media, 7,* 463–479.

Pinkleton, B. E., Austin, E. W., Cohen, M., Chen, Y., & Fitzgerald, E. (2008). Effects of a peer-led media literacy curriculum on adolescents' knowledge and attitudes toward sexual behavior and media portrayals of sex. *Health Communication, 23,* 462–472.

Pinkleton, B. E., Austin, E. W., Cohen, M., Miller, A., & Fitzgerald, E. (2007). A statewide evaluation of the effectiveness of media literacy training to prevent tobacco use among adolescents. *Health Communication, 21,* 23–34.

References

Anderson, P., de Bruijn, A., Angus, K., Gordon, R., & Hastings, G. (2009). Impact of alcohol advertising and media exposure on adolescent alcohol use: A systematic review of longitudinal studies. *Alcohol and Alcoholism, 44,* 229–243.

Aufderheide, P. (1993). *National leadership conference on media literacy.* Conference report. Washington DC: Aspen Institute.

Austin, E. W. (2014). A bicycle riding theory of media literacy. In A. Silverblatt (Ed.), *The Praeger handbook of media literacy, volume 2* (pp. 538–543). Santa Barbara, CA: ABC-CLIO.

Austin, E. W., Chen, Y., Pinkleton, B. E., & Quintero Johnson, J. (2006). The benefits and costs of Channel One in a middle school setting. *Pediatrics, 117,* e-423-e433. Extended abstract, *Pediatrics, 117,* 907–908.

Austin, E. W., Pinkleton, B. E., & Chen, Y. (2015). Processing of sexual media messages improves due to media literacy effects on perceived message desirability. *Mass Communication and Society, 18,* 399–421.

Austin, E. W., Pinkleton, B. E., & Funabiki, R. P. (2007). The desirability paradox in the effects of media literacy training. *Communication Research, 34,* 483–506.

Austin, E. W., Pinkleton, B. E., Hust, S. J. T., & Cohen, M. (2005). Evaluation of an American Legacy Foundation/Washington State Department of Health media literacy pilot study. *Health Communication, 18,* 75–95.

Austin, E. W., Pinkleton, B. E., Radanielina Hita, M., & Ran, W. (2015). The role of parents' critical thinking about media in shaping expectancies, efficacy and nutrition behaviors for families. *Health Communication, 00,* 1–13.

Bandura, A. (1986). *Social foundations of thought and action: A social cognitive theory.* Englewood Cliffs, NJ: Prentice Hall.

Bergsma, L. J., & Carney, M. F. (2008). Effectiveness of health-promoting media literacy education: A systematic review. *Health Education Research, 23,* 522–542.

Chandra, A., Martino, S. C., Collins, R. L., Elliott, M. N., Berry, S. H., Kanouse, D. E., & Miu, A. (2008). Does watching sex on television predict teen pregnancy? Findings from a national longitudinal survey of youth. *Pediatrics, 122,* 1047–1054.

Chen, S. & Chaiken, S. (1999). The heuristic-systematic model in its broader context. In Chaiken, S. & Trope, Y. (Eds.), *Dual-Process Theories in Social Psychology* (pp. 73–96). New York: Guilford Press.

Davis, R. M, Gilpin, E. A., Loken, B., Viswanath, K., & Wakefield, M. A. (2008). *The role of the media in promoting and reducing tobacco use* (tobacco control monograph no. 19). Bethesda, MD: U.S. Department of Health and Human Services, National Institutes of Health, National Cancer Institute.

Fishbein, M., & Cappella, J. N. (2006). The role of theory in developing effective health communications. *Journal of Communication, 56,* S1-S17.

Goldman, M., Brown, S., & Christiansen, B. (1987). Expectancy theory: Thinking about drinking. In H. Blane & D. Leonard (Eds.), *Psychological theories of drinking and alcoholism* (pp. 181–226). New York: Guilford Press.

Hestroni, A. (2007). Three decades of sexual content on prime-time network programming: A longitudinal meta-analytic review. *Journal of Communication, 57,* 318–348.

Hobbs, R. (2011). The state of media literacy: A response to Potter. *Journal of Broadcasting and Electronic Media, 55,* 419–430.

Hobbs, R., & Frost, R. (2003). Measuring the acquisition of media-literacy skills. *Reading Research Quarterly, 38,* 330–355.

Hoffman, E., Pinkleton, B. E., Austin, E. W., & Lei, M. (2012, August). Exploring college students, social media alcohol marketing and associated behaviors. Paper presented to the Mass Communication & Society Division of the Association for Education in Journalism & Mass Communication, Chicago.

Jeong, S., Cho, H., & Hwang, Y. (2012). Media literacy interventions: A meta-analytic review. *Journal of Communication, 62,* 454–472.

Pinkleton, B. E., Austin, E. W., Chen, Y., & Cohen, M. (2012). The role of media literacy in shaping adolescents' understanding of and responses to sexual portrayals in mass media. *Journal of Health Communication, 17,* 460–476.

Pinkleton, B. E., Austin, E. W., Chen, Y., & Cohen, M. (2013). Assessing effects of a media literacy-based intervention on U.S. adolescents' responses to and interpretations of sexual media messages. *Journal of Children and Media, 7,* 463–479.

Pinkleton, B. E., Austin, E. W., Cohen, M., Miller, A., & Fitzgerald, E. (2007). A state-wide evaluation of the effectiveness of media literacy training to prevent tobacco use among adolescents. *Health Communication, 21*, 23–34.

Pinkleton, B. E., Austin, E. W., & Van de Vord, R. (2010). The role of realism, similarity and expectancies in adolescents' interpretation of abuse-prevention messages. *Health Communication, 25*, 258–265.

Potter, W. J. (2010). The state of media literacy. *Journal of Broadcasting and Electronic Media, 54*, 675–696.

8. *Opinion Leader Identification*

Do Kyun Kim,
University of Louisiana at Lafayette
& James W. Dearing,
Michigan State University

Opinion leaders are individuals who influence people in their communication networks and hold the promise of accelerating positive word-of-mouth about and adoption of health interventions. Publications about opinion leadership primarily reside in the diffusion of innovation literature.

Some health innovations are targeted to social systems of health care providers. Others are targeted to social systems of individuals at risk of disease. Both types of social systems typically have people of high informal influence; i.e., opinion leaders. Weimann (1994) reviewed evidence showing that opinion leaders have particular personal, social, and socio-demographic attributes. Personal attributes include innovativeness, individuation combined with social conformity, knowledgeability, familiarity, and interest in the subject/domain, cosmopoliteness, and personal involvement or enduring involvement, while social attributes refer to gregariousness, social activity, centrality (connectedness) in social networks, social accessibility, social recognition, and credibility. Socio-demographic attributes of opinion leaders are not fixed, but vary according to topical domains, cultures, and societies.

Opinion leaders draw the attention of others because followers perceive them to be trustworthy and or expert about a topic. Opinion leaders are influential whether they try to be or not; indeed, much of their credibility likely derives from them not advocating for particular attitudinal and behavioral changes. Followers perceive them to be fair-minded and worthy judges of the pros and cons of innovations such as new health practices or disease prevention programs. Opinion leaders are usually aware of their influence and feel a sense of duty to do what's in the interest of the social system that accords them credibility. A social system may be comprised of the nurses in a hospital, or the teenagers in a high school, or the elderly residents in a town. For example, in the education field, Carlson (1965) investigated the spread of modern math in Allegheny County, Pennsylvania. When modern math was adopted by one school superintendent of modest reputation in 1958, none of 37 other superintendents were interested in adopting it. However, after the three most influential superintendents adopted modern math, all schools, within 4 years, had adopted modern math. Even when they are already aware of an innovation and its advantages, people will often delay adoption of an innovation they consider to be consequential until informal opinion leaders signal approval.

In our age of information abundance, people are swamped with health information through a variety of communication channels including social media, Internet, television, radio, fliers, and real-time unmediated face-to-face interaction. This abundance of information can produce a sense of hesitancy in decision-making because of the many sources available and the uncertain veracity of message content. Opinion leaders bring reasoned judgment to this cacophony. About most innovations opinion leaders are impassive or negative; that is, they function as gatekeepers for the social systems to which they belong. This tendency leads to the rejection of innovations, or very slow and partial diffusion, either of which may be entirely warranted.

Opinion leader–based health intervention strategies (OLS) focus on interpersonal communication by established opinion leaders through existing social networks. Media may be used to augment interpersonal communication, such as in providing detailed descriptive information about an intervention, or detailed evaluative information about how well the intervention works and under which conditions, or supportive examples of how to keep using an intervention by solving problems with its implementation, but the central messaging occurs through interpersonal observation (social modeling) and talk. For the triggering of a diffusion effect, who is doing the talking and whose behavior is being modeled for others to see can make all the difference.

The Stop AIDS Program in San Francisco is a noteworthy example of the OLS approach. When the general public and public health officials first started to recognize the fatal risk of HIV/AIDS in the early 1980s, the gay community in San Francisco recruited opinion leaders among themselves to mobilize and educate others about how to prevent HIV/AIDS. The dense nature of social networks at this time in San Francisco's gay community led to rapid adoption of safe sex practices (Rogers, 2003). Opinion leader–based HIV/AIDS prevention strategy has been adopted by many organizations in different countries. The largest series of studies and subsequent scale-up of their Popular Opinion Leader approach for HIV prevention has been the work of James Kelly and colleagues in studying and then training public health workers about how the identification and training of popular people in bars can accelerate the adoption of safe sex practices (Kelly et al., 1997).

Another example demonstrates how the OLS approach can work well when combined with other intervention components including workshops, skill training, academic detailing, reminders, and feedback. In Latin America, use of evidence-based practices during delivery and childbirth occurs less than 15% of the time. Previous efforts at improving birth attendant performance in Mexico and Thailand by providing access to the latest information about evidence-based practices resulted in no change in what birth attendants do. To increase the use of episiotomy and of prophylactic use of oxytocin during the third stage of labor, Althabe and colleagues (2008) identified and then intervened with opinion leading birth attendants in hospitals. Researchers randomly assigned 19 hospitals in Argentina and Uruguay to receive a multifaceted behavioral intervention, or enhanced standard of care. Desirable practices increased and undesirable practices decreased at the intervention hospitals as compared with control hospitals. At intervention hospitals where opinion leaders had been sociometrically identified by questionnaire and then contacted and recruited to help, the rate of use of prophylactic oxytocin during the third stage of labor increased from 2.1% to 83.6 %. Opinion leading birth attendants were key to the 18-month intervention's success, and they were eager to help by talking with their work colleagues in positive terms about evidence-based birthing practices. Practice changes were sustained for at least 12 months after the end of the study (Althabe, Buekens, Bergel et al., 2008).

Identifying Opinion Leaders

Identification of opinion leaders within a social system can occur through different methods. Here we briefly review two of them: the other-report sociometric method, which produces data for social network analysis, and self-assessment of one's own ability to influence others.

Social network analysis has been used to good effect in health communication research dating back 60 years. Social network analysis investigates relationships among a set of people or other social units by asking whom they seek advice from about a particular topic, such as the improvement of pediatric care if the desired respondents are pediatric care providers (Beck, Bergman, Rahm, Dearing, & Glasgow, 2009) or juvenile justice programs if the desired respondents are judges who preside over such cases (Kim & Dearing, 2013). Social network analysis is a non-probabilistic research method with the capacity to produce estimates of the degree to which opinion leaders may accelerate the diffusion of innovations compared to non-opinion leaders. The results of network data analysis can be presented visually as network maps as well as in statistical form. Figure 1 shows an example of a social network map.

Figure 1. A sociogram of an advice-seeking network.

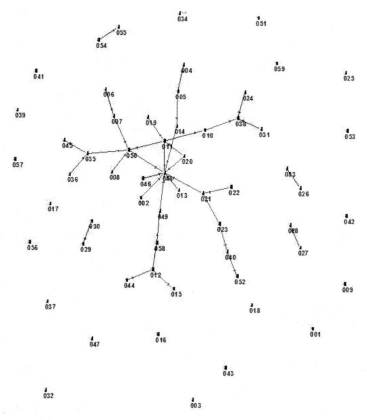

Sociometric questions can be asked at pre-test, to understand who influences whom for a particular topic, and thus whom to recruit into an OLS intervention so that they can be encouraged to discuss an innovation with their peers in the course of normal discussions. Many studies have demonstrated the added benefit of identifying informal opinion leaders and then recruiting them to help in dissemination and resultant diffusion (Lomas et al., 1991; Valente & Pumpuang, 2007) though there are a number of contingencies that can decrease OLS effectiveness (Flodgren et al., 2011), such as correctly identifying opinion leaders but then asking them to behave in ways that they normally do not. In the diffusion literature, change agents and champions function to promote and advocate for change. Opinion leaders, on the other hand, derive their informal status by virtue of their judgment and impartiality, and only promote innovations when they believe the innovation to be of real benefit to the social system in question.

Sociometric questions about advice-seeking that are designed to produce data for social network analysis follow fairly standard formats. Table 1 shows the roster approach for generating such data. This approach is practical when the social system in question is not too large:

Table 1. Sociometric question about advice-seeking.

Physicians learn of innovations in health care delivery through a variety of means, but personal contact is usually required before physicians will try an innovation for themselves. Please select up to 3 people from the following list who you talk to or look to for improving patient care. Just scroll down and click on their names. If you don't see a particular person on the list, feel free to type in their name in the "other" space.

Atkins and his colleges' (2008) study on mental health consultation in low income urban schools provides an example of how well-placed informants can contribute sociometric data. They identified key opinion leaders by asking each teacher who they seek advice from regarding students with academic problems, behavior problems, or curriculum issues and letting the teachers name up to 3 colleagues at their school. This study specified the area of advice-seeking when the researchers ask research subjects' key opinion leaders. This specification is often important to separate people who are generally popular from those more delimited opinion leaders who have more credibility in a certain area, such as school mental health consultations. Table 2 shows typical wording for deriving such data.

Table 2. Specified question with the area of advice-seeking.

Who do you look to for new ideas or better ways of doing things concerning ------?

1. _____

First name   Last name
Organization:_____
Position:_____ _____
I communicate with this person:
5 = daily or more 4 = weekly 3 = monthly 2 = quarterly 1 = yearly

In this instrument, the question about communication frequency is used to analyze and compare the strength of relationships.

Li et al.'s (2013) study on HIV stigma reduction in the medical community demonstrates an integrated method for selecting opinion leaders who can help with the improvement of health services. They combined three identification strategies: (a) hospital stakeholders and department leaders recommended persons known to be socially influential and well respected; (b) during the baseline assessment, randomly selected providers were asked to nominate the three most popular and influential providers in their hospital; and (c) research team members conducted field observations of potential candidates' interactions with their coworkers to verify the popularity of nominees and the nature of their social network (p. 327).

A different approach to identifying opinion leaders is self-assessment via survey measures. This method can be used with larger social systems, including probabilistic sampling as with standard survey research. Self-nomination measures are increasingly used by marketing firms to understand the attitudinal and behavioral characteristics of informal opinion leaders (Goldsmith & DeWitt, 2003). These self-report measures are similar in intent to the Net Promoter Score (Reichheld, 2003), an index that is commonly used in the for-profit sector to assess customer loyalty and a respondent's willingness to advocate on behalf of a product or service. Feick and Price (1987) in marketing research studied "individuals who have information about many kinds of products, places to shop, and other facets of markets, and initiate discussions with consumers and respond to requests from consumers for market information" (p. 85), labeling them mavens.

Boster and colleagues (2011) developed a self-assessment opinion leadership scale that included three constructs—Connectivity, Persuasiveness, and Mavenness—that together comprise a measure of whether an individual functions as highly influential (what they labeled a superdiffuser) in a particular topical domain. Table 3 presents the Boster et al. scale.

Table 3. Self-assessment of opinion leadership scale.

I'm often the link between friends in different groups (C)
I often find myself introducing people to each other (C)
I try to bring people I know together when I think they would find each other interesting (C)
I frequently find that I am the connection between people who would not otherwise know one another (C)
The people I know often know each other because of me (C)
I am good at thinking of multiple ways to explain my position on an issue (P)
When in a discussion, I'm able to make others see my side of the issue (P)
I am able to adapt my method of argument to persuade someone (P)
I can effortlessly offer multiple perspectives on an issue which support my position (P)
More often than not, I am able to convince others of my position during an argument (P)
When I know something about a healthy lifestyle topic, I feel it is important to share that information with others (M)
I like to be aware of the most up-to-date healthy lifestyle information so I can help others by sharing when it is relevant (M)
If someone asked me about a healthy lifestyle issue that I was unsure of, I would know how to help them find the answer (M)
Being knowledgeable enough about healthy lifestyles so that I could teach someone else is important to me (M)
People often seek me out for answers when they have questions about a healthy lifestyle issue (M)

Note: (C): Connectivity, (P): Persuasiveness, and (M) Maven.

Boster and colleagues (2011) found that for healthy lifestyles, mavens were more likely to actively promote health issues. Additional studies by Boster, Carpenter, and Kotowski (2014) of the maven scale demonstrated high construct validity, both for political topics and for health topics. Strong test-retest reliability has also been reported (Boster, 2012). Individuals scoring as political mavens were more politically active and more knowledgeable about politics. Health mavens reported being sought out by others, and that others report that they are good sources of health advice. Across both studies, these authors determined that 8% of subjects exceeded the 75th percentile on each of the connectivity, persuasiveness, and mavenness scales, qualifying them as superdiffusers.

Use of Existing Measures and Future Studies

Both other-report sociometric measures and self-assessment measures show promise for further specification and application in health promotion and disease prevention. In some contexts, the sociometric methods does not work well. This is generally the case for small social systems (of 30 or fewer persons) since the instrumentation can seem intrusive to respondents. Neither does the sociometric method work easily for large social systems (more than 10,000 persons) since those rule out roster survey approaches and present challenges for data-cleaning. The key advantage of the sociometric approach is its inherently relational emphasis, on the structure and content of the ties between individuals, and the outstanding feature of network analysis programs to produce sociograms (as in Figure 1) that graphically describe properties of the system, groups within the system, and individuals. In addition, certain programs enable prospective forecasting for assessing changes to networks, and geo-coding for showing how relationships span geography.

Self-assessment of one's tendency or ability to lead the opinions of others shows great promise for incorporation into standard survey research such as regional and national public opinion surveys. Applying measures of connectedness, persuasiveness, and mavenness to membership surveys of professional associations of public health officials, or any type of homophilous sector such as emergency medical physicians, radiologists, primary care physicians, or executives in health care systems could generate estimates of which individuals (as long as identities are collected) may be most inclined and effective at spreading evidence-based interventions among health care providers. Self-assessment shows the most promise for application to populations that are large, amorphous, yet can be reached to produce sampling frames.

Both of these methods need further research that applies them as strategies in multi-component health promotion and disease prevention interventions. Indeed, an obvious next step is to use these types of measures together in the same studies as a form of methodological triangulation.

Recommended Readings

Boster, F. J., Carpenter, C. J., & Kotowski, M. R. (2014). Validation studies of the maven scale. *Social Influence.* http://dx.doi.org/10.1080/15534510.2014.939224

Goldsmith, R.E., & DeWitt T. (2003). The predictive validity of an opinion leadership scale. *Journal of Marketing Theory and Practice 11*, 28–35.

Kelly, J. A., Murphy, D. A., Sikkema, K. J., McAuliffe T. L., Roffman, R. A., Solomon, L. J., Winett, R. A., & Kalichman, S. C. (1997). Randomized, controlled community-level

HIV prevention intervention for sexual-risk behavior among homosexual men in U.S. cities. *The Lancet, 350,* 1500–1505.

Lomas, J., Enkin, M., Anderson, G. M., Hannah, W. J., Vayda, E., & Singer, J. (1991). Opinion leaders vs audit and feedback to implement practice guidelines. *Journal of the American Medical Association, 265,* 2202–2207.

Valente, T. W., & Pumpuang, P. (2007). Identifying opinion leaders to promote behavior change. *Health Education & Behavior, 34,* 881–896.

References

Althabe, F., Buekens, P., Bergel, E., Belizan, J. M., Campbell, M. K., Moss, N., Hartwell, T., Wright, L. L., for the Guidelines Trial Group. (2008). A behavioral intervention to improve obstetrical care. *New England Journal of Medicine, 358,* 1929–1940.

Atkins, M. S., Frazier, S. L., Leathers, S. J., Graczyk, P. A., Talbott, E., Jakobsons, L., &...Bell, C. C. (2008). Teacher key opinion leaders and mental health consultation in low-income urban schools. *Journal of Consulting and Clinical Psychology, 76*(5), 905–908.

Beck, A., Bergman, D. A., Rahm, A. K., Dearing, J. W., & Glasgow, R. E. (2009). Using implementation and dissemination concepts to spread 21st-century well-child care at a health maintenance organization. *The Permanente Journal, 13*(5), 10–17.

Boster, F. J. (2012). Error of measurement in longitudinal designs: Defining, identifying, and correcting for specific error and transient error. *Communication Research Reports, 29,* 250–256.

Boster, F. J., Carpenter, C. J., Kotowski, M. R. (2014). Validation studies of the maven scale. *Social Influence* http://dx.doi.org/10.1080/15534510.2014.939224

Boster, F. J., Kotowski, M. R., Andrews, K. R., & Serota, K. (2011). Identifying influence: Development and validation of the connectivity, persuasiveness, and maven scales. *Journal of Communication, 61*(1), 178–196.

Feick, L. F., & Price, L. L. (1987). The market maven: A diffuser of marketplace information. *Journal of Marketing, 51,* 83–97.

Flodgren, G., Parmelli, E., Doumit, G., Gattellari, M., O'Brian, M. A., Grimshaw, J., & Eccles, M. P. (2011). Effectiveness of the use of local opinion leaders to promote evidence-based practice and improving patient outcomes. Cochrane Collaboration, August 10.

Goldsmith, R. E., DeWitt, T. (2003). The predictive validity of an opinion leadership scale. *Journal of Marketing Theory and Practice 11*(1), 28–35.

Kelly, J. A., Murphy, D. A., Sikkema, K. J., McAuliffe T. L., Roffman, R. A., Solomon, L. J., Winett, R. A., & Kalichman, S. C. (1997). Randomized, controlled community-level HIV prevention intervention for sexual-risk behavior among homosexual men in U.S. cities. *The Lancet 350,* 1500–1505.

Kim, D. K., & Dearing, J. W. (2013). Communication network analysis for the diffusion of health: Identifying key individuals. In D. K. Kim A. Singhal & G. L. Kreps (Eds), *Health communication strategies for developing global health programs.* New York: Peter Lang, 157–177.

Li, L., Cao, H., Wu, Z., Wu, S., & Xiao, L. (2007). Diffusion of positive AIDS care messages among service providers in China. *AIDS Education & Prevention, 19*(6), 511–518.

Li, L., Guan, J., Liang, L., Lin, C., & Wu, Z. (2013). Popular Opinion Leader intervention for HIV stigma reduction in health care settings. *AIDS Education and Prevention: Official Publication of the International Society for AIDS Education, 25*(4), 327–335.

Lomas, J., Enkin, M., Anderson, G. M., Hannah, W. J., Vayda, E., & Singer, J. (1991). Opinion leaders vs audit and feedback to implement practice guidelines. *Journal of the American Medical Association, 265*(17), 2202–2207.

Reichheld, F. F. (2003). The one number you need to grow. *Harvard Business Review, 81*(12), 46–54.

Rogers, E. M. (2003). *Diffusion of innovations* (5th ed.). New York: Free Press.

Valente, T. W., Pumpuang, P. (2007). Identifying opinion leaders to promote behavior change. *Health Education & Behavior, 34*(6), 881–896.

Weimann, G. (1994). *The influentials: People who influence people.* Albany: State University of New York Press.

9. *Outcome Expectations*

SETH M. NOAR,
University of North Carolina, Chapel Hill
& JESSICA GALL MYRICK,
Indiana University

Health communication campaigns are imperative for the prevention and reduction of indoor tanning, a behavior that is strongly associated with several types of skin cancer, including melanoma (Boniol, Autier, Boyle, & Gandini, 2012). The evidence suggests that UV exposure via indoor tanning at younger ages (i.e., before age 35) may particularly increase the risk of melanoma (Boniol et al., 2012). Thus, the focus of indoor tanning research has primarily been on young people, especially young women who are most likely to engage in this dangerous, cancer-promoting behavior (Centers for Disease Control and Prevention, 2012).

Before messages and campaigns can be developed, however, an understanding of the beliefs that underlie indoor tanning behavior is needed. Studies examining tanning motivations have found attitudes toward indoor tanning, tanning social norms, perceptions of control over tanning, perceptions of skin cancer risk, identification with popular peer crowds, and intentions to tan indoors to be associated with indoor tanning behavior (Hillhouse & Turrisi, 2012; Hillhouse, Turrisi, Holwiski, & McVeigh, 1999; Lazovich et al., 2004). However, previous studies have been limited on a number of fronts. First, many studies have used general attitude measures, single item measures, or measures that have assessed only a relatively narrow set of tanning beliefs. This has limited our ability to comprehensively understand the beliefs that underlie this behavior. Second, previous studies have failed to clearly distinguish among positive and negative sets of beliefs, despite the fact that positive and negative beliefs can play differing roles in the initiation, maintenance, and discontinuation of behavior. Third and finally, while some work in this area has been theory-based, much of it has been atheoretical or has applied theory in an incomplete manner (Hillhouse & Turrisi, 2012).

A comprehensive, multi-dimensional, theory-based measure is needed to garner a more sophisticated understanding of the complex sets of beliefs that underlie the decision to tan indoors. Social Cognitive Theory (SCT) is a comprehensive behavioral theory (Bandura, 1986) that has particular resonance in this area. SCT posits that health behaviors must be understood in the context of reciprocal determinism, or the idea that characteristics of the individual, one's environment, and the behavior interact to determine whether an action is performed.

While SCT posits numerous intrapersonal, interpersonal, and environmental factors to influence behavior, its two core psychosocial determinants are outcome expectations and self-efficacy (Bandura, 2004). Outcome expectations are beliefs about the expected (positive and negative) consequences of engaging in a behavior, and they represent a key motivational factor (i.e., *should* I perform this behavior?). They are theorized to be physical, social, and self-evaluative in nature (discussed in more detail below). While positive expectations incentivize behavior, negative expectations disincentivize it. For instance, a young woman may believe that tanning indoors would be relaxing and make her look great (positive expectations), while she may be somewhat less concerned that the behavior will lead to wrinkles and saggy skin later in life (negative expectations). The balance of positive versus negative expectations influences motivation to perform the behavior (Prochaska et al., 1994).

The second SCT factor is self-efficacy, which refers to one's confidence in performing a behavior across a range of situations. This represents a capability factor (i.e., *can* I perform this behavior?), and scores of studies empirically demonstrate the importance of self-efficacy to behavior (Bandura, 1997). The more one believes in one's ability to perform the behavior, the more likely the person is to engage in that behavior. When the behavior is risky, however, self-efficacy may be more usefully conceptualized as its mirror opposite—temptations (Velicer, DiClemente, Rossi, & Prochaska, 1990). Temptations can promote unhealthy behaviors, and they have been found to predict risky behaviors such as smoking behavior over time (Prochaska, Velicer, Guadagnoli, Rossi, & DiClemente, 1991). They may also be a more intuitive measure for respondents to understand in relation to risky/unhealthy behaviors (i.e., reporting on temptations to engage in the risky behavior rather than on confidence to *not* engage in the risky behavior) (Velicer et al., 1990). In the context of indoor tanning, a young woman may be particularly tempted to tan indoors when a special event is coming up, it's the winter season, or she perceives her skin to be too pale, for instance. Temptations are conceptually distinct from outcome expectations because while outcome expectations are fairly stable *motivational* beliefs, temptations are more about *capability* than motivation (i.e., can I stop myself from tanning?). Also, temptations (like self-efficacy) are specific to situations (e.g., tempted when my friends are going tanning or tempted when it's the winter season).

Measuring Outcome Expectations

Given that both outcome expectations and self-efficacy/temptations are core SCT determinants that are amenable to change, they represent important theoretical factors that can form the basis for prevention messages. We began our program of research by focusing on outcome expectations, as they are viewed as a primary motivator of human behavior. Applied to indoor tanning, physical outcome expectations refer to effects on the body, such as appearance and health effects. Social expectations refer to approval, disapproval, compliments, concerns, and other social reinforcements and punishments. Self-evaluative expectations refer to how engaging in the behavior makes one feel about oneself, such as feeling confident, happy, bad, or guilty. We considered these and other possible domains in the development of the measure (see Table 1).

Table 1. Outcome Expectation Types, Indoor Tanning Topics, and Candidate Items.

Outcome Expectation Types	Indoor Tanning Topics	Positive (If I went indoor tanning…)	Negative (If I went indoor tanning…)
Physical	Appearance	• It would make me more attractive • It would make me look thinner • It would give me a great "glow"	• It would lead to wrinkles later in life • It would make my skin leathery • My tan would look fake
Physical	Health	• It would give me more energy • It would provide my skin with vitamin D • It would clear up acne	• It would lead to skin cancer • It would be addictive • It would be bad for my skin

Outcome Expectation Types	Indoor Tanning Topics	Positive (If I went indoor tanning...)	Negative (If I went indoor tanning...)
Social	Social	• It would be fun to do with my friends • It would prepare me for a vacation or spring break • It would be something that my mom supports	• It would upset people around me • It would upset my dad • It would lead people to worry about my health
Self-Evaluative	Self-evaluative	• It would help lift my spirits • It would improve my mood • It would make me feel more confident	• It would make me feel bad about myself • It would make me feel guilty • It would be an unnecessary luxury
Other	Other	• It would be a way to express myself • It would make me feel proud • It would be a convenient way to get a tan	• It would be a waste of money • It would feel claustrophobic in the tanning booth • It would feel uncomfortably hot and sweaty in the tanning booth

(Note. Response format is (1) *definitely wouldn't*, (2) *probably wouldn't*, (3) *not sure*, (4) *probably would*, (5) *definitely would.*)

In crafting the first comprehensive outcomes expectations measure in this area, we applied a sequential approach to measurement development (Jackson, 1970; Noar, 2003). In order to examine the positive and negative consequences that young women attribute to indoor tanning, we extensively reviewed the research on motivations for indoor tanning, including qualitative, quantitative, and review studies. We grouped types of motivations into topic areas (appearance, health, social, self-evaluative, and other) by valence (positive or negative), with reference to the three types of outcome expectations—physical, social, and self-evaluative. We then wrote multiple items to cover the content domain of each of these areas. Using an iterative process, our research team wrote and reviewed candidate items over the course of several months. We also consulted with a survey expert from our social science research institute who critically reviewed the measure and provided feedback. The intial measure consisted of 70 items. The stem presented before the items stated "*If I went indoor tanning...*" and then each positive expectation item was presented, such as "It would make me look thinner" and "It would be a fast way to get a tan." Then, the same procedure was repeated for the negative expectation items. Participants responded to all items based on the following 5-point scale: 1) *definitely wouldn't*, 2) *probably wouldn't*, 3) *not sure*, 4) *probably would*, 5) *definitely would*. Before the study launched, we pre-tested the measure with 10 individuals from the target audience.

We next launched a survey research study, assessing N=706 young women who were sorority members at a large, public university. Participants answered the 70 candidate items (separately in the positive and negative item groups) as well as numerous additional scales that were included for purposes of validation. We employed maximum likelihood factor analysis with Promax rotation to examine the dimensionality of the outcome expectations scales. We computed factor analyses (separately for positive and negative dimensions), dropped items that cross-loaded (>.30) on multiple factors, re-computed analyses, and re-inspected our output. We repeated this process until a final solution that was both theoretically and empirically interpretable emerged.

Results indicated that positive outcome expectations consisted of 6 reliable dimensions: appearance benefits (α = .92), convenience (α = .88), mood enhancement (α = .95), health improvement (α = .86), social approval (α = .88), and parental approval (r = .76). The negative outcomes expectations consisted of 5 reliable dimensions – health threat (α = .93), psychological/physical discomfort (α = .87), appearance harms (α = .89), social disapproval (α = .88), and parental disapproval (r = .84). We named the scale the Comprehensive Indoor Tanning Expectations (CITE) scale (Noar, Myrick, Morales-Pico, & Thomas, 2014). The full CITE scale is presented in Table 2.

Table 2. The Comprehensive Indoor Tanning Expectations (CITE) Scale.

Positive Outcome Expectations	CITE Subscale	Negative Outcome Expectations	CITE Subscale
1. It would make me look thinner	Appearance benefits	1. It would be dangerous	Health threat
2. It would make me look more toned	Appearance benefits	2. It would increase my chances of getting melanoma	Health threat
3. It would hide my skin imperfections	Appearance benefits	3. It would be bad for my skin	Health threat

Positive Outcome Expectations	CITE Subscale	Negative Outcome Expectations	CITE Subscale
4. It would make me more fashionable	Appearance benefits	4. It would be unhealthy	Health threat
5. It would make me look healthy	Appearance benefits	5. It would lead to skin cancer	Health threat
6. It would make me look great	Appearance benefits	6. It would feel uncomfortably hot and sweaty in the tanning booth	Psychological/physical discomfort
7. It would make me look like a celebrity	Appearance benefits	7. It would feel claustrophobic in the tanning booth	Psychological/physical discomfort
8. It would make me more attractive	Appearance benefits	8. It would be a waste of money	Psychological/physical discomfort
9. It would get me ready for a special event (e.g., a dance)	Convenience	9. It would make me feel bad about myself	Psychological/physical discomfort
10. It would be a fast way to get a tan	Convenience	10. It would be an unnecessary luxury	Psychological/physical discomfort
11. It would be a convenient way to get a tan	Convenience	11. It would be expensive	Psychological/physical discomfort
12. It would prepare me for a vacation or spring break	Convenience	12. It would lead to saggy skin later in life	Appearance harms
13. It would make my tan lines disappear	Convenience	13. It would lead to wrinkles in later life	Appearance harms
14. It would give me a nice base tan	Convenience	14. It would make my skin leathery	Appearance harms
15. It would be enjoyable	Mood enhancement	15. It would lead to premature (early) skin aging	Appearance harms
16. It would reduce stress or tension	Mood enhancement	16. It would make my skin smell bad	Appearance harms
17. It would be relaxing	Mood enhancement	17. It would upset some of my friends	Social disapproval
18. It would improve my mood	Mood enhancement	18. It would upset people around me	Social disapproval

Positive Outcome Expectations	CITE Subscale	Negative Outcome Expectations	CITE Subscale
19. It would help lift my spirits	Mood enhancement	19. It would lead people to worry about my health	Social disapproval
20. It would be healthy for me	Health improvement	20. It would upset my mom	Parental disapproval
21. It would be a safe way to get a tan	Health improvement	21. It would upset my dad	Parental disapproval
22. It would be good for my skin	Health improvement	–	–
23. It would be safer than tanning in the sun	Health improvement	–	–
24. It would lead to compliments from people I date	Social approval	–	–
25. It would make me more desirable to people I date	Social approval	–	–
26. It would lead to compliments from my friends	Social approval	–	–
27. It would be something my mom supports	Parental approval	–	–
28. It would be something my dad supports	Parental approval	–	–

Next, we examined how the CITE subscales were significantly correlated with a set of constructs from the established indoor tanning literature. Zero order correlations indicated that all 11 subscales were significantly ($p<.05$) correlated with the set of measures, including appearance motivation, appearance motivations to tan, and indoor tanning attitudes, norms, temptations, and behavioral intentions. Moreover, all 11 subscales differed significantly ($p<.001$) across three indoor tanner types: non-tanners, former tanners, and current tanners. The pattern of results was such that non-tanners had the most negative and least positive expectations about indoor tanning; current tanners had the most positive and least negative expectations; and former tanners tended to fall in between these 2 groups (see Figure 1).

Figure 1. Mean Levels of CITE Subscales across 3 Tanner Types.

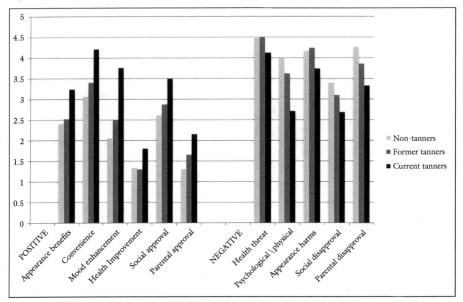

We next sought to confirm the findings of this first study by conducting a second survey research study of sorority members at a large, private university (Noar et al., 2015). We surveyed $N=750$ young women and conducted confirmatory factor analyses of the CITE scale using this independent sample. Results provided additional empirical support for the robustness of the 6 positive and 5 negative CITE subscales, and they revealed that a hierarchical structure fit the data well. This indicated that there is a higher order positive and negative expectation factor, which is made up of 6 and 5 sub-factors, respectively.

We also tested SCT theory-based models to advance a more comprehensive understanding of indoor tanning intentions and behavior. We posed the following hypotheses:

1) Perceived skin type, appearance motivation, general appearance motivations to tan, and media appearance motivations to tan will be associated with both positive and negative expectations about indoor tanning.

2) Positive and negative expectations will be associated with temptations to tan indoors and indoor tanning intentions and behavior.

3) Temptations to tan indoors will be directly and positively associated with indoor tanning intentions and behavior.

After an iterative process of model testing, including removing non-significant paths, we found that the structural equation model predicting *intentions to tan indoors* fit the data well (χ^2 = 3,158.77, p <.001, CFI = .90, RMSEA = .07). As expected, appearance motivation and appearance motivations to tan (general) were significant (p<.05) positive predictors of positive outcome expectations, while perceived skin type and appearance motivation were significant negative predictors of negative outcome expectations. Positive outcome expectations were positively and directly related to temptations to tan indoors and indoor tanning intentions, while negative outcome expectations were a negative predictor of indoor tanning intentions. However, negative outcome expectations were not directly associated with temptations to tan.

We also ran a path model with current tanners (i.e., the subset of the sample that had reported tanning in the past year; n = 207), focusing on predicting *indoor tanning behavior*. This model also fit the data well after an iterative process of model testing, χ^2 = 27.90, p <.001, CFI = .95, RMSEA = .09. Appearance motivation, appearance motivations to tan (general), and appearance motivations to tan (media) were all positively associated with positive outcome expectations, while the only association between these variables and negative outcome expectations was a negative association with appearance motivation. Positive outcome expectations were positively associated with temptations to tan, but there was no direct significant association between positive outcome expectations and indoor tanning behavior. Negative outcome expectations, on the other hand, were not directly associated with temptations but were direct and significant negative predictors of indoor tanning behavior. Temptations did have a positive and significant association with indoor tanning behavior. In summary, the models predicting both intentions to tan indoors and indoor tanning behavior point to the importance of outcome expectations and temptations in understanding and predicting indoor tanning.

Finally, we conducted a third study, which was a longitudinal follow-up add-on to the first two survey research studies (Myrick et al., 2015). We combined the samples used in the exploratory and confirmatory factor analyses to establish a large pool of baseline participants (N = 1,482), and then conducted follow-up web surveys with that sample 6 months later. A total of 553 women participated in both the baseline and follow-up surveys. Using those data, we were able to establish the longitudinal utility of the CITE scale. The scale demonstrated strong test-retest reliability, with positive expectations ranging from r = .55 − .73 (mean = .65 across subscales) and negative expectations ranging from r = .41 to .70 (mean = .56 across subscales). Furthermore, all positive outcome expectations subscales were positively and significantly (p<.001) correlated with Time 2 indoor tanning behavior, while all negative outcome expectation subscales were negatively and significantly ($p<.001$) correlated with Time 2 behavior. Hierarchical logistic regression analyses with all CITE scales entered, and controlling for demographic, skin-type, and skin health history variables, revealed that three CITE subscales were significantly ($p<.05$) associated with Time 2 indoor tanning behavior. Participants who believed that indoor tanning improved their mood and would lead to social approval (positive expectations) were significantly more likely to tan indoors than those who did not hold these beliefs as strongly. Also, participants who believed that indoor tanning would lead to psychological or physical discomfort (negative expectations) were significantly less likely to tan indoors than participants who did not hold these beliefs as strongly.

Use of Existing Measures and Future Studies

The CITE scale has strong psychometric properties and can serve as a valuable tool for advancing indoor tanning research. This scale could be applied in a number of ways in future research. Most notably, work is needed to confirm its reliability and extend evidence for its validity in other samples of young women, including in both cross-sectional and longitudinal studies. For example, do other samples of young women—in other age groups and in other parts of the country—hold similar beliefs about indoor tanning to those found here? To date, the studies reported here are the first studies to develop and test the CITE scale, and further inquiry is needed.

CITE could also be adapted for use with other populations, such as adolescent girls. Adolescents are a critical population as data suggests that adolescence is often when indoor tanning behavior begins (Cokkinides, Weinstock, Lazovich, Ward, & Thun, 2009) and UV radiation is most harmful among those with younger, "immature" skin (Boniol et al., 2012). Application of CITE to adolescents could help us better understand what positive and negative outcome expectations adolescents have *before* they tan indoors the first time, as well as how those beliefs change *after* they tan indoors. This kind of work could lead to better interventions to prevent adolescents from tanning indoors in the first place.

CITE also has key implications for developing messages to deter young women from tanning indoors. Studies can use this scale to inform the development of targeted and tailored messages directed to young women, leading to prevention, reduction, and cessation of this behavior. After anti-tanning messages are developed and pre-tested, the scale could be used in experimental message testing studies to assess whether messages are successful in changing key beliefs. Moreover, given misleading messages coming from the tanning industry, such as the promotion of indoor tanning as a major source of vitamin D (Woo & Eide, 2010), the CITE scale may also be helpful for researchers studying how those messages affect beliefs as well as how to remedy such health misinformation. As there have been numerous calls for a range of health communication interventions to deter young people from indoor tanning (Holman et al., 2013), this is a key priority for future research.

Recommended Readings

Noar, S. M., Myrick, J. G., Morales-Pico, B., & Thomas, N. E. (2014). Development and validation of the comprehensive indoor tanning expectations scale. *JAMA Dermatology, 150*, 512–521.

Noar, S. M., Myrick, J. G., Zeitany, B. S., Kelley, D., Morales-Pico, B., & Thomas, N. E. (2015). Testing a social cognitive theory-based model of indoor tanning: Implications for skin cancer prevention messages. *Health Communication, 30*, 164–174.

References

Bandura, A. (1986). *Social foundations of thought and action: A social cognitive theory.* Englewood Cliffs, NJ: Prentice-Hall.

Bandura, A. (1997). *Self-efficacy: The exercise of control.* New York: W.H. Freeman.

Bandura, A. (2004). Health promotion by social cognitive means. *Health Education & Behavior, 31*, 143–164.

Boniol, M., Autier, P., Boyle, P., & Gandini, S. (2012). Cutaneous melanoma attributable to sunbed use: Systematic review and meta-analysis. *British Medical Journal, 345*, e4757.

Centers for Disease Control and Prevention. (2012). Use of indoor tanning devices by adults – United States, 2010. *Morbidity and Mortality Weekly Report, 61*, 323–326.

Cokkinides, V., Weinstock, M., Lazovich, D., Ward, E., & Thun, M. (2009). Indoor tanning use among adolescents in the US, 1998 to 2004. *Cancer, 115*, 190–198.

Hillhouse, J., & Turrisi, R. (2012). Motivations for indoor tanning: Theoretical models. In C. J. Heckman & S. L. Manne (Eds.), *Shedding light on indoor tanning* (pp. 69–86). New York: Springer.

Hillhouse, J., Turrisi, R., Holwiski, F., & McVeigh, S. (1999). An examination of psychological variables relevant to artificial tanning tendencies. *Journal of Health Psychology, 4*, 507–516.

Holman, D. M., Fox, K. A., Glenn, J. D., Guy, G. P., Jr., Watson, M., Baker, K.,…Geller, A. C. (2013). Strategies to reduce indoor tanning: Current research gaps and future opportunities for prevention. *American Journal of Preventive Medicine, 44*, 672–681.

Jackson, D. N. (1970). A sequential system for personality scale development. In C. D. Spielberger (Ed.), *Current topics in clinical and community psychology* (Vol. 2, pp. 61–96). New York: Academic Press.

Lazovich, D., Forster, J., Sorensen, G., Emmons, K., Stryker, J., Demierre, M.,…Remba, N. (2004). Characteristics associated with use or intention to use indoor tanning among adolescents. *Archives of Pediatrics & Adolescent Medicine, 158*, 918–924.

Myrick, J. G., Noar, S. M., Kelley, D., Zeitany, A. E., Morales-Pico, B. M., & Thomas, N. E. (2015). A longitudinal test of the Comprehensive Indoor Tanning Expectations Scale: The importance of affective beliefs in predicting indoor tanning behavior. *Journal of Health Psychology*. Advanced publication.

Noar, S. M. (2003). The role of structural equation modeling in scale development. *Structural Equation Modeling, 10*, 622–647.

Noar, S. M., Myrick, J. G., Morales-Pico, B., & Thomas, N. E. (2014). Development and validation of the comprehensive indoor tanning expectations scale. *JAMA Dermatology, 150*, 512–521.

Noar, S. M., Myrick, J. G., Zeitany, B. S., Kelley, D., Morales-Pico, B., & Thomas, N. E. (2015). Testing a social cognitive theory-based model of indoor tanning: Implications for skin cancer prevention messages. *Health Communication, 30*, 164–174.

Prochaska, J. O., Velicer, W. F., Guadagnoli, E., Rossi, J. S., & DiClemente, C. C. (1991). Patterns of change: Dynamic typology applied to smoking cessation. *Multivariate Behavioral Research, 26*, 83.

Prochaska, J. O., Velicer, W. F., Rossi, J. S., Goldstein, M. G., Marcus, B. H., Rakowski, W.,…Rosenbloom, D. (1994). Stages of change and decisional balance for 12 problem behaviors. *Health Psychology, 13*, 39–46.

Velicer, W. F., DiClemente, C. C., Rossi, J. S., & Prochaska, J. O. (1990). Relapse situations and self-efficacy: An integrative model. *Addictive Behaviors, 15*, 271–283.

Woo, D. K., & Eide, M. J. (2010). Tanning beds, skin cancer, and vitamin D: An examination of the scientific evidence and public health implications. *Dermatologic Therapy, 23*, 61–71.

10. Outcome Relevant Involvement and Hedonic Relevance

CLAUDE H. MILLER,
University of Oklahoma

Involvement is widely recognized as a key construct central to the arousal, interest, and motivation (Munson & McQuarrie, 1987) of a broad range of research topics within communication, social psychology, and consumer research (Johnson & Eagly, 1989; Ram & Jung, 1989; Zaichkowsky, 1994), and its measurement is essential for a fuller understanding of human decision-making. The broad concept of involvement has been conceptualized and operationalized in various ways across an array of contexts, and has been identified as an important variable in the observation of diverse social phenomena, including: advertising (Greenwald & Leavitt, 1984), interpersonal and social influence (Johnson & Eagly, 1989), message framing (Maheswaran & Meyers-Levy, 1990), message processing (Park, Lee, & Han, 2007), resistance to influence (Pfau et al., 1997), attitude accessibility (Fazio, 1995), and attitude behavior consistency (Cooke & Sheeran, 2004).

Johnson and Eagly (1989) identified three distinct types of involvement—value-relevant, impression-relevant, and outcome-relevant—that are central to the ways in which objects may be conceptually distinguished and identified as having personal relevancy for various anticipated outcomes. It is the measurement of the latter type, outcome relevant involvement (ORI), and particularly its aspect of hedonic relevance (HR), that is the focus of this chapter.

Outcome-relevant involvement has generally been associated with several closely related constructs such as issue involvement (Petty & Cacioppo, 1979), response involvement (Zimbardo, 1960), personal involvement (Zaichkowsky, 1994), and vested interest (Sivacek & Crano, 1982; and see Chapter 26 this volume). Because the manipulations employed in Petty and Cacioppo's (1984) research utilizing the elaboration likelihood model of persuasion (ELM) make salient the outcomes an issue may have on an individual's own goals and desires, ELM research has been characterized by the use of outcome-relevant involvement, the operation of which concerns whether a focus upon an attitude object or issue will have consequential outcomes for the individual, and if so, how much (Johnson & Eagly, 1989). Because of the emphasis on personal consequences, ORI is associated with HR (Miller & Averbeck, 2013), information seeking behaviors (Cho & Boster, 2005; McQuarrie & Munson, 1992), greater elaboration of relevant information (Parse, 1990), and more objective processing (Hubbell, Mitchell, & Gee, 2001).

Measuring Outcome Relevant Involvement and Hedonic Relevance

Cho and Boster (2005) sought to develop and validate scales characterizing involvement as a multidimensional construct following Johnson and Eagly's (1989) notion of value-relevant, outcome-relevant, and impression-relevant involvement, and found their 7-item outcome-relevant involvement subscale to be distinguished from the other two involvement subscales by its strong association with information seeking across topics. In their study, college students made ratings on several topics chosen to have varying levels of involvement (abortion, death penalty, marijuana, jeans, and toothpaste) using 7-point Likert-type scales measured along a strongly disagree/strongly agree continuum (see Table 1). Although the five topics examined appeared to vary in their levels of HR, Cho and Boster (2005) did not attempt to assess the HR construct.

Table 1. Cho and Boster's (2005) Outcome-Relevant Involvement Subscale.

1. Whether [the relevant issue is acted upon] or not has little impact on my life.*
2. All in all, the effect of [the relevant issue] on my life is small.*
3. My life would be changed if [the relevant issue was acted upon].
4. [The relevant issue] has little effect on me.*
5. My life would not change much if [the relevant issue was acted upon].*
6. It is easy for me to think of ways [the relevant issue] affects my life.
7. It is difficult for me to think of ways [the relevant issue] impacts my life.*

Note: Items are measured on a 7-point, Likert-type strongly disagree/strongly agree continuum. Asterisks * designate an item is reversed coded so that higher scores indicate greater involvement.

Based on a review of relevant communication, marketing, psychology, and philosophy literatures, Miller and Averbeck (2013) developed a scale for measuring a bidimensional configuration of ORI made up of subjective

importance (SI)—the cognitive assessment of the perceived personal consequences associated with an object—and HR—the perceived pleasantness versus unpleasantness underlying the motivational force related to that object.
Beyond the pleasure/pain dimension of an attitude object, HR is characterized by the magnitude of perceived personal consequences that object has
for an attitude holder. That is to say, differing topics may or may not have
personal significance for a given receiver; however, only those topics whose
consequences are considered personally relevant should be expected to affect
pertinent behaviors, and it is the combination of these two dimensions—hedonic tone and magnitude of personal consequences—that defines HR.

Miller and Averbeck's (2013) Outcome Relevant Involvement Scale

In their review of value-, outcome-, and impression-relevant involvement,
Cho and Boster (2005) found a number of distinct and valid measures of
involvement; however, they noted that most scales tend to focus on magnitude of arousal rather than the *direction* of arousal relevant to specific goals.
Although there are numerous measures available to capture involvement,
arousal, and the like, none address the more basic notion of HR, nor the
broader notion of ORI. Thus, Miller and Averbeck (2013) sought to develop
a model assessing both the importance/consequentiality and pleasure/pain
dimensions of the construct in a parsimonious fashion, while discriminating
the two aspects of HR and SI that were formerly unexamined and/or indis-
tinguishable using previous measures of importance, involvement, and preference. In short, measures of HR and SI should be capable of discriminating
between the two factors within the broader ORI construct reliably, regardless
of the magnitude, intensity, and/or valance of what is or is not perceived as
hedonically relevant for any given topic or attitude object.

Miller and Averbeck (2013) used logical criterion keying (Craig, 2007) to
develop a list of HR terms based on a literature review covering philosophical,
psychological, physiological, and practical research related articles, chapters,
and books on the concept of HR published over the past 250 years. They then
developed a selection of 15 adjective pairs (see below) conforming to theoretical conceptions of the construct measured along a 7-point semantic differential
continuum. The set of adjective pairs was then subjected to a factor analytic
assessment to obtain the most basic, bidimensional structure of ORI, which
was then used within three studies to assess the characteristics of five different
topics intended to vary in HR (eating, study habits, sex, the environment, and
camera equipment) while being approximately of equal objective importance.

Based on theoretical considerations, the 15 item pairs were used to specify a series of confirmatory factor analysis (CFA) models using maximum likelihood estimation, and those models were further refined and simplified based on fit, parsimony, and unity (i.e., the desire to specify a single model that could fit the data from all five topics) resulting in a final ORI scale consisting of eight item pairs—four retained in the final HR factor: pleasant/unpleasant; pleasurable/unpleasurable; punishing/not punishing; and satisfying/unsatisfying, and four retained in the final *SI* factor: important/unimportant; relevant/irrelevant; significant/insignificant; and consequential/inconsequential.

Miller and Averbeck's (2013) CFA results demonstrated good fit within each of the five content areas tested, and produced two 4-item subscales computed to represent the two latent factors, each of which demonstrated satisfactory internal consistency across topics: HR (4-item α: eating = .84; study = .85; sex = .83; environment = .76; camera = .74); and SI (4-item α: eating = .74; study = .74; sex = .78; environment = .86; camera = .76). Furthermore, the CFA models provided evidence that HR is a unique construct, conceptually distinct from SI within the bidimensional ORI construct. Table 2 provides the final ORI scale divided into HR and SI subscales.

Table 2. HR and SI Subscale Items of the Outcome Relevant Involvement Scale.

Hedonic Relevance		
unpleasant	0 – 1 – 2 – 3 – 4 – 5 – 6	pleasant
unpleasurable	0 – 1 – 2 – 3 – 4 – 5 – 6	pleasurable
not punishing	0 – 1 – 2 – 3 – 4 – 5 – 6	punishing
not satisfying	0 – 1 – 2 – 3 – 4 – 5 – 6	satisfying
Subjective Importance		
unimportant	0 – 1 – 2 – 3 – 4 – 5 – 6	important
irrelevant	0 – 1 – 2 – 3 – 4 – 5 – 6	relevant
insignificant	0 – 1 – 2 – 3 – 4 – 5 – 6	significant
inconsequential	0 – 1 – 2 – 3 – 4 – 5 – 6	consequential

Note: Items dropped from the CFA models on the basis of fit, parsimony, and unity across topics included: painful/not painful; exciting/unexciting; rewarding/unrewarding; interesting/uninteresting; appealing/unappealing: boring/not boring; and personal/impersonal.

Through multiple message topics and media channels (video, text, and Internet), comparisons observed between attitude objects for HR and SI indicated there were significant differences in HR independent of SI. That is to say, HR was perceived to be significantly greater than SI for high HR attitude objects (eating and sex) where there were no significant differences in SI, or where SI levels were in the opposite direction of HR levels. Likewise, there were significant differences in SI independent of HR across low HR attitude objects (study habits, the environment, and camera equipment), where there were no significant differences in HR, or where HR levels were in the opposite direction of SI levels.

Use of the ORI Scale and Future Studies

The parsimonious subscales designed to measure HR and SI within the ORI construct were found to be valid and reliable across different topics of relatively similar importance; and the structure of the scales was internally consistent across studies examining messages using a range of differing language attributes within three different channels (i.e., text, video, and webpage). Across a range of contexts, simply questioning how important an individual considers a topic or attitude object to be may not be sufficient to adequately assess the implications or logical consistency of their involvement, since some topics may be considered more objectively important, or even more subjectively important than others, yet may imply lesser personal consequences as a result of their being assessed as less hedonically relevant. This may be particularly pertinent within health related domains. Therefore, it may be wise to assess both the HR of a topic as well as its perceived SI in cases where an individual's outcome relevant involvement may have a substantial influence on the conclusions being drawn, decisions being made, and actions being taken regarding health-relevant behaviors.

Including an assessment of ORI, and particularly HR, would be useful in a variety of research contexts. For instance, social influence research might especially benefit from a measurement of HR, given that persuasive messages emphasizing the objective importance of an attitude object may produce substantially less behavioral change relative to comparable messages targeting the same attitude object, but emphasizing its hedonic relevancy for the target. Likewise, framing an issue to have great SI without also noting its potential for hedonically relevant personal consequences may result in impressive self-reported attitude-relevant intentions, but inconsistent or wholly absent attitude-relevant behaviors.

Several theory-based programs of research in the health communication domain have focused on the concepts of involvement (e.g., Aldoory, 2001; Petty, Barden, & Wheeler, 2009) and attitude strength (e.g., Green,

2006; Ong et al.,1995) across a variety of topics, and most of these areas of research would benefit by assessing the perceived hedonic relevancy of the issues and actions of concern for the relevant target populations. Attitude research, in general, would gain from an evaluation of attitude objects that vary in HR.

Research using both the ELM and heuristic systematic model of persuasion (HSM) has clearly demonstrated how issues with which individuals are highly involved result in more elaborate and systematic message scrutiny (Eagly & Chaiken, 1993). However, issue involvement considered in terms of objective importance, or even subjective importance, may not capture the narrower, more potent concept of HR, and its potential impact on personal consequentiality that is more reliably predictive of behavior. Hedonic relevance assessed as a conative supplement to the cognitive and affective aspects of social influence can allow researchers to evaluate a more elemental aspect of motivation, thereby improving the effectiveness of health communication across a range of contexts.

Finally, given the pleasure/pain aspect of HR, the assessment of ORI should have obvious implications for a wide variety of health concerns that may be considered subjectively important (i.e., potentially involving severe outcomes) without necessarily acknowledging the immediate hedonically relevant personal consequences involved for an individual. A fuller consideration of and focus on HR would have the effect of boosting the personal stake individuals perceive themselves to have in various topics and issues central to a wide array of health risk behaviors. In addition to subjective importance, assessing and targeting patient perceptions of hedonic relevance within a given health context could greatly enhance the likelihood health practitioners may be able to positively influence their patients with critically important compliance messages.

Recommended Readings

Cho, H., & Boster, F. J. (2005). Development and validation of value-, outcome-, and impression-relevant involvement scales. *Communication Research, 32,* 235–264.

Crano, W. D., & Prislin, R. (2011). *Attitudes and attitude change.* New York: Psychology Press.

Miller, C. H., & Averbeck, J. M., (2013). Hedonic relevance and outcome relevant involvement. *Electronic Journal of Communication, 23* (3), Retrieved November 26, 2014, from http://www.cios.org/www/ejc/v23n34toc.htm#millerfr 2013

References

Aldoory, L. (2001). Making health connections meaningful for women: Factors that influence involvement. *Journal of Public Relations Research, 13,* 163–185.

Cho, H., & Boster, F. J. (2005). Development and validation of value-, outcome-, and impression-relevant involvement scales. *Communication Research, 32,* 235–264.

Cooke, R., & Sheeran, P. (2004). Moderation of cognition-intention and cognition-behavior relations: A meta-analysis of properties of variables from the theory of planned behavior. *British Journal of Social Psychology, 43,* 159–186.

· Craig, R. J. (2007). Developing and validating psychological tests. In P. M. Goldfarb (Ed.), *Psychological tests and testing research trends* (pp. 173–189). Hauppauge, NY: Nova Science Publishers.

Eagly, A. H. & Chaiken, S. (1993). Process theories of attitude formation and change: The elaboration likelihood and heuristic-systematic models. In A. H. Eagly & S. Chaiken, (Eds.), *The psychology of attitudes* (pp. 303–350). Orlando, FL: Harcourt Brace.

Fazio, R. H. (1995). Attitudes as object-evaluation associations: Determinant, consequences and correlates of attitude accessibility In R. E. Petty & J. A. Krosnick (Eds.), *Attitude strength. Antecedents and consequences* (pp. 247–282). Mahwah, NJ: Erlbaum.

Green, M. C. (2006). Narratives and cancer communication. *Journal of Communication, 56,* S163–183.

Greenwald, A. G., & Leavitt, C. (1984). Audience involvement in advertising: Four levels. *Journal of Consumer Research, 11,* 581–592.

Hubbell, A. P., Mitchell, M. M., & Gee, J. C. (2001). The relative effects of timing of suspicion and outcome involvement on biased message processing. *Communication Monographs, 68,* 115–132.

Johnson, B. T., & Eagly, A. H. (1989). Effects of involvement on persuasion: A meta-analysis. *Psychological Bulletin, 106,* 290–314.

Maheswaran, D., & Meyers-Levy, J. (1990). The influence of message framing and issue involvement. *Journal of Marketing Research, 27,* 361–367.

McQuarrie, E. F., & Munson, J. M. (1992). A revised product involvement inventory: Improved usability and validity. In J. F. Sherry & B. Sternthal (Eds.), *Advances in consumer research, 19* (pp. 108–115). Provo, UT: Association for Consumer Research.

Miller, C. H., & Averbeck, J. M., (2013). Hedonic relevance and outcome relevant involvement. *Electronic Journal of Communication, 23* (3), Retrieved November 26, 2014, from http://www.cios.org/www/ejc/v23n34toc.html#millerfr 2013.

Munson, J. M., & McQuarrie, E. F. (1987). The factorial and predictive validities of a revised measure of Zaichkowsky's Personal Involvement Inventory. *Educational and Psychological Measurement, 47,* 773–782.

Ong, L. M. L, de Haes, J. C. J. M., Hoos, A. M., & Lammes, F. B. (1995). Doctor-patient communication: A review of the literature. *Social Science Medicine, 44,* 903–918.

Park, D., Lee, J., & Han, I. (2007). The effect of on-line consumer reviews on consumer purchasing intention: The moderating role of involvement. *International Journal of Electronic Commerce, 11,* 125–148.

Petty, R. E., Barden, J., & Wheeler, S. C. (2009). The elaboration likelihood model of persuasion: Health promotions that yield sustained behavioral change. In R. J. Di-Clemente, R. A. Crosby, & M. Kegler (Eds.), *Emerging theories in health promotion practice and research* (2nd Ed.) (pp. 185–214). San Francisco: Jossey-Bass.

Petty, R. E. & Cacioppo, J. T. (1979). Issue involvement can increase or decrease persuasion by enhancing message-relevant cognitive responses. *Journal of Personality and Social Psychology, 37,* 1915–1926.

Petty, R. E., & Cacioppo, J. T. (1984). The effects of involvement on responses to argument quantity and quality: Central and peripheral routes to persuasion. *Journal of Personality and Social Psychology, 46,* 69–81.

Pfau, M., Tusing, K. J., Lee, W., Godbold, L. C., Koerner, A., Penaloza, L. J., Hong, Y., & Yang, V. S. (1997). Nuances in inoculation: The role of inoculation approach, ego-involvement, and message processing disposition in resistance. *Communication Quarterly, 45,* 461–481.

Ram, S. & Jung, J. (1989). The link between involvement, use innovativeness, and product usage. *Advances in Consumer Research, 16,* 160–166.

Roskos-Ewoldsen, D. R., Ralstin, L. A., & St. Pierre, J. (2002). The quick and the strong: Implications of attitude accessibility for persuasion. In J. P. Dillard & M. Pfau (Eds.), *Persuasion: Developments in theory and practice* (pp. 1–45). Thousand Oaks, CA: Sage.

Sivacek, J., & Crano, W. D. (1982). Vested interested as a moderator of attitude-behavior consistency. *Journal of Personality and Social Psychology, 43,* 210–221.

Zaichkowsky, J. L. (1994). The personal involvement inventory: Reduction, revision, and application to advertising. *Journal of Advertising, 23,* 59–70.

Zimbardo, P. G. (1960). Involvement and communication discrepancy as determinant of opinion conformity. *Journal of Abnormal and Social Psychology, 60,* 86–94.

11. *Patient-Centered Communication*

Melissa B. Wanzer,
Canisius College
& Melanie Booth-Butterfield,
West Virginia University

In the 21st century the concept of "patient-centered communication" is lauded, but constitutes a dilemma. Patients want interaction and at least some control over health care decisions, but they also definitely want to heal and feel better. Health care providers recognize that patients need more than direct physical care, and that providers should address the emotional and psycho-social aspects of the patient through communication as well. But there is far less agreement from either group about how patient-centered care should be accomplished, and how to balance communication interactions to achieve the most positive outcomes (Mahar, 2010).

The drive to embrace patient-centered care has spawned diverse and numerous efforts to inform and train providers; e.g., the *Patient centered Care Improvement Guide*, generated by the Picker Institute (Frampton et al., 2008). Health practitioners are exhorted to communicate in a patient-centered manner. Unfortunately, there are many concerns with what constitutes optimal patient-centered communication, the tension between validated practice and patients' wishes, the manner in which "patient-centered communication" is conceptualized, and subsequently how it can be validly measured (Epstein, et al., 2005).

Certainly patient-centered communication can be taught, but success necessitates both skill training and the motivation to orient and adapt to patient concerns (Levinson, Lesser, & Epstein, 2010). Further, caregivers' behaviors do not assure patient satisfaction. That is, simply because they act in a specified manner doesn't mean it's effective. The assessment of a true patient-centered pattern needs to orient from the patients' perspective, since they are the targets and ultimate interpreters of the intended positive communication.

If patients and their families do not recognize a pattern of patient-centered communication, it ultimately fails.

Therefore, it is paramount to have a clear, validated, efficient-to-use measure of this important yet complex concept. Some measures of patient-centered communication have relied upon more observed communication than self-report (Ledoux, Hilmers, Watson, Baranowski, & O'Connor, 2013), often with elaborate coding schemes. Such attempts often incorporate items without validation, determination of factor structure, or additional supportive data (e.g., Swenson, et al. 2004).

Further, some PCC studies have utilized specific medical contexts, e.g., elderly patients (Wolf & Roter, 2011), oncology (McCormack et al., 2011), or address specific channels such as vocal tones (Williams, Boyle, Herman, Coleman, & Hummert, 2012) or eye contact (Gorawara-Bhat & Cook, 2011). Such assessments perform well within those parameters, but may have moderate cross-situation utility. While these studies serve the specific contextual purpose, they may not always add to the general knowledge of patient-centered communication. Indeed, practitioner-created measures of patient-centered communication sometimes have less-than-optimal outcomes (Dong, Butow, Costa, Dhillon, & Shields, 2014).

Other researchers and practitioners have utilized only selected items from diverse scales, including the Patient-Centered Communication Scale (Wanzer, Booth-Butterfield, & Gruber, 2004) to measure their construct or training outcomes (e.g., Passalacqua & Harwood, 2012). In a similar style, Wrench and Booth-Butterfield (2003) found interrelationships among perceptions of physicians' humor, credibility, and good will, as well as their positive impact on overall patient satisfaction and compliance. But several separate scales were employed for the constructs. It makes sense to employ a more parsimonious, yet validated, self-report approach to the measurement of patient-centered communication (hereafter referred to as PCC).

In the next section of this chapter we offer a definition of PCC and describe the development of the PCCS and research conducted using the PCCS. In the final section of the chapter we offer suggestions for improving the PCCS.

Definition of Patient-Centered Care

Patient-centered care is defined many different ways; however, a common theme in the definitions is the emphasis on the receiver-oriented nature of PCC. For example, in a discussion by Levinson, Lesser, and Epstein (2010) they note that the Institute of Medicine has defined patient-centered care as "respecting and responding to patients' wants, needs and preferences, so that they can make choices in their care that best fit their individual circumstances" (pp. 48–50).

Working from Stewart's (2001) definition of a patient-centered approach to medicine, we define *Patient-centered communication* behaviors as those behaviors with the greatest potential to enhance the quality of the relationship between the health care provider and patient. Communication practices identified as "patient-centered" and included in the PCCS yielded both empirical and experiential support that use of the behavior affected the quality of the health care provider and patient relationship (Wanzer, Booth-Butterfield, & Gruber, 2004).

Measuring Patient-Centered Communication

McCormack et al. (2011) point out a number of problems with both the conceptualization and measurement of PCC. To date, there does not appear to be a comprehensive PCC scale that taps into all aspects of patient-centered care (Epstein et al., 2005). Existing measures or coding schemes used to assess PCC often focus on certain aspects of PCC (i.e., empathy, information sharing, patient involvement) and ignore others. While these measures are useful, they are limited in their ability to measure a wide range of communication behaviors associated with PCC and are often not grounded in theory or a particular model of PCC. Further, they typically measure only the physicians' behaviors (Epstein et al., 2005; McCormack et al., 2011). It is important to assess all care providers' communication practices to understand a patient's experience.

In an attempt to understand the relationship between health care providers' PCC and patient satisfaction, Wanzer, Booth-Butterfield, and Gruber (2004) designed and tested a PCC measure. The PCCS includes six specific communication behaviors enacted by health care providers to reduce uncertainty in health situations, improve interactions and facilitate collaborative patient-provider relationships.

Patients and their family members often report great amounts of anxiety and uncertainly in health care interactions. One way health care providers can reduce uncertainty during these interactions is to use specific communication practices with patients and their family members. A prominent theory that addresses the role of communication in reducing uncertainty is Uncertainty Reduction Theory (URT). According to URT (Berger, 1987; Berger & Calabrese, 1975) people often experience doubts or uncertainties about their ability to predict the outcome of initial encounters, and such uncertainty creates anxiety. The only way uncertainties are reduced is through increased social interaction.

Specifically, Berger advances axioms that explain "the connection between his central concept of uncertainty and eight key variables of relationship development: verbal output, nonverbal warmth, information seeking, self-disclosure, reciprocity, similarity, liking, and shared networks" (Griffin, 2000, p. 137). Wanzer et al., applied axioms 1 and 2 of Berger's URT. Working from axiom 1, the researchers argued that high uncertainty in encounters is reduced primarily through increases in verbal communication between the social interactants. Therefore, information provided by the health care provider (e.g., name, title, or position at the hospital) early in the interaction with the patient and patient's family members reduces patient anxiety and encourages further communication. Similarly, axiom 2 of URT holds that as nonverbal affiliative expressiveness increases, uncertainty levels decrease (Berger, 1975; Griffin, 2000). Thus, health care providers' use of nonverbal immediacy behaviors (e.g., smiling, gestures, and eye contact) will reduce patient anxiety.

Working from a URT perspective, Wanzer et al. developed a measure of PCC that includes the following six communication behaviors: introductions, clarity, empathy, immediacy, humor, and listening.

Introductions

Visiting the doctor's office or hospital can cause significant amounts of anxiety and uncertainty for patients and their families. Health care providers and staff can help reduce patient and family member anxiety by beginning new interactions with appropriate introductions. Health care providers' use of proper introductions can lead to more productive subsequent interaction with patients and patients' family members (Heery, 2000).

Clarity

Another way health care providers can reduce uncertainty for patients or parents of patients is to communicate about procedures, treatments, or illnesses in ways that are clear and direct. It is important for health care providers and staff to communicate clearly in an effort to reduce patient anxiety, avoid misunderstandings, and reduce uncertainty about health-related processes in general (Kreps & Thornton, 1992). A number of existing PCC measures assess physician clarity (Galassi, Schanberg, & Ware, 1992; Little et al., 2001).

Empathy

While empathic communication is not addressed directly in URT theory axioms, it is yet another way health care providers can reduce patient or parent anxiety during social interaction and facilitate collaborative relationships.

A number of researchers and practitioners have pointed out the benefits of health care providers' use of empathic communication in treating patients (Beckman & Frankel, 1984; Mercer, McConnachie, Maxwell, Heaney, & Watt, 2005; Spiro, 1992). Empathic communication is especially important during the medical interview when the physician or health care provider is attempting to obtain a patient's history and understand the meaning of the illness to the patient (Bellet & Maloney, 1991).

Immediacy

The second axiom of URT addresses the inverse relationship between non-verbal affiliative expressiveness and uncertainty levels in initial interaction situations. Nonverbal affiliative behaviors could be said to constitute nonverbal immediacy. Immediate behaviors are those that reduce physical and psychological distance between social interactants; e.g., smiling, eye contact, closer distances, gesturing (Anderson, 1979).

Physicians' use of nonverbal immediacy is associated with greater patient satisfaction and understanding (Larsen & Smith, 1981). When patients perceive their physicians as more immediate they are more satisfied with their physician, generally more satisfied with the medical care they receive, and experience less fear (Richmond et al., 2001). Burgoon et al. (1987) also found that the more contact the patient had with the physician, the more he or she recognized physician's use of immediacy behaviors and that use of these behaviors was correlated with higher levels of patient satisfaction and moderately associated with patient compliance (Burgoon et al., 1987). Thus, similar to empathy, health care providers' use of immediate behaviors can reduce patient uncertainties about their health care provider and enhance these relationships.

Humor

Often when individuals attempt to communicate humorous messages to others they use nonverbal immediacy behaviors (e.g., smiling, gestures, facial expressions, etc.). Thus, humor that is nonverbal in nature could be viewed as one type of nonverbal affiliative behavior with the potential to reduce uncertainty during social interaction. In this context, health care provider's use of appropriate humor could make help make patients feel more at ease in a potentially stressful situation. Again, applying URT, if health care providers use appropriate humor with patients or patients' family members, uncertainty about the situation may be reduced and satisfaction with communication increased.

Listening

Listening is a highly complex and demanding process that "consists of being mindful, hearing, selecting and organizing information, interpreting communication, responding, and remembering" (Wood, 1999; p. 180). Listening has been identified as a social affinity-seeking strategy (Bell & Daly, 1984), and is a skill that health care providers must use daily. From a pragmatic perspective, if physicians do not listen to their patients they may make mistakes leading to medical difficulties and costly malpractice suits. But from a more interpersonal perspective, physicians' willingness to listen is associated with patient satisfaction (Burgoon et al., 1987; Gorawara-Bhat & Cook, 2011).

The Patient-Centered Communication Scale consists of items centered on the previous six areas. Wanzer et al. (2004) created the following items to assess physician, nurse, and staff member use of PCC in a hospital setting. The scale employs a 5-point Likert-type format to assess the extent to which caregivers exhibit the positive behaviors (1 = Never; 2 = Rarely; 3 = Occasionally; 4 = Often; and 5 = Very Often. Also note that items 6 and 11 are reverse coded for analysis.)

1. The physician/nurse/staff member introduced her/himself to me.
2. When the physician/nurse/staff member approached me he/she provided her/his title/position to me.
3. The physician/nurse/staff member used gestures while speaking with me.
4. The physician/nurse/staff member used appropriate humor when communicating with me.
5. The physician/nurse/staff member looked at me while talking to me.
6. The physician/nurse/staff member had a tense body position while talking to me.*
7. The physician/nurse/staff member smiled at me as he/she approached me.
8. The physician/nurse/staff member listened intently during our conversation.
9. The physician/nurse/staff member communicated in a clear and direct manner when talking to me.
10. I felt comfortable expressing any worries or concerns to this physician/nurse/staff member.
11. When I stated any worries or concerns that I had, the physician/nurse/staff member directed the conversation away from my statement.*

12. If I expressed emotions such as anxiety or fear, the physician/nurse/ staff member invited discussions about my concerns.
13. The physician/nurse/staff member asked me to express any concerns that I might have.

To study the relationship between health care providers' use of PCC and satisfaction, Wanzer et al. (2004) distributed the PCCS and satisfaction measure to 195 parents and guardians of children in a children's hospital. Parent/ guardian participants completed separate measures of PCC (clarity, humor, introductions, immediacy, listening, and empathy) for physicians, nurses, and staff and completed brief measures of satisfaction with care and communication. Parent/guardians provided demographic information as well as their length of stay in the hospital.

Similar to previous research that identified a positive correlation between health care providers' use of PCC and satisfaction (Little et al., 2001), Wanzer et al. predicted that parent/guardian perceptions of physician, nurse, and staff use of PCC would correlate with patients' satisfaction with communication. Parents'/guardians' reports of physician, nurse, and hospital staff use of PCC were correlated with satisfaction with communication ($r = .73$, $p = .001$, $r = .61$, $p = .001$, $r = .59$, $p = .001$). Similarly, parents'/guardians' reports of physician and nurse PCC were also correlated with satisfaction with medical care ($r = .67$, $p = .001$, $r = .68$, $p = .001$). Using Cohen's (1988) standards, all of these effect sizes were considered large.

Another important aim of this research was to determine whether certain physician, nurse, or staff PCC behaviors (i.e., clarity, humor, introductions, immediacy, listening, empathy) were stronger predictors of satisfaction than others. Standard multiple regression analyses were conducted to determine which communication practices would have the greatest influence on parent/guardian satisfaction with communication and medical care. Physician *immediacy, listening,* and *empathy* were all significant predictors of parent/ guardian satisfaction with communication. *Empathy* was the only significant predictor of parent/guardian perceptions of satisfaction with communication with nurses. Because patients have somewhat limited interaction with hospital staff members (i.e. admissions, food services, transportation, etc.), only introductions, clarity, and immediacy were examined as potential predictors of parent/guardian satisfaction with communication. Hospital staff *immediacy* and *clarity* emerged as significant predictors of parent/guardian satisfaction with communication.

Similar patterns emerged when examining PCC behaviors that predicted parent/guardian satisfaction of medical care received. For example, physician clarity and listening were significant predictors of parent/guardian satisfaction with medical care. For nurses, introductions and listening were significant predictors of parent/guardian satisfaction with medical care received.

The seminal research by Wanzer et al. (2004) using both a 13 and 7-item version of the PCCS to measure parent/guardian perceptions of physician, nurse, and staff PCC was promising. The 13-item PCCS proved to be a reliable estimate of physician PCC (α = .86) and nurse (α = .82) communication practices. A shortened 7-item PCCS was a reliable measure of hospital staff communication practices (α = .79). Parent/guardian reports of physician (M = 57.10, SD = 7.82) and nurse (M = 57.51, SD =6.18) PCC were very similar and quite high.

The PCCS was modified and used in a follow-up study to measure nurses' perceptions of physician communication practices. To gain another perspective on health care providers' use of PCC, Wanzer, Wojtaszczyk, and Kelly (2009) asked 205 nurses to complete a modified version of the PCCS. Nurses indicated how often the physician used targeted behaviors in their work interactions (i.e., clarity, humor, etc.) and how often they observed physicians engaging in PCC with patients and families. The 10-item version of the PCCS employed in this study to measure nurse-centered communication (hereafter referred to as NCC) and PCC performed reliably (α = .88 for both versions of the revised scale). As predicted, nurses' perceptions of NCC were associated with satisfaction with communication, relationship satisfaction, job satisfaction, and collaboration at work. Nurses' perceptions of NCC were correlated with perceptions of PCC. Finally, nurses viewed the physicians as engaging in the PCC behaviors more often than the NCC behaviors.

Use of Existing Measures and Future Studies

Collectively, these studies shed light on how self and other report measures can be used to reliably assess PCC. The PCCS is not without flaws as it has not been extensively validated, may not include all possible patient-centered communication practices, and may reflect patients' general reactions to their care rather than specific health care provider behaviors (Epstein et al., 2005). Additional research is needed on the PCCS to address measurement concerns expressed with other PCC measures. Future PCC studies might employ focus groups or interviews to determine an array of different types of health care behaviors viewed as PCC. In addition, researchers should study the role that concordance plays in determining the quality of interactions between care providers and patients.

At this point, the Patient-Centered Communication Scale represents a sound self-report instrument to assess how patients recognize and interpret care givers' communication. It is appropriately related to satisfaction, has been successfully administered in several formats, and reliably addresses the concept of patient-centered communication.

Recommended Readings

Epstein, R., Franks, P., Fiscella, K. Cleveland, S., Melsrum, S., Kravitz, R. & Duberstein, P. (2005). Measuring patient-centered communication in patient-physician consultations: Theoretical and practical issues. *Social Science & Medicine, 61*, 1516–1528.

Levinson, W., Lesser, S., & Epstein, R. (2010). Developing physician communication skills for patient-centered care. *Health Affairs, 29*, 1310–1318.

Wanzer, M. B., Booth-Butterfield, M., & Gruber, K. (2004). Perceptions of health care providers: Communication relationships between patient-centered communication and satisfaction. *Health Communication, 16*, 363–384.

Wanzer, M. B. Wojtaszczyk, A. M , & Kelly, J. (2009). Nurses' perceptions of physicians' communication: The relationship among communication practices, satisfaction, and collaboration. *Health Communication, 24*, 683–691.

References

Anderson, J. F. (1979). Teacher immediacy as a predictor of teaching effectiveness. In D. Nimmo (Ed.), *Communication Yearbook 3,* 543–559. New Brunswick, NJ: Transaction Books.

Beckman, H. B., & Frankel, R. M. (1984). The effect of physician behaviour on the collection of data. *Annals of Internal Medicine, 101*, 692–696.

Bell, R., & Daly, J. A. (1984). The affinity-seeking function of communication. *Communication Monographs, 51*, 91–115.

Bellet, P. S., & Maloney, M. J. (1991). The importance of empathy as an interviewing skill in medicine. *Journal of the American Medical Association, 266*, 1831–1832.

Berger, C. (1987). Communicating under Uncertainty. In M. Roloff & G. Miller (Eds.), *Interpersonal Processes: New Directions in Communication Research* (pp. 39–62). Newbury Park, CA: Sage.

Berger, C., & Calabrese, R. (1975). Some explorations in initial interaction and beyond: Toward a developmental theory of interpersonal communication. *Human Communication Research, 1*, 99–112.

Burgoon, J. K., Pfau, M., Parrott, R., Birk, T., Coker, R., & Burgoon, M. (1987). Relational communication, satisfaction, compliance-gaining strategies, and compliance in communication between physicians and patients. *Communication Monographs, 54*, 307–324.

Cohen, J. (1988). *Statistical power analysis for the behavioral sciences* (2nd ed.). Hillsdale, NJ: Erlbaum.

Dong, S., Butow, P. N., Costa, D., Dhillon, H. M., & Shields, C. G. (2014). The influence of patient-centered communication during radiotherapy education sessions on post-consultation patient outcomes. *Patient Education & Counseling, 95,* 305–312.

Epstein, R., Franks, P., Fiscella, K. Cleveland, S., Melsrum, S., Kravitz, R., & Duberstein, P. (2005). Measuring patient-centered communication in patient-physician consultations: Theoretical and practical issues. *Social Science & Medicine, 61,* 1516–1528.

Frampton, S., Guastello, S., Brady, C., Hale, M., Horowitz, S., Bennett Smith, S., & Stone, S., (2008). *Patient-centered care improvement guide.* Picker Institute, Inc. Retrieved from http://pickerinstitute.org/publications-and-resources

Galassi, J. P. Schanberg, R., & Ware, W. B. (1992). The patient reactions assessment: A brief measure of the quality of the patient-provider medical relationship. *Psychological Assessment, 4,* 346–351.

Gorawara-Bhat, R. & Cook, M. A. (2011). Eye contact in patient-centered communication. *Patient Education and Counseling, 82,* 442–447. doi: 10.1016/j.pec.2010.12.002.

Griffin, E. (2000). *A First Look at Communication Theory* (4th ed). New York: McGraw Hill.

Heery, K. (2000). Straight talk about the patient interview. *Nursing, 30,* 66–67.

Kreps, G., & Thornton, B. (1992). *Health Communication and Policy.* Prospect Heights, IL: Waveland Press.

Larsen, K. M., & Smith, C. K. (1981). Assessment of nonverbal communication in the patient-physician interview. *Journal of Family Practice, 12,* 481–488.

Ledoux, T., Hilmers, A., Watson, K., Baranowski, T., & O'Connor, T. M., (2013). Development and feasibility of an objective measure of patient-centered communication fidelity in a pediatric obesity intervention. *Nutrition & Behavior, 45,* pp. 349–354. doi: 10.1016/j.jneb.2012.10.006.

Levinson, W., Lesser, S., & Epstein, R. (2010). Developing physician communication skills for patient-centered care. *Health Affairs, 29,* 1310–1318. doi: 10.1377/hlthaff.2009.0450.

Little, P., Everitt, H., Williamson, I., Warner, G., Moore, M., Gould, C., Ferrier, K., & Payne, S. (2001). Observational study of effect of patient centeredness and positive approach on outcomes of general practice consultations. *British Medical Journal, 323,* 908–911.

Mahar, M. (2010). *What does don berwick mean by "patient-centered" care? (ezra klein confuses the enemy).* Retrieved from http://www.healthbeatblog.com/2010/07.

McCormack, L. A., Treiman, K., Rupert, D., Williams-Piehota, P., Nadler, E., Arora, N. K., Lawrence, W., & Street, R. L. (2011). Measuring patient-centered communication in cancer care: A literature review and the development of a systematic approach. *Social Science & Medicine, 72,* 1085–1095.

Mercer, S. W., McConnachie, A., Maxwell, M., Heaney, D., & Watt, G. C. (2005). Relevance and practical use of the consultation and relational empathy (care) measure in general practice. *Family Practice, 22,* 328–334.

Passalacqua, S. A., Harwood, J. (2012). VIPS communication skills training for paraprofessional dementia caregivers: An intervention to increase person-centered dementia care. *Clinical Gerontologist, 35,* 425–445. doi: 10.1080/07317115.2012.702655.

Richmond, V. P., Smith, R. S., Heisel, A. D., & McCroskey, J. C. (2001). Nonverbal immediacy in the physician/patient relationship. *Communication Research Reports, 18,* 211–216.

Spiro, H. (1992). What is empathy and can it be taught? *Annals of Internal Medicine, 116,* 843–846.

Stewart, M. (2001). Towards a global definition of patient centered care: The patient should be the judge of patient centered care. *British Medical Journal, 322,* 444–445.

Swenson, S., Buell, S., Zettler, P., White, M., Ruston, D., & Lo, B. (2004). Patient-centered communication: Do patients really prefer it? *Journal of General Internal Medicine, 19,* 1069–1079. doi: 10.1111/j.1525-1497.2004.30384.x.

Wanzer, M. B., Booth-Butterfield, M., & Gruber, K. (2004). Perceptions of health care providers' communication: Relationships between patient-centered communication and satisfaction. *Health Communication, 16,* 363–384.

Wanzer, M. B. Wojtaszczyk, A. M., & Kelly, J. (2009). Nurses' perceptions of physicians' communication: The relationship among communication practices, satisfaction, and collaboration. *Health Communication, 24,* 683–691. DOI: 10.1080/10410230903263990.

Williams, K. N., Boyle, D. K., Herman, R. E., Coleman, C. K., & Hummert, M. L. (2012). Psychometric analysis of the emotional tone rating scale: a measure of person-centered communication. *Clinical Gerontologist, 35,* 376–389. doi: 10.1080/07317115.2012.702648.

Wolf, J. L., & Roter, D. L. (2011). Older adults' mental health function and patient-centered care: Does the presence of a family companion help or hinder communication? *Journal of General Internal Medicine, 27,* 661–668. doi: 10.1007/s11606-011-1957-5.

Wood, J. T. (2004). *Interpersonal communication: Everyday encounters* (4th ed.). Belmont, CA: Wadsworth.

Wrench, J., & Booth-Butterfield, M. (2003). Increasing patient satisfaction and compliance: An examination of physician humor orientation, compliance-gaining strategies, and perceived credibility. *Communication Quarterly, 51,* 482–503.

12. Perceived Argument Strength

Xiaoquan Zhao,
George Mason University
& Joseph N. Cappella,
University of Pennsylvania

Health communication research often involves the use of persuasive messages to increase awareness, enhance knowledge, change attitudes, and modify behavior. A key variable in message construction and evaluation is argument strength. Although many studies have used self-reported measures of argument strength, or broader measures of message effectiveness, rarely are these measures based on careful theoretical explication and rigorous empirical validation (Yzer, LoRusso, & Nagler, 2015). This chapter presents a scale of perceived argument strength that draws on relevant persuasion theories, shows desirable psychometric properties, and promises ease of use and wide applicability across populations and contexts.

The importance of argument strength is most well-known within the theoretical framework of the elaboration likelihood model (ELM, Petty & Cacioppo, 1986). According to ELM, messages featuring strong versus weak arguments will lead to different persuasive outcomes depending on the audience's motivation and ability to process the message. ELM researchers have traditionally relied on an empirical procedure called "thought listing" to determine argument strength (Cacioppo & Petty, 1981). Typically, potential arguments are presented to a sample of the target audience who then write down their thoughts while reading or hearing those arguments. Arguments that elicit more favorable than unfavorable thoughts are deemed to be relatively strong and those eliciting more unfavorable than favorable thoughts are considered to be relatively weak.

The validity of thought listing is well accepted and it is widely used in health communication research. However, thought-listing also has some limitations (Cacioppo, von Hippel, & Ernst, 1997). It is a relatively inefficient procedure—it takes time to complete the task and additional coding is often necessary before the data can be used. The procedure can be difficult to administer to populations with limited cognitive ability (e.g., children) or literacy skills (e.g., immigrants). In situations where sensitive topics are involved, motivation to report accurately may be low, compromising the completeness and quality of the data generated.

To complement thought listing, a self-reported measure of perceived argument strength offers advantages in terms of ease of administration, suitability for different populations, and the potential to cover a wide range of theoretical perspectives and topic domains. The cognitive response approach taken by ELM has traditionally focused on valence profiling of the generated thoughts. But other theories have also offered insights that can enrich the understanding of argument strength and inform the construction of measurement tools. Of note, Morley's work (1987) approached argument strength from the perspective of the "cognitive operations" that recipients perform in processing information including ones perceived to be plausible, important, and novel. When these three perceptions occur, belief change tends to follow.

Behavior change research in health contexts has employed expectancy value approaches, specifically the reasoned action approach to behavior prediction and change (Fishbein & Ajzen, 2010). Arguments in health persuasion often highlight particular behavioral outcomes underlying attitudes toward the target behavior. From the reasoned action perspective, the strength of such arguments is primarily determined by the perceived probability and subjective appeal of the outcome. To assess perceived argument strength, thus, it is important to include indicators of both the perceived truth value of the argument and perceived desirability of the featured outcome.

The broader reasoned action framework also emphasizes the importance of self-efficacy or behavioral control in the actual performance of behavior. A vast amount of literature in health communication and intervention provides supportive evidence that a sense of efficacy or confidence in enacting a recommended health behavior is a critical determinant of eventual behavior adoption. A measure of perceived argument strength for use in health communication research, thus, may also benefit from the inclusion of a component that assesses the argument's potential to enhance recipients' confidence in enacting the target behavior.

Measuring Perceived Argument Strength

A self-reported measure of perceived argument strength was developed based on considerations as discussed above (for a fuller account of the scale development research, see Zhao, Strasser, Cappella, Lerman, & Fishbein, 2011). This scale includes several theoretically motivated components: thought valence, plausibility, importance, confidence, and overall persuasiveness. Although each of these components could be developed into multi-item subscales, only one or two items are used to assess each component for the sake of scale brevity and suitability for both adult and non-adult populations. The preliminary version of the scale also included a novelty component. But this latter component failed to load adequately on the latent construct in repeated testing and was removed from the final scale, which is presented in Table 1.

Table 1. Perceived argument strength scale.

---

1. The statement is a reason for ___ that is believable.
2. The statement is a reason for ___ that is convincing.
3. The statement gives a reason for ___ that is important to me.
4. The statement helped me feel confident about how best to ___.
5. The statement would help my friends ___.
6. The statement put thoughts in my mind about wanting to___.
7. The statement put thoughts in my mind about not wanting to___.
8. Overall, how much do you agree or disagree with the statement?
9. Is the reason the statement gave for _____ a strong or weak reason?

Instructions: Fill in the blanks with the target behavior for the persuasive argument. Use a 5- or 7-point Likert scale (strongly disagree to strongly agree) to score items 1–8. Use a 5- or 7-point Likert type scale (very weak to very strong) to score item 9. Reverse code item 7 before constructing summary score.

A series of studies were conducted to test the factorial structure, internal consistency, and construct validity of the scale. In two studies, one targeting adolescents and the other adult smokers, arguments used in a large number of real world anti-drug and anti-smoking campaign PSAs were carefully extracted and evaluated using the perceived argument strength scale. In both studies, confirmatory factor analysis of the scale with a single-factor structure provided adequate fit to the data. Factor loadings showed strong relationships between the individual scale items and the underlying factor (range = .62 to .83 and .55 to .85, respectively). The scale also exhibited excellent internal consistency (range = .75 to .92 and .82 to .96, respectively, for individual arguments). In both studies, average perceived argument strength score for individual participants (who evaluated a random subset of all the arguments) correlated significantly with subsequent behavioral intention (r = .35 and -.44, respectively) and other behavioral antecedents, providing evidence of predictive validity. In one of the studies, need for cognition was also measured for the purpose of testing discriminant validity. According to ELM, need for cognition should not influence assessment of argument strength because it is only supposed to affect level of argument elaboration. The data supported this prediction, showing no relationship between need for cognition and perceived argument strength ratings (r = -.03).

Convergent validity of the scale was tested using a classic ELM design. Strong vs. weak arguments in support of a senior comprehensive exam policy were culled from previous literature and shown to a group of undergraduate students. The student participants completed thought listing for a random half of the arguments and rated the other half using the perceived argument strength scale. Thus, for each argument, two separate indicators of argument strength were obtained, one based on thought favorability, the other the self-reported scale. These two indicators correlated strongly (r = .77), providing evidence of convergence between the traditional thought listing procedure and the perceived argument strength scale.

The scale has been used (or adapted) in many empirical health communication studies. Further evidence of its validity is now available. Some studies have used the scale to identify messages with varying argument strength that are then used to test theoretically motivated hypotheses about message processing and effects. Research in this area has shown consistent evidence that the scale can successfully differentiate between strong versus weak messages. Of particular interest, one study showed that anti-smoking ads with strong arguments elicited stronger physiological reaction (heart rate and skin conductance) in adult smokers than those with weaker arguments (Strasser et al., 2009). Another recent study found that anti-drug PSAs identified as strong versus weak using the scale generated different brain responses consistent with theory-based understanding of information processing (Weber, Huskey, Mangus, Westcott-Baker, & Turner, 2015). A study by Wang et al. (2013) showed not only stronger intentions and attitudes to quit smoking for the stronger arguments but also reduced cotinine levels one month later in response to the stronger arguments. These outcomes were predicted by activation of specific brain regions. Falcone et al. (2011) reported specific genetic factors linked to central processing of message features including argument strength measured with the scale presented here. These physiological, genetic, and neuroimaging data provide important new evidence for the validity of the scale.

Other studies use the perceived argument strength scale primarily as a measure of message evaluation or persuasive outcome (e.g., Zhao & Nan, 2010). These studies have shown a consistent pattern of congruence between perceived argument strength ratings and other message responses, such as liking, message-evoked emotions, attitude, and intention. An extension of this line of research treats perceived argument strength as a mediator between message exposure and actual message effectiveness. A recent study in this area found that aggregate perceived argument strength scores for anti-smoking PSAs across the sample (as opposed to individual ratings) were able to predict smoking cessation intentions on the individual level (Bigsby, Cappella, & Seitz, 2013). This evidence is unique because it removes the potential confounding influence of individual characteristics on perceived argument strength ratings and behavioral intentions. As such, it offers a clearer causal interpretation of the relationship between perceived argument strength and subsequent outcomes of persuasion. It also suggests that the perceived argument strength scale is indeed measuring perceptions of argument strength rather than individual predispositions, thus lending further credence to the measure's validity.

Use of Existing Measures and Future Studies

Argument strength is arguably the cornerstone of persuasion, which in turn is a central activity in many health communication efforts. This chapter presents a brief, self-reported measure of perceived argument strength. Built upon relevant persuasion and behavioral theories, this scale has a clear conceptual foundation and has been subjected to systematic and careful empirical validation. Evidence so far suggests that this scale has good psychometric properties and practical utility. As a complementary tool to the thought listing procedure, this scale has potential to be useful in a wide variety of health communication contexts where the manipulation and/or assessment of argument strength is necessary.

It should be noted that this scale is called *perceived* argument strength. This reflects a measurement approach that focuses on audience reactions to persuasive arguments. An alternative approach to argument strength is to focus on relevant message characteristics that are known to increase or decrease argument quality (O'Keefe & Jackson, 1995). Objective definitions of strong arguments in advance of their testing are still remote even though some recent conceptual developments are promising (O'Keefe, 2013). It is for this reason that measurement techniques based on cognitive response, such as thought listing and the scale proposed here, have important utility in persuasion and health communication research. Having said the above, it is still critical to be mindful of the differences between the two approaches. It is generally inadvisable to refer to the current scale and the ratings it generates simply as argument strength (as opposed to perceived argument strength). Imprecise use of terminology could result in much confusion regarding the nature and usefulness of the scale.

As with any self-report measure, subjectivity is an important limitation of the perceived argument strength scale. That is, individual ratings can reflect not only the influence of message characteristics, but also personal predispositions, such as current attitude and intention. One way to ameliorate this problem, as shown in Bigsby et al. (2013), is to use aggregate ratings based on a large sample (and preferably an independent sample) to ascertain perceived argument strength. When this is not possible, however, researchers are encouraged to be sensitive to the subjective nature of the ratings when interpreting their data.

This scale was developed within the framework of ELM and focuses on argument strength. Arguments are the building blocks of messages, and argument strength fundamentally decides message effectiveness. For this reason, researchers interested in the strength and effectiveness of entire messages should also find utility in this scale. Indeed, many empirical studies have adapted this scale to measure perceived message effectiveness, and the adaption is relatively straightforward (mostly by replacing the word "statement" with "message" or other appropriate terms).

Thus far, the perceived argument strength scale has only been used in a limited number of health communication contexts, mostly drug use and smoking. Future research should extend its use to other health domains to further test its validity and usefulness. It should also be noted that the perceived argument strength scale is not the only measure of its kind in the literature. What distinguishes this scale from other existing measures is its clear theoretical foundation and systematic empirical validation. Although these characteristics should afford this scale advantages in measurement quality, direct comparison of this scale with other alternative measures has not been conducted. Future research may look to pursue this agenda.

Recommended Readings

Kang, Y., Cappella, J., & Fishbein, M. (2006). The attentional mechanism of message sensation value: Interaction between message sensation value and argument quality on message effectiveness. *Communication Monographs, 73,* 351–378

Weber, R., Huskey, R., Mangus, J. M., Westcott-Baker, A., & Turner, B. O. (2015). Neural predictors of message effectiveness during counterarguing in antidrug campaigns. *Communication Monographs, 82,* 4–30.

Zhao, X., & Nan, X. (2010). Influence of self-affirmation on responses to gain- versus loss-framed antismoking messages. *Human Communication Research, 36,* 493–511.

Zhao, X., Strasser, A., Cappella, J. N., Lerman, C., & Fishbein, M. (2011). A measure of perceived argument strength: Reliability and validity. *Communication Methods and Measures, 5,* 48–75.

Zhao, X., Villagran, M. M., Kreps, G. L., & McHorney, C. (2012). Gain versus loss framing in adherence-promoting communication targeting patients with chronic diseases: The moderating effect of individual time perspective. *Health Communication, 27,* 75–85.

References

Bigsby, E., Cappella, J. N., & Seitz, H. H. (2013). Efficiently and effectively evaluating public service announcements: Additional evidence for the utility of perceived effectiveness. *Communication Monographs, 80,* 1–23. doi:10.1080/03637751.2012.739 706.

Cacioppo, J. T., & Petty, R. E. (1981). Social psychological procedures for cognitive response assessment: The thought-listing technique. In T. V. Merluzzi, C. R. Glass, & M. Genest (Eds.), *Cognitive assessment* (pp. 309–342). New York: Guilford Press.

Cacioppo, J. T., von Hippel, W., & Ernst, J. M. (1997). Mapping cognitive structures and processes through verbal content: The thought-listing technique. *Journal of Consulting and Clinical Psychology, 65,* 928–940.

Falcone, M., Jepson, C., Sanborn, P., Cappella, J. N., Lerman, C., & Strasser, A. A. (2011). Association of BDNF and COMT genotypes with cognitive processing of antismoking PSAs. *Genes, Brain & Behavior, 10,* 862–867. http://dx.doi.org/10.1111/j.1601-183X.2011.00726.x

Fishbein, M., & Ajzen, I. (2010). *Predicting and changing behavior: The reasoned action approach* (1st ed.). New York: Psychology Press.

Morley, D. D. (1987). Subjective message constructs: A theory of persuasion. *Communication Monographs, 54,* 183–203.

O'Keefe, D. J. (2013). The relative persuasiveness of different forms of arguments-from-consequences: A review and integration. In C.T. Salmon (Ed.), *Communication Yearbook 36* (pp. 109–135). New York: Routledge.

O'Keefe, D. J., & Jackson, S. (1995). Argument quality and persuasive effects: A review of current approaches. In S. Jackson (Ed.), *Argumentation and values: Proceedings of the ninth SCA/AFA conference on argumentation* (pp. 88–92). Annandale, VA: Speech Communication Association.

Petty, R. E., & Cacioppo, J. T. (1986). *Communication and persuasion: Central and peripheral routes to attitude change.* New York: Springer-Verlag.

Strasser, A. A., Cappella, J. N., Jepson, C., Fishbein, M., Tang, K. Z., Han, E., & Lerman, C. (2009). Experimental evaluation of antitobacco PSAs: Effects of message content and format on physiological and behavioral outcomes. *Nicotine & Tobacco Research, 11,* 293–302. doi:10.1093/ntr/ntn026.

Wang, A. L., Loughead, J. W., Strasser, A. A., Ruparel, K., Romer, D. R., Blady, S. J.,... Langleben, D. D. (2013). Content matters: Neuroimaging investigation of brain and behavioral impact of televised anti-tobacco public service announcements. *Journal of Neuroscience, 33,* 7420–7427. doi:10.1523/JNEUROSCI.3840-12.2013.

Weber, R., Huskey, R., Mangus, J. M., Westcott-Baker, A., & Turner, B. O. (2015). Neural predictors of message effectiveness during counterarguing in antidrug campaigns. *Communication Monographs, 82,* 4–30. doi:10.1080/03637751.2014.971414.

Yzer, M., LoRusso, S., & Nagler, R. H. (2015). On the conceptual ambiguity surrounding perceived message effectiveness. *Health Communication, 30,* 125–134. doi:10.1080/10410236.2014.974131.

Zhao, X., & Nan, X. (2010). Influence of self-affirmation on responses to gain- versus loss-framed antismoking messages. *Human Communication Research, 36,* 493–511. doi:10.1111/j.1468-2958.2010.01385.x.

Zhao, X., Strasser, A., Cappella, J. N., Lerman, C., & Fishbein, M. (2011). A measure of perceived argument strength: Reliability and validity. *Communication Methods and Measures, 5,* 48–75. doi:10.1080/19312458.2010.547822.

13. Perceived Attributes of Innovations

DO KYUN KIM,
University of Louisiana At Lafayette
& JAMES W. DEARING,
Michigan State University

Research about the diffusion of innovations investigates the determinants of the adoption of an idea, practice, program, technology, or object by an individual, organization, or social system, and other issues such as the role of social influence on adoption, imitative behavior, the fidelity of implementation of innovations, the quality of adaptations made by implementers, and sustained use of innovations, and the unintended consequences of diffusion processes (Rogers, 2003). The diffusion model forms a part of the basis for dissemination and implementation science, a particular recent emphasis by researchers in public health (Brownson, Colditz, & Proctor, 2012) and health care (Berwick, 2003). The parameters of diffusion research are expansive. Diffusion study is conducted by researchers in international development, sociology, management and marketing, political science, education, agriculture, public health and health services, as well as communication and its related fields of journalism, telecommunication, and new media studies.

Health communication researchers studying diffusion have tended to focus either on public health campaigns where individuals at risk are the potential adopters of a message and its related behavioral actions (such as how mothers can correctly fasten mosquito nets over beds to reduce cases of malaria among infants and the elderly), or efforts to encourage medical staff to adopt evidence based practices in clinical settings (for example to reduce the percent of infections contracted by patients while they are in a hospital for medical treatment). In both public health and health care diffusion research, researchers have often studied the factors that influence the adoption of health innovations. The present chapter introduces a scale that measures how a health innovation is perceived by the unit of adoption (whether that unit is an individual or a group of people in an organization).

An innovation in the context of health communication can be understood as anything that change agents promote to target populations, whether those targets are individuals at risk or those intermediaries who provide services to them, such as K–12 teachers acting on behalf of low-income children. Government agencies such as the U.S. Agency for Research on Healthcare Quality, quality assurance associations, state or provincial health departments, community-based nonprofit organizations, school clinics, for-profit firms, and research teams can all function as change agencies and employ change agents. Target population members may not perceive themselves as a strata, group, or population (as with bicycle-riding children in the Twin Cities in Minnesota, or nurses in Arizona's public clinics) yet their shared characteristics enable change agents to identify them as a sampling frame, develop messages that can be pretested with representative members, and then efficiently reach and communicate with them. The diffusion of innovations among such populations is partly determined by the efficacy of the innovation(s) in question, and by strategies that consider the entire over-time process of diffusion.

A common strategy of intervention developers who have knowledge of the diffusion model is to structure messages and interventions based on what has been shown to affect adoption. One of the critical elements that determine the adoption of an innovation is the set of characteristics or "attributes" that categorize and reflect how target population members perceive the innovation. The importance of perceived attributes stems from the well-established research finding that the way in which a potential adopter perceives an innovation can explain considerable variance in explaining their adoption of the innovation. Everett M. Rogers, the leading figure in conducting diffusion research and synthesizing the model across multiple academic fields, devoted one chapter of each of his five editions of his book *Diffusion of Innovations* (2003) to these perceived pros and cons.

Rogers (2003) grouped research about attributes into five categories: (1) relative advantage, 2) compatibility, 3) complexity, 4) trialability, and 5) observability. Relative *advantage* refers to how much better or worse an innovation is perceived in comparison to previous or alternative innovations that serve the same purpose. Subsequent researchers have divided this construct into two: *Cost*, as in how costly an innovation is perceived either monetarily or in other resources such as time, and *Effectiveness*, as in how well and how regularly an innovation achieves its objectives. *Compatibility* is the extent to which an innovation fits with the existing values, routines, and needs of potential adopters. *Complexity* and its converse *Simplicity* is the extent to which an innovation is perceived to be easy to understand and use. *Trialability* refers to the degree to which an innovation can be conveniently experienced, so the potential adopters reduce their uncertainty in committing to the innovation. *Observability* is the extent to which an innovation's results are visible. Numerous studies over several decades have shown that the higher the relative advantage (with perceived lower cost and higher effectiveness), compatibility, simplicity, trialability, and observability, the higher the likelihood of unit-level adoption and, thus, system-level diffusion.

Since there is considerable variance in innovations (from ideas to technologies to policies) and many topical areas (from automobile manufacturing to health promotion), some innovations have special properties and, thus, unique attributes that reflect those properties. For example, the effectiveness of engineering and biological innovations to remediate hazardous waste depends greatly on variations in soil, water, and temperature. What is quite effective at a contaminated Midwest site may be wholly ineffective at a mountainous location in the West. Since these types of innovations require large investments to bring to the field, potential adopters will prominently consider the risk involved in adoption. Thus, perceived risk and other attributes such as robustness or generalizability can be as important as any of the standard innovation attributes categorized by Rogers (2003) in these cases. The measurement of innovation attributes, like a number of the measures reviewed in the present book, is often customized to better fit particular topical domains.

Measuring Perceived Attributes of an Innovation

Aiming to investigate potential adopters' perceptions on an innovation, various researchers have developed scales to measure perceived attributes. One important study was conducted by Moore and Benbasat (1991) on scale development to measure the perceptions of adopting an information technology, specifically, Personal Work Stations (PWS). Although it is not in the context of health communication research, their systemic scale development exemplified how to develop an instrument to measure perceived attributes of innovations for different research purposes. As a result of repeated tests of theory-based questions, Moore and Benbasat settled on 31 items measuring 5 perceived attributes and 13 items for 3 other constructs of voluntariness, image, and result demonstrability. They also selected 22 items from their full measure for a short version of the instrument, with 15 of those items assessing the standard Rogers attributes (Moore & Benbasat, 1991, p. 216). Factor loadings ranged from 0.45 to 0.86. Cronbach's alpha of the eight subscales (by factors) were also acceptable (r = 0.71) to high (r = 0.95). The 15 items for the 5 perceived attributes are in Table 1.

Table 1. Moore & Benbasat's (1991) Scale to Measure the 5 Perceived Attributes.

(Relative Advantage)

1. Using a PWS enables me to accomplish tasks more quickly.

2. Using a PWS improves the quality of work I do.

3. Using a PWS makes it easier to do my job.

4. Using a PWS enhances my effectiveness on the job.

5. Using a PWS gives me greater control over my work.

(Compatibility)

1. Using a PWS is compatible with all aspects of my work.

2. I think that using a PWS fits well with the way I like to work.

3. Using a PWS fits into my work style.

(Ease of Use—Complexity)

1. My interaction with a PWS is clear and understandable.

2. I believe that it is easy to get a PWS to do what I want it to do.

3. Overall, I believe that a PWS is easy to use.

4. Learning to operate a PWS is easy for me.

(Visibility—Observability)

1. In my organization, one sees PWS on many tasks.

2. PWS are not very visible in my organization.

(Trialability)

1. Before deciding whether to use any PWS applications, I was able to properly try them out.

Applying Moore and Benbasat's scale to the health communication context, Pankratz, Hallfors, and Cho's (2002) study on the diffusion of a federal drug prevention policy, *Principles of Effectiveness (PE)*, has served as a foundational referent for many health communication studies. The Principles of Effectiveness was designed to reduce illegal drug use, violence, and disruptive behavior in schools and recipients of Safe and Drug Free Schools (SDFS) funds. The target population of this study were 107 SDFS coordinators in 12 states. Using a 5-point Likert scale, their instrument had 17 items (See *Table 1* in Pankratz, Hallfors, & Cho, 2002, p. 319). After conducting a principle component factor analysis with a varimax rotation and a promax rotation, 3 items were eliminated. As a result, 14 items remained, assessing relative advantage, compatibility, complexity, and observability.

As Table 2 shows, this study combined relative advantage and compatibility together as one factor, although questions 1 and 2 were originally designed for compatibility. Pankratz, Hallfors, and Cho explained this with reasons based on real-world situations. For example, the prevention coordinators think of the Principles of Effectiveness' relative advantage in the same way that they think of compatibility; the two constructs are one for this policy innovation. A similar result was found in another important study done by Atkinson (2007). This instrument did not produce a statistically significant measure for traialability. The 3 domains (relative advantage/compatibility, complexity, and observability) with 14 valid items presented acceptable Cronbach's alphas, ranging from $r = 0.71$ to $r = 0.89$.

Table 2. Pankratz, Hallfors, and Cho's (2002) instrument to measure the perceived attributes of a federal health promotion policy.

1. Using the PE is compatible with the substance use coordination activities in my school district. (Relative Advantage / <u>Compatibility</u>)

2. I think that using the PE fits well with the way I like to work. (Relative Advantage / <u>Compatibility</u>)

3. I believe that using the PE would require my school district to make substantial changes to our present substance use prevention program. (Complexity)

4. It will be difficult to train teachers and staff to implement the PE. (Complexity)

5. Overall, I believe that it will be complicated to implement the PE. (Complexity)

6. Parents will not be able to see any changes in student behavior if the PE are implemented. (Observability)

7. Teachers will like the changes if the PE are implemented. (Observability)

8. Using the PE will enhance my effectiveness on the job. (<u>Relative Advantage</u> / Compatibility)

9. Using the PE will increase my ability to get non-SDFS substance use prevention funds for my school district. (<u>Relative Advantage</u> / Compatibility)

10. Using the PE will increase the quality of substance use prevention programs in my district. (<u>Relative Advantage</u> / Compatibility)

11. Using the PE will have no effect on student substance use rates. (<u>Relative Advantage</u> / Compatibility)

12. The PE require more work than can be done with current SDFS funding. (Complexity)

13. Even if SDFS did not encourage the use of these Principles, I would like to implement them in my school district. (<u>Relative Advantage</u> / Compatibility)

14. Overall, I find using the PE to be advantageous for my school district. (<u>Relative Advantage</u> / Compatibility)

(* Items 3, 4, 5, 6, 11, & 12 need to be reverse coded in analysis.)

Atkinson's (2007) study was conducted with the purpose of designing a questionnaire to assess perceived attributes of eHealth innovations. This study used *HealthQuest*, a multimedia CD-ROM-based computer application designed for personal health classes at universities, for this test. Using both confirmatory factor analysis and exploratory factor analysis, Atkinson found that factors were loaded by each perceived attribute. However, as mentioned above for the explanation of Pankratz, Hallfors, and Cho's (2002) scale, the attribute of compatibility only achieved a low factor score (Table 4 in Atkinson, 2007, p. 618). The Cronbach's alphas for the 4 scales in the 4 factors presenting relative advantage, complexity, trialability, and observability were acceptable, ranging from $r = 0.75$ to $r = 0.91$. The final valid questions that were identified through this study appear in Table 3.

Table 3. Atkinson's (2007) Questionnaire Items.

(Relative Advantage)
1. *HealthQuest* is better than using workbooks or paper and pencil tests for learning about health.
2. *HealthQuest* is more interesting than other materials I have used as part of a course.
3. Using *HealthQuest* made learning about health a better experience than I would have otherwise.
(Simplicity)
I had no difficulty finding the information that I wanted.
I had no difficulty understanding how to get around in *HealthQuest*.
I had no difficulty understanding how *HealthQuest* technically worked.
I had no difficulty getting the program to work on a CD-ROM.
I had no difficulty in getting the activities to work.
(Trialability)
Being able to try out *HealthQuest* was important in my deciding whether or not to buy it.

(Observability)
Other students seemed interested in *HealthQuest* when they saw me using it.

Although some studies did not find compatibility to be its own construct, Windsor and colleagues (2013) developed an instrument that validly identified all 5 attributes. Their study aimed to diffuse a smoking cessation and reduction in pregnancy treatment (SCRIPT) to a statewide prenatal care program directors and providers in West Virginia. This study concerned organizational rather than the individual level of adoption. In addition, while other studies included factors other than the 5 perceived attributes, this study solely focused on the 5 attributes.

After checking the validity of the instrument with expert reviewers for face validity and confirmatory factor analysis, Windsor and his colleagues' initial 43 items were reduced to a 28-item instrument covering the 5 perceived attributes. Cronbach's alphas for the scales ranged from acceptable ($r = 0.71$) to excellent ($r = 0.88$). Their instrument is presented in Table 4:

Table 4. Windsor and His Colleagues' (2013) 28 Item Instrument.

(Relative Advantage)	
1.	The use of the SCRIPT program has clear advantages over other interventions for pregnant smokers.
2.	Use of the SCRIPT program will help to improve pregnancy outcomes of RFTS (West Virginia Right From The Start) clients.
3.	If I use all the steps in the SCRIPT program, my client will more likely quit smoking.
4.	Using the SCRIPT program with my clients increases my productivity.
5.	The SCRIPT program is an evidence-based method for helping pregnant women quit smoking.
6.	Successful implementation of the SCRIPT program with clients by DCCs (designated care coordinators) will improve the status of our region in the State Health Department.
7.	Overall, I think using the SCRIPT program to be advantageous for my region.
8.	Using the SCRIPT program enhances my effectiveness in counseling my clients to quit smoking.
9.	The SCRIPT program improves overall quality of RFTS home visits.

(Compatibility)

1. The steps in the SCRIPT program can be easily integrated into other practice activities during my home visits.

2. The SCRIPT program meets my need to counsel my clients to quit smoking.

3. The SCRIPT program will help DCCs reach RFTS goals and objectives.

4. The SCRIPT program is compatible with the current RFTS counseling policies.

(Complexity)

1. Implementing the SCRIPT program regularly with my client at a home visit is too complex.

2. The RFTS home visit is the optimal time and place to deliver the SCRIPT program.

3. I have difficulty talking with my clients about smoking in their house.

4. The steps listed in the RFTS Policy-Procedures Manual are too complex. They need to be simplified.

5. Patient assessment of tobacco use can be easily done in the SCRIPT program.

6. Trying to remember all the components of the SCRIPT program is hard.

(Observability)

1. My RCC is totally supportive of the SCRIPT program.

2. The effectiveness of the SCRIPT program will be hard to document.

3. I recommend the use of the SCRIPT program to other DCCs and prenatal care providers in West Virginia.

4. The DCCs in my region do not really support the routine use of the SCRIPT program.

(Trialability)

1. I am confident that I can demonstrate the SCRIPT program procedures to other DCCs.

2. DCCs need more time and practice to use the SCRIPT program with their clients.

3. I need more training to use the SCRIPT program effectively.

4. I have not had enough training to use the CO monitor.

5. RFTS in my region provides DCCs with the resources needed to adopt the SCRIPT program in regular practice.

Use of Existing Measures and Future Studies

This chapter reviewed scales that have been used in a number of research projects to measure innovation attributes. Many studies have cited and built upon Moore and Benbasat's (1991) study as foundational to develop their scale.

A recent meta-analysis of Rogers' innovation attributes concludes that from analysis of 226 published studies, averaged p-values showed relative advantage and compatibility to be statistically significant and positively related to adoption. Complexity, as expected, was negatively associated with adoption with statistical significance. The evidence supporting the attributes of trialability and observability was more varied, which is a finding consistent with Rogers' original review and many others (Kapoor, Dwivedi, & Williams, 2014).

In choosing a scale and/or developing a new scale, a researcher should carefully consider additional referents that best fit in terms of the research agenda. For example, Windsor and colleagues' study of a tobacco treatment program (SCRIPT) additionally reviewed studies dealing with scales on tobacco prevention, such as Steckler and colleagues (1992), and similar studies like Pankratz, Hallfors, and Cho's (2002) study on a federal drug prevention policy and Goldman's (1994) study on perceptions of innovations of a national health education campaign.

Specific to the five attributes identified by Rogers (2003), some studies have inverted complexity to simplicity (Atkinson, 2007) or ease of use (Moore and Benbasat, 1991). Other diffusion scholars have argued for disentangling the omnibus attribute of relative advantage into two attributes of cost and effectiveness (Dearing & Kreuter, 2010). Among the five perceived attributes, complexity is the only attribute that requires reverse coding unless one divides relative advantage into cost and effectiveness, in which case the attribute of cost also requires reverse coding. All other attributes operate as the higher the degree of an attribute, the higher the likelihood of adoption of the innovation in question. Therefore, in order to make all measurement consistent and interpretation more convenient, it is recommended for a researcher to make modifications for reverse coding.

Finally, while eHealth has been popularized and the object of much app development, only a few studies, such as Atkinson (2006) and Hellström and her colleagues (2009), have investigated the perceived attributes of an eHealth innovation. It is encouraged that future studies pay attention to the perceived attributes of eHealth innovations, which will greatly contribute to diffusion studies for public health and health care in the 21st century.

Recommended Readings

Kapoor, K. K., Dwivedi, Y. K., & Williams, M. D. (2014). Rogers' innovation adoption attributes: A systematic review and synthesis of existing research. *Information Systems Management, 31*, 74–91.

Kim, D-K., Dinu, L. F., & Wonjun, C. (2013). Online games as a component of school textbooks: a test predicting the diffusion of interactive online games designed for the textbook reformation in South Korea. *International Journal of Information & Communication Technology Education, 9*, 52–65.

Moore, G. C., & Benbasat, I. (1991). Development of an instrument to measure the perceptions of adopting an information technology innovation. *Information Systems Research, 2*, 192–222.

Windsor, R., Cleary, S., Ramiah, K., Clark, J., Abroms, L., & Davis, A. (2013). The Smoking Cessation and Reduction in Pregnancy Treatment (SCRIPT) adoption scale: Evaluating the diffusion of a tobacco treatment innovation to a statewide prenatal care program and providers. *Journal of Health Communication, 18*, 1201–1220.

References

Atkinson, N. (2007). Developing a questionnaire to measure perceived attributes of eHealth innovations. *American Journal of Health Behavior, 31*(6), 612–621.

Berwick, D. M. (2003). Disseminating innovations in health care. *Journal of the American Medical Association, 289* (15), 1969–1975.

Brownson, R., Colditz, G., & Proctor, E. (2012). *Dissemination and implementation research in health: Translating science to practice.* New York: Oxford University Press.

Dearing, J. W., & Kreuter, M. W. (2010). Designing for diffusion: How can we increase uptake of cancer communication innovations? *Patient Education & Counseling, 81*(S),100–110.

Goldman, K. (1994). Perceptions of innovations as predictors of implementation levels: The diffusion of a nationwide health education campaign. *Health Education Quarterly, 21*, 433–445.

Hellström, L., Waern, K., Montelius, E., Astrand, B., Rydberg, T., & Petersson, G. (2009). Physicians' attitudes towards ePrescribing–evaluation of a Swedish full-scale implementation. *BMC Medical Informatics and Decision-making, 9*, 37–46.

Kapoor, K. K., Dwivedi, Y. K., Williams, M. D. (2014). Rogers' innovation adoption attributes: A systematic review and synthesis of existing research. *Information Systems Management, 31*, 74–91.

Moore, G. C., & Benbasat, I. (1991). Development of an instrument to measure the perceptions of adopting an information technology innovation. *Information Systems Research, 2*, 192–222.

Pankratz, M. M., Hallfors, D. D., & Cho, H. H. (2002). Measuring perceptions of innovation adoption: The diffusion of a federal drug prevention policy. *Health Education Research, 17*, 315–326.

Rogers, E. M. (2003). *Diffusion of innovations* (5th ed.). New York: Free Press.

Steckler, A., Goodman, R., McLeroy, K., Davis, S., & Koch, G. (1992). Measuring the diffusion of innovative health promotion programs. *American Journal of Health Promotion, 6,* 214–224.

Windsor, R., Cleary, S., Ramiah, K., Clark, J., Abroms, L., & Davis, A. (2013). The Smoking Cessation and Reduction in Pregnancy Treatment (SCRIPT) adoption scale: evaluating the diffusion of a tobacco treatment innovation to a statewide prenatal care program and providers. *Journal of Health Communication, 18,* 1201–1220.

14. Perceived Message Effectiveness, Attitude Toward Messages, and Perceived Realism

Jounghwa Choi,
Hallym University
& Hyunyi Cho,
Purdue University

Message evaluation is an important aspect of formative research for health campaigns. By assessing audience reaction to prototype messages, formative research on messages allows health communication practitioners to identify effective message ideas or components and strengths and weakness of health campaign messages (Atkin & Freimuth, 2013; Hyunyi Cho & Choi, 2010). While there can be various aspects of message evaluation (i.e., production quality, attention, comprehensibility, readability, sensation value, etc.), assessing how audiences evaluate message content has an important practical implication as it is indicative of actual message effects (Dillard, Shen, & Vail, 2007; Dillard, Weber, & Vail, 2007). In this chapter, we discuss three theoretical constructs related to message evaluation: assessing audience's perception of message effectiveness, assessing audience's attitude toward messages, and perception about message realism.

Review of Conceptualization

Perceived Message Effectiveness

One of the most frequently discussed concepts of message evaluation is perceived message effectiveness (PME). Dillard et al. (2007) defined perceived message effectiveness as "an estimate of the degree to which a persuasive message will be favorably evaluated—in terms of its persuasive potential—

by recipients of that message" (p. 617). It concerns individuals' subjective evaluation of a message as a whole, thus it is differentiated from perception of argument strength or quality, which concerns evaluating specific arguments as components of a message (Dillard, Weber et al., 2007).

PME has a theoretical and practical significance because it is expected to be related to actual message effectiveness. Fishbein and colleagues (Fishbein, Hall-Jamieson, Zimmer, von Haeften, & Nabi, 2002) argued that judgment of effectiveness would be a necessary though not sufficient condition for actual effect. Consistent with this argument, Dillard and colleagues (Dillard, Shen et al., 2007; Dillard, Weber et al., 2007) found that PME is positively related to actual effects such as attitude and behavioral intention: Dillard, Weber et al.'s (2007) meta-analysis revealed a moderate correlation ($r = .41$) between perceived and actual message effectiveness; Dillard, Shen et al.'s (2007) study showed evidence for a causal relationship from perceived effectiveness to actual effectiveness (AE). Additional evidence has been provided by Bigsby, Capella, and Seitz (2013). These findings suggest that the use of PME can be an efficient approach for formative research diagnosing the actual effectiveness of a message. In addition to its practical implication for formative research, scholars also suggest that persuasive effectiveness could serve as a persuasion strategy: since PME is related to actual effectiveness, manipulating message recipients' judgment of a message could serve as a useful technique for persuasive campaigns (Dillard, Shen et al., 2007). Hyunyi Cho and Boster (2008) suggested that a component of intervention could be designed in a way to elicit interpersonal communication concerning a perceived effect so that it can affect actual outcomes of the campaign.

The term PME has been often referred to as "perceived message quality"(e.g., Hullett, 2002). For example, Hyunyi Cho and Choi (2010) defined perceived message quality as "the judgment of the effectiveness of the message in fulfilling its intended outcome in the intended audience (p. 304)." Studies that embraced these terminologies have used the measurement items such as "compelling," "plausible," and "believable" (e.g., Hullett, 2002; La France & Boster, 2001). Therefore, perceived message quality is considered to be the same concept as perceived message effectiveness that Dillard and colleagues used (Dillard, Shen et al., 2007; Dillard, Weber et al., 2007).

Studies in the research tradition of perceived message quality (e.g., Hullett, 2004; Lavine & Snyder, 1996) also provide support for the role of PME in persuasion, showing a positive relationship between the construct and attitude toward behavior. For example, Hullett (2004, study1) reports that increased perception of message strength of a health advocacy message is positively related to attitude toward getting tested for genital herpes, in turn predicting behavioral intention. Similar findings have been reported in the domain of health behavior (Hyunyi Cho & Choi, 2010) and political behavior (Lavine & Snyder, 1996).

Attitude Toward Messages

Attitude toward message(A_{msg}) can be conceptualized as the overall evaluation of a message under consideration (A. A. Mitchell & Olson, 1981). Scholars borrowed the concept of A_{msg} from the concept of attitude toward advertisement (A_{ad}) (Hyunyi Cho & Choi, 2010; Dillard & Peck, 2000, 2001). While Dillard and his colleagues developed their idea about PME from the concept of A_{ad} in advertising research, they conceived that this concept cannot be directly applied to Public Service Announcements (PSA) messages, thus reconceptualizing it as PME. In their rationale, the logic that "liking for one should lead to liking for the other" is not applicable because PSAs frequently deal with social ills (Dillard, Shen et al., 2007, p. 468). However, when PSAs deal with social ills, what is being advocated in PSAs is not the social ills themselves but the solutions for social ills. In this sense, it is intuitively reasonable to expect that liking PSAs should lead to liking the solutions to social ills presented in the PSAs, at least in certain circumstances. Slater (2006) suggested that we collectively consider A_{ad} theory for health communication research and intervention. While he acknowledged that the relationship between A_{ad} and health behavior could be tricky for negative appeal messages, this would not mean that the concept of A_{ad} is not applicable for health messages. Keeping the conceptual definition of A_{ad} in advertising research, Hyunyi Cho and Choi (2010) directly adopted the concept of A_{ad} and applied it to PSA messages.

According to Hyunyi Cho and Choi (2010), A_{msg} represents a subjective evaluation of messages that is drawn from internal cues, whereas PME or perceived message quality is more objective as it is drawn more from external cues. Put differently, while PME is deemed a measure of cognition-based evaluation, attitude toward message is considered to be a measure of affect-based message evaluation (Hyunyi Cho & Choi, 2010). This conceptualization of A_{msg} corresponds to the unidimensional view of A_{ad}, which considers A_{ad} as purely affective in nature (e.g., Lutz, 1985). Further, Hyunyi Cho and Choi's (2010) conceptual distinction between PME and A_{msg} is consistent with the long tradition of advertising research that differentiates affective and cognitive evaluations of advertisements. Following Shimp's (1981) proposition, a number of advertising researchers have argued for multidimensionality of A_{ad} in terms of cognitive and affective dimensions. In the studies adopting this view (Burton & Lichtenstein, 1988; Hyongoh Cho & Stout, 1993; Olney, Holbrook, & Batra, 1991), the affective dimension was measured with items such as pleasant/unpleasant, attractive/unattractive, and enjoyable/not enjoyable. On the other hand, the cognitive dimension was measured with items such as informative/uninformative, persuasive/nonpersuasive, convincing/unconvincing, and ineffective/effective, which are similar to PME measures (e.g., convincing, compelling, effective, etc. in Dillard, Shen et al. 2007). This supports the rationale to differentiate affect-based message evaluation (i.e., A_{msg}) from cognition-based message evaluation (i.e., PME). As the cognitive dimension of message evaluation is likely to be captured by PME, in this chapter we conceptualize A_{msg} in terms of affective evaluation.

Predictive Utility of Perceived Message Effectiveness and Attitude toward Messages

It is important to distinguish A_{msg} from PME because they are likely related to differential message and behavioral variables. Hyunyi Cho and Choi (2010) showed that PME and A_{msg} are differentially related to message characteristics and outcome variables. First, A_{msg} was predicted by positive affect while PME was predicted by the elicited affect that the message intended, either positive or negative. That is, the valence of the message affect did not differentially influence PME while A_{msg} depended on the magnitude of positive affect elicited by the message. Furthermore, their study showed that actual effectiveness (i.e., attitude toward behavior) was more likely predicted by A_{msg} rather than PME for positively valenced messages; whereas for negatively valenced messages, actual effectiveness was more influenced by PME rather than A_{msg}, although this relationship was attenuated after employing control variables. These findings suggest that the utility of A_{msg} may be limited to evaluating positive messages, whereas PME can be used for both positive and negative messages.

Perceived Realism

Perceived realism is defined as subjective judgment of the extent to which the narrative world is reflective of the real world (Gerbner & Gross, 1976). This is an important aspect of narrative persuasion, which attempts to influence people's beliefs, attitudes, and behaviors through stories such as entertainment education media contents (Hyunyi Cho, Shen, & Wilson, 2014).

Perceived realism is found out to be an important factor determining PME and A_{msg}. Specifically, extant theoretical literature suggests perceived realism produce positive message effects by influencing emotional involvement with messages (Busselle & Bilandzic, 2008; Green, 2004; Larkey & Hecht, 2010), identification with characteristics/context in messages (Larkey & Hecht, 2010; Potter, 1986) and perceived effectiveness of messages (Hyunyi

Cho & Boster, 2008; Fishbein et al., 2002). As PME and A$_{msg}$ are predictors of the actual effectiveness of messages and PME can serve as a strategy to increase persuasive power of messages, understanding the role of perceived realism in message evaluation is important.

Perceived realism has been often treated as unidimensional (e.g., Fishbein et al., 2002) while at the same time it has been deemed to be a multidimensional construct (Busselle & Greenberg, 2000; Hall, 2003; Pouliot & Cowen, 2007). Recently, an attempt to empirically explore and test the structure of the construct has been done by Hyunyi Cho et al. (2014), based on Hall's (2003) synthesis of previous conceptualizations. A five dimensional model of perceived realism that includes plausibility, typicality, factuality, narrative consistency, and perceptual quality was proposed. Three of the dimensions address the likelihood of occurrence of the story in reality (Hyunyi Cho et al., 2014). Specifically, plausibility was conceptualized as the degree to which events or behaviors portrayed in narratives are perceived to possibly occur in the real world. Typicality is the degree to which events or characteristics in narratives are perceived to be common in real life. Factuality refers to the degree to which representations of events or behaviors in narratives agree with the specifics in the real world that the narratives are supposed to portray. The other two dimensions concern the quality of the story itself (Hyunyi Cho et al., 2014). While narrative consistency concerns perceptions of internal and structural consistency of a story and its elements, perceptual quality is related to perception of the quality of manufactured elements of a media narrative. Hyunyi Cho et al.'s (2014) empirical test supported the model and showed that these five dimensions are differentially related to mediators and outcomes of narrative persuasion (Hyunyi Cho et al., 2014).

Measuring the Effectiveness of Health Messages

Perceived Message Effectiveness

There has been no formal systematic research on scale development for PME, probably because the construct is viewed as possessing an intuitive meaning on its own terms (Dillard, Shen et al., 2007). There is no definite set of measurement items and the items used differ by study. For example, Dillard and Peck (2000, 2001) used two 7-point semantic differential scales (i.e., not at all/very persuasive, not at all/very convincing; α = .95). Mitchell (2000) used one item (not persuasive—very persuasive) as a mean for an induction check for her experiment. Among studies that used multiple items, a few studies (e.g., Hullett, 2002; M. Mitchell, Brown, Morris-Villagran, & Villagran, 2001) reported conducting a confirmatory factor analysis (CFA) to test validity and reliability along with other variables. M. Mitchell et al.'s (2001) CFA results reported unidimensionality of eight items used (α = .94) and a part of the items available included "the message was compelling" and "the message was dumb." In the case of Hullett (2002), three out of seven items were retained (α = .78) as a result of confirmatory factor analysis but the information regarding the items used in the analysis is not available. Examples of measurement items from previous studies are presented in Table 1.

Table 1. Examples of measurement items for perceived message effectiveness.

Dillard, Shen et al. (2007)* (α = .78~.96)	Fishbein et al. (2002)** (α = .78~.92)	Cesario et al. (2004)* (α = .83~.93)
believable/not believable compelling/not compelling convincing/not convincing effective/ineffective forgettable/memorable important/unimportant misleading/straightforward not at all/very persuasive right/wrong sensible/not sensible wise/foolish	Was the message convincing? Would it be helpful for (target audience) in (performing a behavior)? Would (target audience) be more or less likely to (perform a behavior) after seeing the ad? How confident did the ad make you feel about (doing a behavior)?	coherent compelling convincing effective influential persuasive

* Multiple studies described used different set of items respectively.
** Questionnaires are presented with revision so that they can be usable in other contexts.

As an aspect of measurement, Dillard, Weber et al. (2007) suspected that the relationship between perceived and actual effect may depend on the style of measurement of PME. They differentiated impact measurement (e.g., Hullett, 2004) from attribute measurement (e.g., Cesario, Grant, & Higgins, 2004) in terms of style. In the impact measurement style, PME is measured in terms of a message's likely outcome (e.g., persuasive, effective, convincing, etc.), while in the attribute measurement style, it is measured in terms of specific message features (e.g, "how reasonable were the views expressed by the author" (Reid, Gunter, & Smith, 2005, p. 199). Many of the studies were classified by Dillard, Weber et al. as using an amalgam of impact and attribute measures (e.g., Lavine et al., 1999; M. M. Mitchell, 2000). Their meta-analysis results suggest that an impact-attribute combination measure may have greater effect compared to the impact-only measure. The effect of measurement style was detected in the regression analysis while it was not in the correlational analysis: That is, stronger correlations between PME and actual effectiveness were detected for the combination measure. With caution, this finding could be interpreted to suggest that such an impact-attribute combination measure may serve as a more sensitive assessment because it was more strongly related to actual effectiveness, taking into consideration other research artifacts such as novelty of topics or focus of the advocacy.

Attitude Toward Messages

Similar to perceived message effectiveness, there is no definite set of measurement items for attitude toward messages. In advertising research, A_{ad} is usually measured with a set of semantic differential scales utilizing pairs of bipolar adjectives. In general, frequently used items include good/bad, favorable/unfavorable, pleasant/unpleasant, positive/negative, etc. For example, MacKenzie and Lutz (1989) used three items of good/bad, pleasant/unpleasant, and favorable/unfavorable (α = .88~89), which were also used in Lord et al. (1995). In Hyunyi Cho and Choi (2010), to assess A_{msg} of PSA advertisements, two pairs of bipolar adjectives were used: good/bad and positive/negative (r = .65, p <.001). Mitchell and Olson (1981) used the four items (good/bad, dislike/like, not irritating/irritating, uninteresting/interesting; α = .87) out of seven items as a result of exploratory factor analysis. Advertising research on A_{ad} has often employed items that may capture both affective and cognitive dimensions without differentiating the factor structure. For example, Henthorne et al. (1993) used the items such as "good" and "interesting" along with "informative," "appropriate," "easy to understand," "objective" (α = .77). However, as we discussed above, affective and cognitive dimensions can be conceptually differentiated and may play different roles in communication. Therefore we recommend future research use measures with a focus on the affective dimension to measure A_{msg}. Examples of A_{msg} measures (often referred to as attitude toward advertisement in studies), which we think meet this criterion and are used in the context of risk and health communication, are provided in Table 2.

Table 2. Examples of measurement items for attitude toward message.

Hyunyi Cho & Choi (2010) ($\alpha = .95$)	Slater et al. (2002)* ($\alpha = .87 \sim .90$)
Good/bad Positive/negative	Enjoyable Likeable Not irritating

Perceived Realism

With a unidimensional approach, Fishbein et al. (2002) employed four 4-point Likert scale items, which ask if a message is (1) believable, (2) honest, (3) if a real person would act like the person in the message, and (4) if the situation is likely to happen in real life ($\alpha = .86$). This measure has been used in several other studies such as Hyunyi Cho and Boster (2008, $\alpha = .92$).

As aforementioned, the five factor multidimensional model, proposed and tested by Hyunyi Cho et al. (2014), received empirical support. Hyunyi Cho et al.'s (2014) confirmatory factor analysis of the data provided evidences in favor of the first-order five-factor model over the first-order single factor model and the second-order single factor model. Reliability of the items for each factor ranged from .82 to .90 (see Table 3). More importantly, these factors were differentially related to indicators of persuasion process variables including emotional involvement, identification, and message evaluation. Specifically, plausibility was related only to emotional involvement and typicality was related only to identification. Narrative consistency and perceptual quality were directly related to message evaluation (i.e., perceived message effectiveness) whereas other realism dimensions indirectly influence message evaluation through plausibility or identification. Because differential dimensions of perceived realism prime different routes to persuasion, future formative evaluation of messages and persuasive communication efforts would benefit from distinguishing and utilizing differential realism dimensions to enhance message effectiveness.

Table 3. Items for the Perceived Realism Scale by Hyunyi Cho et al. (2014).

Items	Reported Reliability
Plausibility 1. The ad showed something that could possibly happen in real life. 2. The event in the ad portrayed possible real-life situations. 3. The story in the ad could actually happen in real life. 4. Never in real life would what was shown in the ad happen. 5. Real people would not do the things shown in the ad.	$\alpha = .90$
Typicality 1. Not many people are likely to experience the event portrayed in the ad. 2. The ad portrayed an event that happens to a lot of people. 3. What happened to the people in the ad is what happens to people in the real world.	$\alpha = .84$
Factuality 1. The ad was based on facts. 2. The ad showed something that had really happened. 3. What was shown in the ad had actually happened.	$\alpha = .89$
Narrative Consistency 1. The ad showed a coherent story. 2. The story portrayed in the ad was consistent. 3. Parts of the ad were contradicting each other. 4. The story portrayed in the ad made sense. 5. The event in the ad had a logical flow.	$\alpha = .82$
Perceptual Quality 1 The visual elements of the ad were realistic. 2. The audio elements of the ad were realistic. 3. The acting in the ad was realistic. 4. The scenes in the ad were realistic. 5. I felt that the overall production elements of the ad were realistic.	$\alpha = .90$

Use of Existing Measures and Future Studies

Understanding how audiences may evaluate health messages has an important implication because it can help health campaign planners to assess whether conceptual and executional aspects of the message strategy will be effective.
The three constructs reviewed in this chapter have communality in that they
concern evaluation of messages. That can be utilized as a tool for formative

evaluation. As discussed above, each construct may tap into different aspects of messages thus researchers and practitioners should think about which construct would be better to evaluate messages under consideration. On the basis of extant research we offer the following recommendations.

First, measuring PME rather than A_{msg} might be more useful for formative research if the messages being tested are likely to elicit negative emotions (e.g., fear appeal message or loss-framed message), because actual effect (e.g., attitude toward behavior) is more likely to be related to PME than A_{msg} for this type of message (Hyunyi Cho & Choi, 2010). Additionally, measuring PME, researchers or practitioners may want to specify referents as related to their own specific research. Using no specific frame of referents in measuring PME was an issue raised by Dillard, Weber et al. (2007). An approach to remedy this limitation would be considering the findings from third person effect studies. For example, given that people tend to have a first-person perception for prosocial messages (Hyunyi Cho & Boster, 2008), health practitioners may want to use third-person referents to measure PME in order to conduct more strict formative research. If the messages are targeting those who already engage in risky behaviors and pretesting is taking place among this population, measuring PME with the in-group referents (e.g., self or friends) rather than out-group referents could be a more conservative assessment because of the underestimation of message effects on in-group members (Hyunyi Cho & Boster, 2008).

Second, A_{msg} might be a better tool than PME if the messages being tested elicit positive emotions (e.g., gain-framed message or positive emotion appeal messages), as A_{msg} rather than PME was more predictive to actual message effect for this type of messages (Hyunyi Cho & Choi, 2010). Also, it is advised to employ measurement items that tap the affective dimension solely in order to disentangle its effect from PME effects.

Finally, perceived realism would be a useful tool to evaluate health messages with narratives. In particular, when formative research is done with a diagnostic purpose, using perceived realism over PME, especially with a multidimentional measure, is recommended because it will allow researchers to examine which aspects of narratives should be improved.

Health message evaluation could be considered in various aspects and not limited to the constructs reviewed in this chapter. Depending on the nature of the message under evaluation and the purpose of evaluation, researchers may want to consider additional theoretical constructs such as perceived message cognition value (Lane, Harrington, Donohew, & Zimmerman, 2006) or perceived message sensation value (Palmgreen, Stephenson, Everett, Baseheart,

& Francies, 2002), or attitudes toward message recommendation (Shen, 2014).

As aforementioned, Dillard et al. (2007) raised an issue regarding the frame of reference for PME. As most studies that employed PME did not specify a referent, little is known about the frame of reference people use when they make PME judgments and how that affects their judgment (Dillard, Weber et al., 2007). More research is needed to examine how referent manipulation of PME measures affects individuals' responses and the relationships of PME with its predictors and outcomes. Additionally, further investigation is necessary to verify the different roles of PME and A_{msg} in persuasion by including both measures. Beyond Hyunyi Cho and Choi's (2010) exploration of gain- and loss-framing messages, for example, researchers could investigate it in the context of emotional appeals. As for perceived realism, more empirical tests for Hyunyi Cho et al.'s (2014) five dimensional model of perceived realism are suggested. Additional validation of the scale among different populations in different research contexts would be beneficial, too.

Recommended Readings

Cho, H. (Ed.). (2011). *Health communication message design: Theory and practice.* Thousand Oaks, CA: Sage.

Cho, H., & Choi, J. (2010). Predictors and the role of attitude toward the message and perceived message quality in gain- and loss-frame antidrug persuasion of adolescents. *Health Communication, 25*(4), 303–311. doi: 10.1080/10410231003773326.

Cho, H., & Friley, L. (2014). Narrative communication of risk: Toward balancing accuracy and acceptance. In H. Cho, T. O. Reimer, & K. A. McComas (Eds.), *The SAGE handbook of risk communication* (pp. 180–192). Thousand Oaks, CA: Sage.

Cho, H., Shen, L., & Wilson, K. (2014). Perceived realism: Dimensions and roles in narrative persuasion. *Communication Research, 41*(6), 828–851. doi: 10.1177/0093650212450585.

Dillard, J. P., Weber, K. M., & Vail, R. G. (2007). The relationship between the perceived and actual effectiveness of persuasive messages: A meta-analysis with implications for formative campaign research. *Journal of Communication, 57*(4), 613–631. doi: 10.1111/j.1460-2466.2007.00360.x.

References

Atkin, C. K., & Freimuth, V. (2013). Guidelines for formative evaluation research in campaign design. In R. E. Rice & C. K. Atkin (Eds.), *Public communication campaigns* (4th ed., pp. 53–68). Thousand Oaks, CA: SAGE Publications, Inc.

Bigsby, E., Cappella, J. N., & Seitz, H. H. (2013). Efficiently and effectively evaluating public service announcements: Additional evidence for the utility of perceived effectiveness. *Communication Monographs, 80*(1), 1–23. doi: 10.1080/03637751. 2012.739706.

Burton, S., & Lichtenstein, D. R. (1988). The effect of ad claims and ad context on attitude toward the advertisement. *Journal of Advertising, 17*(1), 3–11. doi: 10.2307/4188659.

Busselle, R. W., & Bilandzic, H. (2008). Fictionality and perceived realism in experiencing stories: A model of narrative comprehension and engagement. *Communication Theory, 18*(2), 255–280.

Busselle, R. W., & Greenberg, B. S. (2000). The nature of television realism judgments: A reevaluation of their conceptualization and measurement. *Mass Communication & Society, 3*(2–3), 249–268.

Cesario, J., Grant, H., & Higgins, E. T. (2004). Regulatory fit and persuasion: Transfer from "feeling right." *Journal of Personality and Social Psychology, 86*(3), 388.

Cho, H., & Boster, F. J. (2008). First and third person perceptions on anti-drug ads among adolescents. *Communication Research, 35*(2), 169–189. doi: 10.1177/0093650207313158.

Cho, H., & Choi, J. (2010). Predictors and the role of attitude toward the message and perceived message quality in gain- and loss-frame antidrug persuasion of adolescents. *Health Communication, 25*(4), 303–311. doi: 10.1080/10410231003773326.

Cho, H., Shen, L., & Wilson, K. (2014). Perceived realism: Dimensions and roles in narrative persuasion. *Communication Research, 41*(6), 828–851 doi: 10.1177/0093650212450585.

Cho, H., & Stout, P. A. (1993). An extended perspective on the role of emotion in advertising processing. *Advances in Consumer Research, 20*(1), 692–697.

Dillard, J. P., & Peck, E. (2000). Affect and persuasion emotional responses to public service announcements. *Communication Research, 27*(4), 461–495.

Dillard, J. P., & Peck, E. (2001). Persuasion and the structure of affect. *Human Communication Research, 27*(1), 38–68. doi: 10.1111/j.1468-2958.2001.tb00775.x.

Dillard, J. P., Shen, L., & Vail, R. G. (2007). Does perceived message effectiveness cause persuasion or vice versa? 17 consistent answers. *Human Communication Research, 33*(4), 467–488. doi: 10.1111/j.1468-2958.2007.00308.x.

Dillard, J. P., Weber, K. M., & Vail, R. G. (2007). The relationship between the perceived and actual effectiveness of persuasive messages: A meta-analysis with implications for formative campaign research. *Journal of Communication, 57*(4), 613–631. doi: 10.1111/j.1460-2466.2007.00360.x.

Fishbein, M., Hall-Jamieson, K., Zimmer, E., von Haeften, I., & Nabi, R. (2002). Avoiding the boomerang: Testing the relative effectiveness of antidrug public service announcements before a national campaign. *American Journal of Public Health, 92*(2), 238–245. doi: 10.2105/AJPH.92.2.238.

Gerbner, G., & Gross, L. (1976). Living with television: The violence profile. *Journal of Communication, 26*(2), 172–194.

Green, M. C. (2004). Transportation into narrative worlds: The role of prior knowledge and perceived realism. *Discourse Processes, 38*(2), 247–266.

Hall, A. (2003). Reading realism: Audiences' evaluations of the reality of media texts. *Journal of Communication, 53*(4), 624–641.

Henthorne, T. L., LaTour, M. S., & Nataraajan, R. (1993). Fear appeals in print advertising: an analysis of arousal and ad response. *Journal of Advertising, 22*(2), 59–69.

Hullett, C. R. (2002). Charting the process underlying the change of value-expressive attitudes: The importance of value-relevance in predicting the matching effect. *Communication Monographs, 69*(2), 158–178. doi: 10.1080/714041711.

Hullett, C. R. (2004). Using functional theory to promote sexually transmitted disease (std) testing: The impact of value-expressive messages and guilt. *Communication Research, 31*(4), 363–396. doi: 10.1177/0093650204266103.

La France, B. H., & Roster, F. J. (2001). To match or mismatch? That is only one important question. *Communication Monographs, 68*(3), 211–234.

Lane, D. R., Harrington, N. G., Donohew, L., & Zimmerman, R. S. (2006). Dimensions and validation of a perceived message cognition value scale. *Communication Research Reports, 23*(3), 149–161. doi: 10.1080/08824090600796369.

Larkey, L. K., & Hecht, M. (2010). A model of effects of narrative as culture-centric health promotion. *Journal of health communication, 15*(2), 114–135.

Lavine, H., Burgess, D., Snyder, M., Transue, J., Sullivan, J. L., & Haney, B. (1999). Threat, authoritarianism, and voting: An investigation of personality and persuasion. *Personality and Social Psychology Bulletin, 25*(3), 337–347.

Lavine, H., & Snyder, M. (1996). Cognitive processing and the functional matching effect in persuasion: The mediating role of subjective perceptions of message quality. *Journal of Experimental Social Psychology, 32*(6), 580–604. http://dx.doi.org/10.1006/jesp.1996.0026

Lord, K. R., Lee, M.-S., & Sauer, P. L. (1995). The combined influence hypothesis: Central and peripheral antecedents of attitude toward the ad. *Journal of Advertising, 24*(1), 73–85.

Lutz, R. J. (1985). Affective and cognitive antecedents of attitude toward the ad: a conceptual framework. In L. F. Alwitt & A. A. Mitchell (Eds.), *Psychological processes and advertising effects: Theory, research and application* (pp. 45–63). Hillsdale, NJ: Lawrence Erlbaum Associates, Publishers.

MacKenzie, S. B., & Lutz, R. J. (1989). An empirical examination of the structural antecedents of attitude toward the ad in an advertising pretesting context. *Journal of Marketing, 53*(2), 48–65.

Mitchell, A. A., & Olson, J. C. (1981). Are product attribute beliefs the only mediator of advertising effects on brand attitude? *Journal of Marketing Research, 18*(3), 318–332. doi: 10.2307/3150973.

Mitchell, M., Brown, K., Morris-Villagran, M., & Villagran, P. (2001). The effects of anger, sadness and happiness on persuasive message processing: A test of the negative state relief model. *Communication Monographs, 68*(4), 347–359.

Mitchell, M. M. (2000). Able but not motivated? The relative effects of happy and sad mood on persuasive message processing. *Communications Monographs, 67*(2), 215–226.

Olney, T. J., Holbrook, M. B., & Batra, R. (1991). Consumer responses to advertising: The effects of ad content, emotions, and attitude toward the ad on viewing time. *Journal of Consumer Research, 17*(4), 440–453. doi: 10.2307/2626838.

Palmgreen, P., Stephenson, M. T., Everett, M. W., Baseheart, J. R., & Francies, R. (2002). Perceived message sensation value (PMSV) and the dimensions and validation of a PMSV scale. *Health Communication, 14*(4), 403–428. doi: 10.1207/S15327027HC1404_1.

Potter, W. J. (1986). Perceived reality and the cultivation hypothesis. *Journal of Broadcasting & Electronic Media, 30*(2), 159–174. doi: 10.1080/08838158609386617.

Pouliot, L., & Cowen, P. S. (2007). Does perceived realism really matter in media effects? *Media Psychology, 9*(2), 241–259.

Reid, S. A., Gunter, H. N., & Smith, J. R. (2005). Aboriginal self-determination in Australia. *Human Communication Research, 31*(2), 189–211.

Shen, L. (2014). Antecedents to psychological reactance: The impact of threat, message frame, and choice. *Health Communication*(ahead-of-print), 1–11.

Shimp, T. A. (1981). Attitude toward the ad as a mediator of consumer brand choice. *Journal of Advertising, 10*(2), 9–48.

Slater, M., Karan, D., Rouner, D., & Walters, D. (2002). Effects of threatening visuals and announcer differences on responses to televised alcohol warnings. *Journal of Applied Communication Research, 30*(1), 27–49.

Slater, M. D. (2006). Specification and misspecification of theoretical foundations and logic models for health communication campaigns. *Health Communication, 20*(2), 149–157.

15. Perceived Norms and Health Behavior

NICK CARCIOPPOLO,
University of Miami

Social norms represent behavior that is accepted and expected in a given situation based on shared cultural or systematic values (Myers, 2012; Rokeach, 1973). The motivation to comply with perceived norms can influence an immensity of health related intentions, decisions, and behavior. In many respects, we are all behaviorally adrift on a sea of normative influence. Consider this example, which makes the preceding sentence appear more apt than exaggeration. In the summer of 2014, people began challenging friends, family, co-workers, and celebrities to do one of two things: donate one-hundred dollars for amyotrophic lateral sclerosis (ALS) research, or pour a bucket of ice water over their head while on camera, known as the "ice bucket challenge." This campaign resulted in $115 million in donations over two months, compared to the $19 million ALS received during the entire previous year (ALS, 2014; Steel, 2014). While this challenge proved to be a successful fundraising strategy, a curious phenomenon arose: rather than choosing either to donate or dump a bucket of ice water over one's head, many participants chose to do *both*. Although some dismissed this behavior as an attention-seeking form of vanity, it may be more appropriately described through the lens of normative influence. When friends, family, and celebrities are witnessed enacting a socially desirable behavior, such as raising money and awareness for charity, it can motivate others to enact the behavior as well to tangibly associate themselves with the desirable target. As writing a check for ALS research was not a highly visible action, one way to demonstrate participation was to pour a bucket of ice water over one's head, post proof of this action to social media, and then write the check. The ALS campaign outcome demonstrates the extent to which normative perceptions can guide our behavior, often without explicit awareness. The current chapter will conceptually and operationally define different types of social norms, describe theoretical frameworks that include normative components, and suggest future possibilities for measurement of normative constructs.

Types of Social Norms

Descriptive norms are conceptually defined as our perceptions of others' behavior in a given situation (Borsari & Carey, 2003). This perception can often influence our own behavioral choices to be more consistent with the perceived norm. If one believes that others are enacting a particular behavior, such as drinking alcohol at a social gathering, he or she may be more likely to drink as well to conform to the perceived norms of that situation. Health behavior researchers have observed that college students consistently overestimate their peers' drinking behavior relative to their own (Borsari & Carey, 2003). If the perceived drinking norm is greater than the actual drinking norm, one may feel social pressure to drink more to conform to the perceived norm. One meta-analysis found that after accounting for predictors included in the theory of planned behavior, descriptive norms account for about five percent of the variance in behavioral intentions (Rivis & Sheeran, 2003)

Subjective norms refer to the perception of what others think you should do in a given situation (Ajzen, 1991). In the case of drinking behavior, subjective norms are perceptions of whether important others would consider drinking appropriate in that social setting. An important distinction is that the same individual can hold competing perceptions of the subjective norm. For instance, one may perceive that other party guests think that one should drink alcohol, and also believe that a police officer or concerned parent may disapprove. In these instances, behavior will be most influenced by the salience of a particular normative perception (Ajzen & Fishbein, 1980). A meta-analysis found that on average, perceptions of subjective norms account for about twelve percent of the variance in behavioral intentions, but caution that the use of single-item indicators of subjective norms in many studies may suppress the effect (Armitage & Conner, 2001).

Injunctive norms refer to perceived social approval of a behavior in a particular situation (Cialdini, Reno, & Kallgren, 1990). This definition appears conceptually similar to subjective norms. Indeed, some researchers do not make conceptual or operational distinctions between subjective and injunctive norms (Boer & Westhoff, 2006; Fishbein, 2008; Lapinski & Rimal, 2005), however research using confirmatory factor analysis suggests that they may be best modeled as separate constructs (Park & Smith, 2007). As with subjective norms, people can hold competing injunctive normative perceptions, and will likely be most influenced by whichever perception is most salient given the situation.

Theoretical Frameworks

Much health communication research focuses on highlighting the disconnect between perceived and actual norms in an effort to reduce problematic health behaviors, called social norms marketing (SNM) research (for examples, see DeJong et al., 2003; Wechsler et al., 2003). SNM campaigns take a harm-reduction approach to reduce problematic drinking behavior by highlighting the difference between one's perceived norm in a given situation and the actual norm (DeJong et al., 2003). Generally, this is done by conducting formative research among the target population to identify the actual behavioral norm. In the context of drinking behavior, this may involve a representative survey of a college student body to determine the average number of drinks students consume when they go to a party. Next, the actual drinking norm is presented in intervention materials to heavy drinkers (perhaps Greek members) to highlight the difference between one's own drinking behavior and the actual norm on campus. The goal of these interventions is to encourage problematic drinkers to reduce their drinking behavior to be more reflective of the actual drinking norms on campus. Although a meta-analysis found that students tend to overestimate actual descriptive and injunctive university drinking norms (Borsari and Carey, 2003), researchers are nevertheless divided concerning the overall effectiveness of these interventions (see Campo, Cameron, Brossard, & Frazer, 2004; Campo & Cameron, 2006). As some suggest, SNM campaigns work well to align perceptions of norms with actual norms, but may not adequately affect behavior (Borsari & Carey, 2003). Social distance from the normative reference group can function to moderate the relationship between normative beliefs and outcomes. As an example, it may be a point of pride among some fraternity members to highlight how much more they drink than the average student on campus. Thus instead of attenuating risky drinking behavior, presenting normative drinking information to certain high-risk groups may function to validate or commemorate their own drinking behavior. Considering this, some studies suggest developing interventions that target and challenge small-group norms, such as a fraternity as opposed to a university, can be successful (Far & Miller, 2003) and that normative appeals should focus on small-group normative perceptions to better address heavy-drinking behavior (Borsari & Carey, 2003; Cho, 2006). Others suggest that the inconsistencies witnessed in previous research stem from failure to identify and account for other potential moderators of the norm-behavior relationship (Lapinski &

Rimal, 2005), which subsequent research using the theory of normative social behavior (TNSB, Rimal & Real, 2005) seeks to address.

The TNSB assesses the extent to which various normative mechanisms serve as mediators and moderators of the relationship between descriptive drinking norms and drinking behavior (Rimal & Real, 2005, Rimal, 2008). In particular, the theory suggests that the relationship between descriptive drinking norms and drinking behavior may be both mediated and moderated by injunctive normative perceptions and outcome expectations, and moderated by beliefs about group identity (Rimal & Real, 2005; Rimal, 2008). Outcome expectations measured in the model include perceived benefits to oneself, perceived benefits to others, and anticipatory socialization—the tendency to view alcohol as a social lubricant. Group identity assesses the extent to which perceived similarity to others on campus and aspiration to be like others on campus moderate the relationship between perceived descriptive norms and drinking intentions and behavior. Although this framework was developed specifically for the context of college student drinking it should be applied and amended for use with other health behaviors that have strong normative components.

Perhaps the most widely used theories that address normative motivations are the family of theories developed by Fishbein and Ajzen, including the theory of reasoned action (TRA; Fishbein & Ajzen, 1975), theory of planned behavior (TPB; Ajzen, 1991), and the integrative model (Fishbein, 2008). The TRA/TPB both include subjective norms and motivation to comply with those norms as predictors of intentions and behavior. The integrative model updates the TRA/TPB framework and assesses only descriptive and injunctive norms as well as motivation to comply with those norms as predictors of intentions and behavior (Fishbein, 2008; Yzer, 2012). Motivation to comply is a crucial component of normative perceptions. If a person does not feel compelled to comply with a given norm, it is less likely to influence his or her decision. The TRA/TPB and integrative model explicitly operationalize an interaction between normative perceptions and motivations to comply, however it is not uncommon to see research that only measures normative perceptions without considering motivation to comply.

Measuring Social Norms

Below are three scales developed by Park and colleagues (2009) to measure descriptive, subjective, and injunctive university drinking norms. All items are assessed on 5-point Likert scales. Along with the scales listed below, the authors also measured U.S. descriptive and U.S. injunctive norms, conducting a confirmatory factor analysis to assess scale validity. The analysis supported a five-factor solution, suggesting national and university drinking norms as distinct factors, that may be differentially related to health behaviors, and potentially moderate the association between other psychosocial predictors and subsequent outcomes.

Table 1. Descriptive, Subjective, and Injunctive Drinking Norms Measures.

Descriptive Drinking Norms

1. Most [university] students limit their alcohol consumption to zero to four drinks when they party.

2. Most [university] students do not go over four drinks in one occasion when they party.

3. Most [university] students have zero to four drinks when they party.

Subjective Drinking Norms

1. Most people who are important to me think that I should limit my alcohol consumption to zero to four drinks the next time that I party.

2. Most people whose opinion I value believe that I should limit my alcohol consumption to zero to four drinks the next time that I party.

3. Most people who matter a lot to me expect me to limit my alcohol consumption to zero to four drinks the next time that I party.

Injunctive Drinking Norms

1. Most [university] students would approve of my limiting my alcohol consumption to zero to four drinks when I party.

2. Most [university] students would endorse my limiting my alcohol consumption to zero to four drinks when I party.

3. Most [university] students would support my limiting my alcohol consumption to zero to four drinks when I party.

Note: Measures from Park, Klein, Smith, & Martell, 2009.

The following measures (Table 2) are taken from a study on handwashing in a child care center. Lapinski and colleagues (2013) used the TNSB to determine how normative perceptions can influence handwashing behavior among people who work with children. All items were measured on a 5-point Likert scale from strongly disagree to strongly agree and scales were subjected to confirmatory factor analysis to verify factor structure. In this study, injunctive norms were significantly related to handwashing behavior, as was the interaction between descriptive and injunctive norms. Motivation to comply was not significantly associated with handwashing behavior, nor was the interaction between motivation to comply and descriptive norms. The authors suggest that this may be due to the fact that employees were more motivated by children's perceptions of them rather than their peers, whereas the study was focused on the normative influence of other workers.

Table 2. Descriptive and Injunctive Handwashing Norms and Motivation to Comply.

Injunctive Norms

1. Thorough handwashing is something that most coworkers in my classroom think you should do.
2. The coworkers who usually work in my classroom endorse thorough handwashing.
3. Coworkers in my classroom may judge me based on whether or not I wash my hands thoroughly.
4. I feel like coworkers in my classroom would think less of me if I didn't wash my hands thoroughly.

Descriptive Norms

1. Most coworkers in my classroom wash their hands thoroughly.
2. Most of the coworkers in my classroom engage in thorough handwashing.
3. Most of the coworkers in my classroom wash their hands as thoroughly as they are supposed to.
4. The majority of the people in my classroom wash their hands thoroughly.

Motivation to Comply

1. (coworkers) It is important for me to do what my coworkers at my Center think I should do.
2. (parents) What parents at my Center think I should do is important to me.
3. (lead teachers) What the lead teachers at the Center think about what I do is important to me.
4. (children) What children at the Center think about my behaviors is important to me.

Note: Measures from Lapinski, Anderson, Shugart, & Todd, 2013.

Use of Existing Measures and Future Studies

With the exception of the measures detailed above, little factor analysis work has been conducted establishing validated scales to assess normative influence.

However a few other studies have performed confirmatory factor analyses on normative measures, including studies conducted in the context of descriptive condom use norms (Noar, Zimmerman, Palmgreen, Lustria, & Horosewski, 2006), descriptive drinking norms (Neighbors, Larimer, & Lewis, 2004), descriptive water conservation norms (Lapinski, Rimal, DeVries, & Lee, 2007), perceived handwashing norms among college students (Lapinski, Maloney, Braz, & Shulman, 2013), and subjective norms regarding physical activity (Motl, et al., 2002).

Despite the validated normative measures that currently exist, there is nevertheless opportunity for researchers to develop and validate normative measures in other health contexts. For example, there is a growing body of literature that points to normative influence as a substantial contributor to indoor tanning bed use (Hillhouse, Turrisi, & Shields, 2007). Currently, there has been little interventional research to explore this topic. Additionally, more work may be necessary to develop and validate normative measures in the contexts of smoking cigarettes, drug use, and "sexting" among adolescents. Among college students, normative research should explore the ways in which norms influence nooptropic drug use (e.g., Adderall, modafinil, racetams), as well as to understand how norms within some Greek social organizations can lead to sexual violence and exploitation. Another largely unexplored area where normative perceptions may guide behavior is in the context of workplace health interventions. Many workplaces have instituted incentives for fitness, weight-loss, and/or preventive health screening (Seaverson, Grossmeier, Miller, & Anderson, 2009). Sometimes these incentives are team-based, where employees work together to achieve health and fitness goals as a group. There is likely a strong normative component that affects the performance and maintenance of these various health behaviors that is largely unexplored in contemporary health communication research.

There is also an opportunity for researchers to explore different types of normative measures. To illustrate, some preliminary research suggests that historical drinking norms—perceptions of traditional, ritualistic descriptive norms over time—may influence drinking behavior (Carcioppolo & Jensen, 2012). More work in this area should be conducted to develop and validate measures of historical normative perceptions concerning behaviors that are steeped in customs or tradition. Another approach that researchers could explore is to develop measures of perceived normative pressure. An example of this can be seen in Noar and colleagues, (2014) measure of outcome expectations concerning indoor tanning bed use. This measure includes six items that address positive and negative outcome expectations regarding social approval of indoor tanning bed use, including items like, indoor tanning "would lead to compliments from people I date," "would make me more desirable to people I date," and "would lead people to worry about my health" (Noar et al., 2014, p. 517). These outcome expectations assess factors that can lead one to comply with perceived normative pressure.

One can conceptualize the relationship between social norms and perceived normative pressure similarly to the relationship between self-efficacy and perceived barriers. While variance in self-efficacy may account for barriers one perceives to enacting a behavior, measuring self-efficacy alone does not inform researchers about the specific barriers that affect behavior. Relatedly, variance in subjective or injunctive norms may account for perceived normative pressures (i.e., outcome expectation relevant to norms), but does not measure explicit pressures that one may feel from others. It is possible that measures of perceived normative pressure can allow researchers to determine discrete social phenomena that contribute to the performance of health behaviors while simultaneously addressing normative perceptions, and in doing so, identify potential targets for future interventional research. Future research in this area should assess the comparative effectiveness of measures of perceived normative pressure compared to standard measures of descriptive, injunctive, and subjective norms.

Recommended Readings

Ho, S. S., Liao, Y., & Rosenthal, S. (2014). Applying the theory of planned behavior and media dependency theory: Predictors of public pro-environmental behavioral intentions in Singapore. *Environmental Communication, 9*(1), 77–99.

Lapinski, M. K., Anderson, J., Shugart, A., & Todd, E. (2013). Social influence in child care centers: A test of the theory of normative social behavior. *Health Communication, 29,* 219–232.

Park, H. S., Klein, K. A., Smith, S., & Martell, D. (2009). Separating subjective norms, university descriptive and injunctive norms, and U.S. descriptive and injunctive norms for drinking behavior intentions. *Health Communication, 24,* 746–751.

Park, H. S., & Smith, S. W. (2007). Distinctiveness and influence of subjective norms, personal descriptive and injunctive norms, and societal descriptive and injunctive norms on behavioral intent: A case of two behaviors critical to organ donation. *Human Communication Research, 33,* 194–218.

Yun, D., & Silk, K. J. (2011). Social norms, self-identity, and attention to social comparison information in the context of exercise and healthy diet behavior. *Health Communication, 26,* 275–285.

References

Ajzen, I. (1991). The theory of planned behavior. *Organizational Behavior and Human Decision Processes, 50,* 179–211.

Ajzen, I., & Fishbein, M. (1980). *Understanding attitudes and predicting social behavior.* Englewood Cliffs, NJ: Prentice-Hall.

ALS (2014, September, 22nd). *Ice bucket challenge enthusiasm translates to support of ALS activities.* Retrieved from: http://www.alsa.org/news/archive/ice-bucket-chal lenge-092214.html

Armitage, C. J., & Conner, M. (2001). Efficacy of the theory of planned behaviour: A meta-analytic review. *The British Journal of Social Psychology, 40,* 471–499. doi: 10.1348/014466601164939.

Boer, H., & Westhoff, Y. (2006). The role of positive and negative signaling communi-cation by strong and weak ties in the shaping of safe sex subjective norms of ado-lescents in South Africa. *Communication Theory, 16,* 75–90. doi: 10.1111/j.1468-2885.2006.00006.x.

Borsari, B., & Carey, K. B. (2003). Descriptive and injunctive norms in college drinking: A meta-analytic integration. *Journal of Studies on Alcohol, 64,* 331–341.

Carcioppolo, N., & Jensen, J. D. (2012). Perceived historical drinking norms and current drinking behavior: Using the theory of normative social behav-ior as a framework for assessment. *Health Communication, 27,* 766–775. doi: 10.1080/10410236.2011.640973.

Cho, H. (2006). Readiness to change, norms, and self-efficacy among heavy-drinking college students. *Journal of Studies on Alcohol and Drugs, 67,* 131–138.

Cialdini, R. B., Reno, R. R., & Kallgren, C. A. (1990). A focus theory of normative conduct: Recycling the concept of norms to reduce littering in public places. *Journal of Per-sonality and Social Psychology, 58,* 1015–1026. doi: 10.1037/0022-3514.58.6.1015.

DeJong, W., Schneider, S. K., Towvim, L. G., Murphy, M. J., Doerr, E. E., Simonsen, N. R.,...Scribner, R. A. (2003). A multisite randomized trial of social norms mar-keting campaigns to reduce college student drinking: A replication failure. *Substance Abuse, 30,* 127–140. doi: 10.1080/08897070902802059.

Far, J., & Miller, J. (2003). The small group norms challenging model: Social norms in-terventions with targeted high risk groups. In H. W. Perkins (Ed.), *The social norms approach to preventing school and college age substance abuse: A handbook for educators, counselors, clinicians* (pp. 111–132). San Francisco: Jossey-Bass.

Fishbein, M. (2008). A reasoned action approach to health promotion. *Medical Deci-sion-making, 28,* 834–844. doi: 10.1177/0272989x08326092.

Fishbein, M., & Ajzen, I. (1975). *Belief, attitude, intention, and behavior: An introduction to theory and research.* Reading, MA: Addison-Wesley.

Hillhouse, J., Turrisi, R., & Shields, A. L. (2007). Patterns of indoor tanning use: Implications for clinical interventions. *Archives of Dermatology, 143*, 1530–1535. doi: 10.1001/archderm.143.12.1530.

Lapinski, M. K., Anderson, J., Shugart, A., & Todd, E. (2013). Social influence in child care centers: A test of the theory of normative social behavior. *Health Communication, 29*, 219–232. doi: 10.1080/10410236.2012.738322.

Lapinski, M. K., Maloney, E. K., Braz, M., & Shulman, H. C. (2013). Testing the effects of social norms and behavioral privacy on hand washing: A field experiment. *Human Communication Research, 39*, 21–46. doi: 10.1111/j.1468-2958.2012.01441.x.

Lapinski, M. K., & Rimal, R. N. (2005). An explication of social norms. *Communication Theory, 15*, 127–147. doi: 10.1111/j.1468-2885.2005.tb00329.x.

Lapinski, M. K., Rimal, R. N., DeVries, R., & Lee, E. L. (2007). The role of group orientation and descriptive norms on water conservation attitudes and behaviors. *Health Communication, 22*, 133–142. doi: 10.1080/10410230701454049.

Motl, R. W., Dishman, R. K., Saunders, R. P., Dowda, M., Felton, G., Ward, D. S., & Pate, R. R. (2002). Examining social-cognitive determinants of intention and physical activity among Black and White adolescent girls using structural equation modeling. *Health Psychology, 21*, 459–467. doi: 10.1037/0278-6133.21.5.459.

Myers, D. G. (2012). *Social psychology* (11th ed.). New York: McGraw-Hill.

Neighbors, C., Larimer, M. E., & Lewis, M. A. (2004). Targeting misperceptions of descriptive drinking norms: Efficacy of a computer-delivered personalized normative feedback intervention. *Journal of Consulting and Clinical Psychology, 72*, 434. doi: 10.1037/0022-006X.72.3.434.

Noar, S. M., Myrick, J., Morales-Pico, B., & Thomas, N. E. (2014). Development and validation of the comprehensive indoor tanning expectations scale. *JAMA Dermatology, 150*, 512–521. doi: 10.1001/jamadermatol.2013.9086.

Noar, S. M., Zimmerman, R. S., Palmgreen, P., Lustria, M., & Horosewski, M. L. (2006). Integrating personality and psychosocial theoretical approaches to understanding safer sexual behavior: Implications for message design. *Health Communication, 19*, 165–174. doi: 10.1207/s15327027hc1902_8.

Park, H. S., Klein, K. A., Smith, S., & Martell, D. (2009). Separating subjective norms, university descriptive and injunctive norms, and U.S. descriptive and injunctive norms for drinking behavior intentions. *Health Communication, 24*, 746–751. doi: 10.1080/10410230903265912.

Park, H. S., & Smith, S. W. (2007). Distinctiveness and influence of subjective norms, personal descriptive and injunctive norms, and societal descriptive and injunctive norms on behavioral intent: A case of two behaviors critical to organ donation. *Human Communication Research, 33*, 194–218. doi: 10.1111/j.1468-2958.2007.00296_2.x.

Rimal, R. N. (2008). Modeling the relationship between descriptive norms and behaviors: A test and extension of the theory of normative social behavior (TNSB). *Health Communication, 23*, 103–116. doi: 10.1080/10410230801967791.

Rimal, R. N., & Real, K. (2005). How behaviors are influenced by perceived norms: A test of the theory of normative social behavior. *Communication Research, 32*, 389–414. doi: 10.1177/0093650205275385.

Rivis, A., & Sheeran, P. (2003). Descriptive norms as an additional predictor in the theory of planned behaviour: A meta-analysis. *Current Psychology, 22*, 218–233. doi: 10.1007/s12144-003-1018-2.

Rokeach, M. (1973). *The nature of human values.* New York: The Free Press.

Seaverson, E. L. D., Grossmeier, J., Miller, T. M., & Anderson, D. R. (2009). The role of incentive design, incentive value, communications strategy, and worksite culture on health risk assessment participation. *American Journal of Health Promotion, 23*, 343–352. doi: 10.4278/ajhp.08041134.

Steel, E. (2014, August 21). 'Ice bucket challenge' donations for A.L.S. research top $41 million. *The New York Times,* pp. B2.

Wechsler, H., Nelson, T. E., Lee, J. E., Seibring, M., Lewis, C., & Keeling, R. P. (2003). Perception and reality: A national evaluation of social norms marketing interventions to reduce college students' heavy alcohol use. *Journal of Studies on Alcohol, 64,* 484–494.

Yzer, M. (2012). The integrative model of behavioral prediction as a tool for designing health messages. In H. Cho (Ed.) *Health communication message design: Theory and practice* (pp. 21–40). Thousand Oaks, CA: Sage Publications.

16. *Planned Behavior*

Lee Ann Kahlor,
University of Texas at Austin
& Ming-Ching Liang,
Metropolitan State University

The theory of planned behavior (TPB) (Ajzen, 1988; Ajzen, 1991; Ajzen & Fishbein, 2005) suggests that behaviors can be explained by three social-cognitive factors: (1) favorable and unfavorable evaluations of the behavior, manifest as attitudes toward the behavior; (2) perceived social pressure to perform or not perform the behavior, manifest as subjective norms regarding the behavior; and (3) perceived ability to perform the behavior, manifest as perceived behavioral control (Ajzen, 1988, 1991, 2002; Ajzen & Manstead, 2007). These three social-cognitive factors contribute to the generation of behavioral intention, which is a direct antecedent to actual behavior. The relationship between intention and behavior, however, is influenced by actual control over behavior. Figure 1 shows a visual depiction of the overall framework and relationships among its concepts.

Figure 1. The theory of planned behavior.

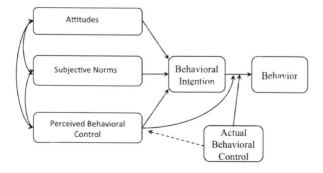

The theory has been tested over the past several decades across myriad behaviors and contexts. Within the realm of health behaviors specifically, the TPB has helped explain variance in intentions to perform health behaviors ranging from physical activity (Armitage, 2005) to sunscreen use (Allom, Mullan, & Sebastian, 2013). According to a 2011 meta-analysis of studies that applied the TPB to health behaviors between 1982 and 2010, the model accounted for, on average, 19 percent of the variance in behavior and 44 percent of the variance in behavior intention across studies during that time frame (McEachan, Conner, Taylor, & Lawton, 2011).

Measuring Planned Behaviors

Measurement of the constructs that are key to accessing TPB concepts and relationships among those concepts has evolved over time, and scale development has been well-detailed by Ajzen and colleagues (c.f., Ajzen, n.d.; Ajzen, 2005; Fishbein & Ajzen, 2010). For example, Fishbein and Ajzen (2010) suggest that scale development should be preceded by a clear definition of the behavior of interest, as well as the specific action targeted, context for the action, and a specific time frame for the action. Once defined clearly, behaviors then can be assessed with objective or self-reported measures. It should be noted, however, that research suggests that the TPB explains variability in self-reported behaviors better than in objectively measured behaviors (McEachan et al., 2011).

Measures of behavioral intention (BI), which precede behavior in the model, should correspond to the action, target, context, time, and criteria of the actual behavior—this reflects what Ajzen and Fishbein (1980) label the principle of compatibility. Behavior intentions are typically measured with Likert-style items using response options such as extremely unlikely/extremely likely, disagree/agree, and impossible/possible (Fishbein & Ajzen, 2010, p. 44).

The three belief-based concepts—attitudes toward the behavior, subjective norms, and perceived behavioral control also are measured consistent with the action, target, etc., defined in the early stages of scale development.

Attitudes toward behavior (Att), including cognitive (instrumental attitudes) and affective (experiential attitudes) evaluation of the behavior, are primarily measured with semantic differential items. These items prompt respondents to indicate their attitudinal positions related to the behavior on a bipolar evaluative adjective scale (Fishbein & Ajzen, 2010). Common adjectives used for instrumental attitudes including bad-good and harmful/beneficial, while unpleasant/pleasant and boring/interesting frequently have been used to indicate experiential attitudes toward behavior.

Subjective norms (SN) measures consist of two elements: injunctive and descriptive norms (Cialdini, Reno, & Kallgren, 1990). Injunctive norms are associated with the individual's perceptions of what should be done, and descriptive norms refer to the perceptions of others' engagement in the behavior of interest (Fishbein & Ajzen, 2010, p.131). Subjective norms scales consist of items measuring the perceptions of important referents' behaviors (descriptive norms) and beliefs about the action (injunctive norms). For example, "most people who are important to me think I *should-should not* perform behavior X" (injunctive); "most people who are important to me *do-do not* perform behavior X" (descriptive) (Fishbein & Ajzen, 2010).

Perceived behavior control (PBC) involves the perceptions of skills, opportunities, resources, and barriers associated with the behavior (Fishbein & Ajzen, 2010). This construct can be measured in semantic differential items or in the Likert format. Typical items include: "I am confident that I can perform behavior X," "my performance of X behavior is completely up to me," "I could perform behavior X if I really wanted to," and "performing X behavior is under my control."

Providing a sample standard questionnaire (Table 1), Fishbein and Ajzen (2010) noted some further considerations when developing measurements for Att, SN, and PBC. First, the principle of compatibility should be applied to the three motivational factors of TPB. That is, the behavior associated with the attitudes, subjective norms, and the perceived control should correspond to the specificity of the behavior and behavioral intention. Second, these three variables can be measured indirectly with behavioral beliefs and belief strength, normative beliefs and motivation to comply, and control beliefs and power of control factors.

Table 1. Sample questionnaire items adapted from Fishbein & Ajzen (2010).

Construct	Sample Items	Format
Att	My performing X behavior is… Good-Bad Unpleasant-Pleasant Harmful-Beneficial Interesting-Boring	7-point semantic differential

Construct	Sample Items	Format
SN	Most people who are important to me think I should perform X behavior. Most people whose opinion I value would approve of my performance of X behavior. Most people I respect and admire will perform X behavior. Most people like me have performed X behavior.	7-point semantic differential or Likert with agree-disagree, likely-unlikely, or true-false
PBC	I am confident that I can perform X behavior. My performance of X behavior is completely up to me. If I really wanted to, I could perform X behavior. For me to perform X behavior is under my control.	7-point semantic differential or Likert with agree-disagree, likely-unlikely, or true-false
BI	I intend to perform X behavior. I will perform X behavior. I am willing to perform X behavior. I plan to perform X behavior.	7-point semantic differential or Likert with agree-disagree, likely-unlikely, or true-false
Behavior (after Y timeframe)	In the past Y timeframe, how often have you performed X behavior? I have performed X behavior in the past Y timeframe.	7-point semantic differential or Likert with never-almost always, or true-false

An interesting discussion of validity issues related to the TPB can be found in Ajzen's 2011 editorial in *Psychology of Health* (Ajzen, 2011). There he addresses criticism and debate about the theory's ability to explain human behavior. That criticism is not entirely within the scope of this chapter, but should be read by anyone intending to use the theory as a framework for their research. In that same editorial, Ajzen also discusses the findings of a meta-analysis of the theory applied to health behaviors; this meta-analysis also should be a must-read for anyone interested in applying the theory to information- or communication-related behaviors (McEachan et al., 2011).

Use of Existing Measures and Future Studies

Given the robustness of the TPB and the validity and reliability of its requisite measures as described by Ajzen, and the theory's applicability to health-related behaviors, it is a promising approach for the study of health information related behaviors. Indeed, the model's concepts have been applied to one specific health information behavior—information seeking—with notable success in the context of health and risk information-seeking behaviors (Kahlor, 2007; Kahlor, 2010; Liu, Doucette, Farris, et al., 2005; Ross, Kohler, Grimley et al., 2007; Yoo & Robbins, 2008).

Reflecting on Table 1 above, researchers interested in applying the TPB to information-related health behaviors can create a TPB instrument with simple tailoring of the items in that table. For example, to measure attitude toward seeking HIV information online in the next month, the first block of items can begin, "For me, seeking information online about HIV is..." The response options would be presented exactly as listed in the table, as 7-point semantic differential items featuring "good-bad," etc.

Scholars also have attempted to incorporate additional variables to expand the TPB to explain information behaviors. The founders of TPB left open the possibilities to add in the model more factors that substantially increase predictive power (Ajzen & Fishbein, 1980). The planned risk information seeking model (PRISM, Kahlor, 2010) represents an effort to integrate additional elements in TPB. Based on various models in health communication, PRISM incorporates risk perception, perceived knowledge insufficiency, and affective reactions with the TPB model to predict risk information seeking intention. PRISM was based on the Griffin et al. (1999) risk information seeking and processing model.

Kahlor (2010) proposed the PRISM as a framework to predict general health information seeking intention. In that study, PRISM explained a significantly larger proportion of the variances in information seeking intention and exhibited a better model fit than the TPB and the risk information seeking and processing model (Griffin, Dunwoody, & Neuwirth, 1999). In the context of cancer risk information seeking, a recent study (Hovick, Kahlor, & Liang, 2014) introduced source beliefs, past search, and outcome expectancies to the PRISM model, but concluded that the original PRISM fit the data better.

In addition to predicting health information seeking, the TPB has been used to design intervention programs that facilitate interpersonal discussions of health information. For example, a study found that subjective norms, attitudes toward behavior, and emotional reactions predicted college female students' intention for conversations with partners about condom use; behavioral control, however, did not significantly increase the variance explained in behavioral intention (Chan & Fishbein, 1993).

Overall, the TPB has been frequently applied to explain behaviors, including information behaviors in the context of health communication. To ensure measurement quality, compatibility among TPB variable measures should be emphasized. Scholarly attempts to incorporate additional factors in the TPB model to explain health information behavior reinforce the usefulness of the theory. Future research should extend the focus to predicting changes in health communication behaviors.

Recommended Readings

Eastin, M. S., Kahlor, L. A., Liang, M. C., & Abi Ghannam, N. (2015). Information-seeking as a precaution behavior: exploring the role of decision-making stages. *Human Communication Research* (Forthcoming).

Griffin, R. J., Dunwoody, S., & Yang, Z. J. (2012). 15 linking risk messages to information seeking and processing. *Communication Yearbook 36*, 323–361.

Ho, S. S., Detenber, B. H., Rosenthal, S., & Lee, E. W. (2014). Seeking information about climate change: effects of media use in an extended PRISM. *Science Communication*, (Forthcoming).

Hovick, S. R., Kahlor, L., & Liang, M.-C. (2014). Personal cancer knowledge and information seeking through prism: the planned risk information seeking model. *Journal of Health Communication, 19*(4), 512–524.

Kahlor, L. (2010). PRISM: A planned risk information seeking model. *Health communication, 25*(4), 345–356.

References

Ajzen (n.d.). *Constructing a theory of planned behavior questionnaire.* http://people.umass.edu/aizen/pdf/tpb.measurement.pdf

Ajzen, I. (2005). Laws of human behavior: Symmetry, compatibility, and attitude-behavior correspondence. In A. Beauducel, B. Biehl, M. Bosniak, W. Conrad, G. Schönberger, & D. Wagener (Eds.), *Multivariate research strategies* (pp. 3–19). Aachen, Germany: Shaker Verlag.

Ajzen, I. (2011). The theory of planned behaviour: reactions and reflections. *Psychology & Health, 26*(9), 1113–1127. doi: 10.1080/08870446.2011.613995.

Ajzen, I. (2014). The theory of planned behaviour is alive and well, and not ready to retire: A commentary on Sniehotta, Presseau, and Araújo-Soares. *Health Psychology Review*, 1–7. doi: 10.1080/17437199.2014.883474.

Ajzen, I., & Fishbein, M. (1980). *Understanding attitudes and predicting social behaviour.* Englewood Cliffs, NJ: Prentice-Hall.

Allom, V., Mullan, B., & Sebastian, J. (2013). Closing the intention–behaviour gap for sunscreen use and sun protection behaviours. *Psychology & Health, 28*(5), 477–494. doi: 10.1080/08870446.2012.745935.

Armitage, C. J. (2005). Can the theory of planned behaviour predict the maintenance of physical activity? *Health Psychology, 24*(3), 235–245. doi: 10.1037/0278-6133.24.3.235.

Chan, D. K. S., & Fishbein, M. (1993). Determinants of college women's intentions to tell their partners to use condoms. *Journal of Applied Social Psychology, 23*(18), 1455–1470. doi: 10.1111/j.1559-1816.1993.tb01043.x.

Cialdini, R. B., Reno, R. R., & Kallgren, C. A. (1990). A focus theory of normative conduct: Recycling the concept of norms to reduce littering in public places. *Journal of Personality and Social Psychology, 58*(6), 1015–1026. doi: 10.1037/0022-3514.58.6.1015.

Fishbein, M., & Ajzen, I. (2010). *Predicting and changing behavior: The reasoned action approach*. New York: Taylor & Francis.

Griffin, R. J., Dunwoody, S., & Neuwirth, K. (1999). Proposed model of the relationship of risk information seeking and processing to the development of preventive behaviors. *Environmental Research, 80*(2), S230–S245. doi:10.1006/enrs.1998.3940.

Hovick, S. R., Kahlor, L., & Liang, M.-C. (2014). Personal cancer knowledge and information seeking through PRISM: The planned risk information seeking model. *Journal of Health Communication, 19*(4), 512–524. doi: 10.1080/10810730.2013.821556.

Kahlor, L. A. (2007). An augmented risk information seeking model: The case of global warming. *Media Psychology, 10*(3), 414–435. doi: 10.1080/15213260701532971.

Kahlor, L. (2010). PRISM: A planned risk information seeking model. *Health communication, 25*(4), 345–356. doi: 10.1080/10410231003775172.

Liu, Y., Doucette, W. R., Farris, K. B., & Nayakankuppam, D. (2005). Drug information–seeking intention and behavior after exposure to direct-to-consumer advertisement of prescription drugs. *Research in Social and Administrative Pharmacy, 1*(2), 251–269. doi:10.1016/j.sapharm.2005.03.010.

McEachan, R. R. C., Conner, M., Taylor, N. J., & Lawton, R. J. (2011). Prospective prediction of health-related behaviours with the theory of planned behaviour: A meta-analysis. *Health Psychology Review, 5*(2), 97–144. doi: 10.1080/17437199.2010.521684.

Ross, L., Kohler, C. L., Grimley, D. M., & Anderson-Lewis, C. (2007). The theory of reasoned action and intention to seek cancer information. *American Journal of Health Behavior, 31*(2), 123–134. http://dx.doi.org.ezproxy.lib.utexas.edu/10.5993/AJHB.31.2.2

Sniehotta, F. F., Presseau, J., & Araújo-Soares, V. (2014). Time to retire the theory of planned behaviour. *Health Psychology Review, 8*(1), 1–7. doi: 10.1080/17437199.2013.869710.

Yoo, E.-Y., & Robbins, L. S. (2008). Understanding middle-aged women's health information seeking on the web: A theoretical approach. *Journal of the American Society for Information Science and Technology, 59*(4), 577–590. doi: 10.1002/asi.20766.

17. Psychological Reactance

Brian L. Quick,
University of Illinois at Urbana-Champaign
& Tobias Reynolds-Tylus,
University of Illinois at Urbana-Champaign

Described as an aversive motivational state following a threatened or elimi-nated freedom, psychological reactance emerged onto the scene as a popular construct more than five decades ago for explaining resistance to persuasion (for a review, see Brehm, 1966; Brehm & Brehm, 1981). Despite the pop-ularity of psychological reactance theory, the operationalization of reactance both as a psychological state and as an individual difference variable remained underdeveloped until recently. In the current chapter we set out to offer read-ers a validated conceptualization and operationalization of psychological re-actance both as a state and trait. Additionally, evidence in support of recent operationalizations will also be provided. We begin with an overview of psy-chological reactance theory followed by scale development with respect to reactance as both a psychological state and an individual difference variable. We conclude the chapter by highlighting opportunities for scale application and modification in the future.

Brehm and Brehm (1981) conceptualized psychological reactance as a "motivational state that is hypothesized to occur when a freedom is eliminated or threatened with elimination" (Brehm & Brehm, 1981, p. 37). Thus, implicit in their definition is that psychological reactance is a two-step process consist-ing of a freedom threat followed by reactance. Brehm (1966) articulated four principles to guide reactance research. First, reactance can only be aroused if individuals believe they have freedom to choose among alternatives. Second, as the threatened freedom increases in importance, psychological reactance also increases. Third, as the number of freedom threats increases, reactance also increases. Finally, as implied threats are presented, reactance arousal increases (Brehm, 1966). Support for these principles emerged in the literature (for a review, see Brehm & Brehm, 1981) although the tenability of these findings were limited without a validated measure for psychological reactance.

Despite the clarity of their conceptualization and frequent attention given to psychological reactance theory among psychologists, attempts at measuring reactance remained understudied until the late 20th century. In fact, it was not until Burgoon, Alvaro, Broneck, Miller, Grandpre, Hall, and Frank's spirited review of reactance theory that communication researchers began to apply Brehm's (1966) theory within the persuasion context and in health campaigns in particular. Their comprehensive review of the theory's illustrious past provided communication researchers with a glimpse of the remarkable heuristic value of psychological reactance theory. Perhaps the most important unanswered question pertained to the measurement of reactance. Historically speaking, reactance had been measured via its antecedents and outcomes (Quick, Shen, & Dillard, 2012).

Measuring Psychological Reactance

Spearheading the effort to operationalize psychological reactance was Dillard and Shen (2005) who argued that reactance could be measured through cognitions and affect. More specifically, within the context of meningitis and responsible alcohol consumption, they tested the effectiveness of measuring reactance as (a) purely negative cognitions, (b) purely anger, (c) both anger and negative cognitions, and (d) an intertwined model featuring both anger and negative cognitions. Across both contexts, the intertwined model proved to be the most empirically acceptable operationalization. Following Dillard and Shen's (2005) seminal study, Quick and associates (Quick & Considine, 2008; Quick & Stephenson, 2008) began to encourage reactance researchers to model reactance as a two-step process featuring a freedom threat induction followed by reactance, measured with the intertwined model promulgated by Dillard and Shen a few years earlier. The instruments to assess freedom threat perceptions, anger, and negative cognitions are presented below in Table 1.

Table 1. State Reactance Measures.

Freedom Threat Measure (Dillard & Shen, 2005)
1. The message tried to make a decision for me.
2. The message tried to pressure me.
3. The message threatened my freedom to choose.
4. The message tried to manipulate me.

Anger Measure (Dillard & Shen, 2005)

1. Did you feel angry while viewing this message?

2. Did you feel annoyed while viewing this message?

3. Did you feel irritated while viewing this message?

4. Did you feel aggravated while viewing this message?

Negative Cognitions (Dillard & Shen, 2005)

Relevant negative cognitions void of emotions serve as the indicator for negative cognitions.

These measures continue to withstand the passing of time as researchers have employed Dillard and Shen's (2005) measure of psychological reactance across a host of contexts (for a review, see Quick et al., 2012). Throughout these studies, researchers have discovered message features (e.g., domineering, vivid language) arousing freedom threat perceptions as well as features (e.g., empathy, narratives, message novelty) that mitigate reactance from arising. Equally important, from these studies, researchers have demonstrated a variety of outcomes associated with psychological reactance including unfavorable message (Grandpre, Alvaro, Burgoon, Miller, & Hall, 2003) and source appraisals (Miller, Lane, Deatrick, Young, & Potts, 2007), attitudes (Dillard & Shen, 2005; Quick, 2012), and intentions (Rains & Turner, 2007) toward an advocated behavior. Together the measurement advances for psychological reactance as a psychological state have certainly advanced the field forward.

With the burgeoning popularity of psychological reactance theory, researchers have begun to reassess the validity of Dillard and Shen's (2005) psychological reactance measure. For starters, Quick (2012) set out to evaluate their measure vis-à-vis Lindsey's (2005) reactance measure, which had grown in popularity among communication researchers since its inception (e.g., Reinhart, Marshall, Feeley, & Tutzauer, 2007). Lindsey (2005) developed a four-item measure incorporating anger, freedom threat perceptions, and negative cognitions into a unidimensional construct. With two instruments in use, Quick evaluated both measures with respect to their reliability and validity. Each measure formed an acceptable reliability (Quick, 2012). Validity was examined by evaluating both measures in a nomothetic network featuring a freedom threat as an antecedent and three endogenous variables including attitudes, motivations, and source appraisal. Results demonstrated Dillard and Shen's (2005) measure was superior to Lindsey's (2005) instrument with respect to model fit. Specifically, Quick concluded Dillard and Shen's measure was superior with respect to reliability and validity. Moreover, conceptually speaking, it was more congruent with Brehm's (1966) notion that reactance follows freedom threats. More recently, Rains' (2013) meta-analysis ($K = 20$, $N = 4,942$) offered additional evidence in support of measuring reactance as an amalgamation of anger and negative cognitions following exposure to a freedom threat. In addition to conceptualizing and operationalizing reactance as a psychological state, a growing number of researchers consider reactance to be an individual difference variable as well.

Although Brehm's (1966) original formulation of psychological reactance theory did not specifically discuss reactance as an individual trait, he did acknowledge the possibility of individual differences in reactions to persuasive stimuli. Later work by Brehm and Brehm (1981) acknowledged that the notion of reactance as an individual difference variable is consistent with the theory's original formulations. Specifically, the conceptualization of reactance as a personality trait is consistent with the idea that individuals vary in their needs for autonomy and self-determination (Wicklund, 1974). Work by Dowd and colleagues (Dowd et al., 1994; Seibel & Dowd, 2011) has shown that a high trait reactant individual has a personality style characterized by resistance for rules and regulations, high autonomy, low concern for social norms, and high defensiveness. Accordingly, high trait reactant individuals have been found to experience higher freedom threats, and therefore are more resistant to persuasive attempts (Quick, Scott, & Ledbetter, 2011; Quick & Stephenson, 2008). Likewise, high trait reactant individuals have been found to be more likely to engage in risky health behaviors than low trait reactant individuals, thereby making this a promising segmentation variable for health campaigners (Miller et al., 2006).

Several authors have proposed conceptualizations of trait reactance (Dowd, Milne, & Wise, 1991; Hong & Page, 1989; Merz, 1983), albeit with disagreements on the underlying dimensions. Merz (1983) was the first to develop a self-report measure of trait reactance, which was later translated into English by Tucker and Byers (1987) and Hong and Ostini (1989). However, due to the psychometric instability of Merz's (1983) scale (Donnell, Thomas, & Buboltz, 2001; Hong & Ostini, 1989; Tucker & Byers, 1987), two additional scales have been developed to measure trait reactance: the Therapeutic Reactance Scale (Dowd et al., 1991) and the Hong Reactance Scale (Hong, 1992; Hong & Faedda, 1996; Hong, Giannakopoulos, & Williams, 1994; Hong & Page, 1989).

In response to the limitations of Merz's (1983) scale, Dowd and colleagues (1991) developed the Therapeutic Reactance Scale as a measure of trait reactance. In their formulation of trait reactance, Dowd and colleagues (1991) proposed that trait reactance has two underlying dimensions: (a) *behavioral reactance* (e.g., "If I am told what to do, I often do the opposite"), and (c) *verbal reactance* (e.g., "I enjoy debates with other people"). Although Dowd and colleagues (1991) initially provided some evidence for the reliability and validity of their scale, more recently the Therapeutic Reactance Scale has been criticized for being psychometrically unstable (Buboltz, Thomas, & Donnell, 2002).

The most commonly used scale to measure trait reactance comes from the work of Hong and colleagues (Hong, 1992; Hong & Faedda, 1996; Hong et al., 1994; Hong & Page, 1989). Dillard and Shen (2005) have argued that the Hong scale has the most favorable psychometric properties and the greatest conceptual correspondence with psychological reactance theory. The most current conceptualization of the Hong Reactance Scale (Hong & Faedda, 1996) proposes that trait reactance is best conceptualized with four dimensions: (a) *emotional responses to restricted choice*, (b) *reactance to compliance*, (c) *resisting influence from others*, and (d) *reactance to advice and recommendations*. Recent work by Shen and Dillard (2005) has suggested that the Hong Reactance Scale is unidimensional at the second order; therefore the use of a single score by treating the dimensions as subscales is both theoretically sound and empirically justifiable. Hong and Faedda's (1996) reactance scale is presented in Table 2.

Table 2. Hong's (1996) Psychological Reactance Scale Items.

1.	Regulations trigger a sense of resistance in me.
2.	I find contradicting others stimulating.
3.	When something is prohibited, I usually think "that's exactly what I am going to do."
4.	I consider advice from others to be an intrusion.
5.	I become frustrated when I am unable to make free and independent decisions.
6.	It irritates me when someone points out things which are obvious to me.
7.	I become angry when my freedom of choice is restricted.
8.	Advice and recommendations usually induce me to do just the opposite.
9	I resist the attempts of others to influence me.
10.	It makes me angry when another person is held up as a model for me to follow.
11.	When someone forces me to do something, I feel like doing the opposite.
12.	The thought of being dependent on others aggravates me.*

13. It disappoints me to see others submitting to society's standards and rules.*

14. I am contented only when I am acting on my own free will.*

(Note: * = Items not included in the 11-item scale.)

Use of Existing Measures and Future Studies

Laboratory studies have demonstrated the utility of measuring reactance as both a psychological state and an individual difference variable. As we look ahead to future psychological reactance theory studies, the heuristic value of the theory is ripe as a framework for message design as well as an audience segmentation variable. For starters, an abundance of research identifies message strategies successfully reducing reactance arousal within a variety of heath contexts. The time has come for researchers to apply findings from laboratory studies into local, statewide, regional, and national campaigns. A recent study by Quick, Kam, Morgan, Montero-Liberona, and Smith (2015) found that radio ads featuring a freedom-restoration postscript (e.g., It's up to you. Your decision can save lives) did not significantly reduce freedom threat perceptions among adults. Although this lone study did not support continued use of freedom restoration postscripts, more research testing the effectiveness of professionally produced messages aimed at heterogeneous audiences is warranted. To date, the vast majority of reactance studies have recruited from college student or adult samples from individualistic cultures (for an exception, see Quick & Kim, 2009). Additionally, future research should apply Dillard and Shen's (2005) reactance measure to entertainment education messages. Although a few noteworthy studies demonstrate the ability for narratives to decrease psychological reactance among viewers, research employing the measures discussed in this chapter would enhance the generalizability of these findings. In doing so, researchers should seek to refine approaches to garner negative cognitions. As others have noted elsewhere (e.g., Quick et al., 2012), the thought listing procedure is cumbersome, subsequently limiting the theory's application to projects conducted outside of the laboratory.

Similarly to reactance as a psychological state, the heuristic value of reactance as an individual difference variable is also rich. As observed earlier, the personality characteristics (e.g., autonomy, rebelliousness, sensation seeking) positively associated with trait reactance are noteworthy from a public health standpoint. For example, Miller and Quick's (2010) research supports segmenting audiences along these psychographics given their propensity to use tobacco products and to engage in risky sex. To date, the authors are unaware of health campaigners bifurcating audiences along this personality dimension. Certainly, with an understanding of the repertoire of effective message features to minimize reactance from occurring among the most reactant prone individuals, public health practitioners are poised to create more theoretically sophisticated messages.

Recommended Readings

Dillard, J. P., & Shen, L. (2005). On the nature of reactance and its role in persuasive health communication. *Communication Monographs, 72*, 144–168.

Quick, B. L. (2012). What is the best measure of psychological reactance? An empirical test of two measures. *Health Communication, 27*, 1–9.

Quick, B. L., & Kim, D. K. (2009). Examining reactance and reactance restoration with Korean adolescents: A test of psychological reactance within a collectivist culture. *Communication Research, 36*, 765–782.

Quick, B. L., & Stephenson, M. T. (2008). Examining the role of trait reactance and sensation seeking on reactance-inducing messages, reactance, and reactance restoration. *Human Communication Research, 34*, 448–476.

Rains, S. A. (2013). The nature of psychological reactance revisited: A meta-analytic review. *Human Communication Research, 39*, 47–73.

References

Brehm, J. W. (1966). *A theory of psychological reactance.* New York: Academic Press.

Brehm. J. W., & Brehm, S. S. (1981). *Psychological reactance: A theory of freedom and control.* San Diego, CA: Academic Press.

Buboltz Jr., W. C., Donnell, A. J., & Thomas, A. (2002). Evaluating the factor structure and internal consistency reliability of the Therapeutic Reactance Scale. *Journal of Counseling & Development, 80*(1), 120–125.

Burgoon, M., Alvaro, E., Grandpre, J., & Voulodakis, M. (2002). Revisiting the theory of psychological reactance: Communicating threats to attitudinal freedom. In J. P. Dillard and M. Pfau (Eds.), *The persuasion handbook: Developments in theory and practice* (pp. 213–232). Thousand Oaks, CA: Sage.

Dillard, J. P., & Shen, L. (2005). On the nature of reactance and its role in persuasive health communication. *Communication Monographs, 72*(2), 144–168. doi: 10.1080/03637750500111815.

Donnell, A. J., Thomas, A., & Buboltz Jr., W. C. (2001). Psychological reactance: Factor structure and internal consistency of the questionnaire for the measurement of psychological reactance. *The Journal of Social Psychology, 141*(5), 679–687. doi: 10.1080/00224540109600581.

Dowd, E. T., Milne, C. R., Wise, S. L. (1991). The Therapeutic Reactance Scale: A measure of psychological reactance. *Journal of Counseling and Development, 69*, 541–545.

Dowd, E. T., Wallbrown, F., Sanders, D., & Yesenosky, J. M. (1994). Psychological re-actance and its relationship to normal personality variables. *Cognitive Therapy and Research, 18*(6), 601–612.

Hong, S. M. (1992). Hong's Psychological Reactance Scale: A further factor analytic val-idation.*Psychological Reports, 70,* 512–514.

Hong, S. M., & Faedda, S. (1996). Refinement of the Hong Psychological Reactance Scale. *Educational and Psychological Measurement, 56,* 173–182.

Hong, S. M., Giannakopoulos, E., Laing, D., & Williams, N. A. (1994). Psychological reactance: Effects of age and gender. *Journal of Social Psychology, 134,* 223–228.

Hong, S. M., & Ostini, R. (1989). Further evaluation of Merz's psychological reactance scale. *Psychological Reports, 64*(3), 707–710.

Hong, S. M., & Page, S. (1989). A psychological reactance scale: Development, factor structure and reliability. *Psychological Reports, 64,* 1323–1326.

Merz, J. (1983) Fragebogen zur Messung der psychologischen Reaktanz [A questionnaire for the measurement of psychological reactance]. *Diagnostica, 29,* 75–82. From *Psychological Abstracts,* 1983, 70, No. 93531.

Miller, C. H., Burgoon, M., Grandpre, J. R., & Alvaro, E. M. (2006). Identifying princi-pal risk factors for the initiation of adolescent smoking behaviors: The significance of psychological reactance. *Health Communication, 19,* 241–252.

Miller, C. H., & Quick, B. L. (2010). Sensation seeking and psychological reactance as health risk predictors for an emerging adult population. *Health Communication, 25,* 266–275.

Quick, B. L. (2012). What is the best measure of psychological reactance? An empirical test of two measures. *Health Communication, 27,* 1–9. doi: 10.1080/10410236.2011.567446.

Quick, B. L., & Considine, J. R. (2008). Examining the use of forceful language when designing exercise persuasive messages for adults: A test of conceptualiz-ing reactance arousal as a two-step process. *Health Communication, 23,* 483–491. doi:10.1080/10410230802342150.

Quick, B. L., Kam, J. A., Morgan, S. E., Montero Liberona, C. A., & Smith, R. A. (2015). Prospect theory, discrete emotions, and freedom threats: An extension of psycho-logical reactance theory. *Journal of Communication, 65*(1), 40–61. doi: 10.1111/jcom.1213

Quick, B. L., & Kim, D. K. (2009). Examining reactance and reactance restoration with Korean adolescents: A test of psychological reactance within a collectivist culture. *Communication Research, 36,* 765–782. doi:10.1177/009365020346797.

Quick, B. L., Scott, A. M., & Ledbetter, A. M. (2011). A close examination of trait reac-tance and issue involvement as moderators of psychological reactance theory. *Journal of Health Communication, 16*(6), 660–679. doi: 10.1080/10810730.2011.551989.

Quick, B. L., Shen, L., & Dillard, J. P. (2013). Reactance theory and persuasion. In J. P. Dillard and L. Shen (Eds.), *The SAGE handbook of persuasion: Advances in theory and research* (2nd ed., pp. 167–183). Los Angeles: Sage.

Quick, B. L., & Stephenson, M. T. (2007). Further evidence that psychological reactance can be modeled as a combination of anger and negative cognitions. *Communication Research, 34,* 255–276. doi: 10.1177/0093650207300427.

Quick, B. L., & Stephenson, M. T. (2008). Examining the role of trait reactance and sensation seeking on reactance-inducing messages, reactance, and reactance restoration. *Human Communication Research, 34,* 448–476. doi:10.1111/j.1468-2958.2008.00328.x.

Rains, S. A. (2013). The nature of psychological reactance revisited: A meta-analytic review. *Human Communication Research, 39,* 47–73. doi:10.1111/j.1468-2958.2012.01443.x.

Rains, S. A., & Turner, M. (2007). Psychological reactance and persuasive health communication: A test and extension of the intertwined model. *Human Communication Research, 33,* 241–269. doi: 10.1111/j.1468-2958.2007.00298.x.

Reinhart, A. M., Marshall, H. M., Feeley, T. H., & Tutzauer, F. (2007). The persuasive effects of message framing in organ donation: The mediating role of psychological reactance. *Communication Monographs, 74,* 229–255.

Seibel, C. A., & Dowd, E. T. (2001). Personality characteristics associated with psychological reactance. *Journal of Clinical Psychology, 57*(7), 963–969.

Shen, L., & Dillard, J. P. (2005). Psychometric properties of the Hong psychological reactance scale. *Journal of Personality Assessment, 85*(1), 74–81.

Tucker, R. K., & Byers, P. Y. (1987). Factorial validity of Merz's psychological reactance scale. *Psychological Reports, 61*(3), 811–815.

Wicklund, R. A. (1974). *Freedom and reactance.* Hillsdale, NJ: Lawrence Erlbaum Associates, Inc.

18. Risk Behavior Diagnosis

CRAIG TRUMBO,
Colorado State University
& SE-JIN KIM,
Colorado State University

Health communication has long occupied a position that serves not only the scientific investigation of how information affects human health behaviors but also the practical concerns of the execution of information delivery to achieve positive health outcomes. In this manner health communication researchers have an opportunity to participate in important translational work that can place effective diagnostic tools in the hands of professional health communicators.

That was the primary goal for the development of the Risk Behavior Diagnosis Scale (Witte, Cameron, McKeon, & Berkowitz, 1996). At the time of the scale's original publication, health communication researchers had already been strongly involved in an examination of how fear appeal messages motivate behavior and behavior change. One of the interesting discoveries in this work was the very real possibility of a fear-based message precipitating a reverse, or boomerang, effect in which the message recipient would become motivated to control the feeling of fear rather than motivated to control the threat. In some cases it was seen that harmful behavior, such as smoking, could actually become more entrenched under this response condition.

That was an observation made by Witte and colleagues in their extensive development of the Extended Parallel Process Model (EPPM)(Witte & Allen, 2000). What they found was that a carefully considered mix of message elements could motivate desired health behavior and mitigate against an undesired reverse effect. And in this work they identified the need for a simple assessment tool to characterize individuals or audiences relative to given health threats and protective actions, as well as to assess message effects in the development of health communication materials. Thus the RBD Scale was created.

The scale includes four components, each with 3 measurement items, for a total length of 12 items. Response efficacy measures the degree to which the individual perceives the recommended health response to be actually effective. Self-efficacy measures the degree to which the individual feels able to perform the recommended health response. These combine to capture the dimension of efficacy. The degree to which the individual feels susceptible to the health threat and the degree to which the individual perceives the health threat as severe combine to capture the dimension of threat.

To make the scale amenable to clinical and field use the researchers conceptualized a single summary measure derived from the four elements to represent a "critical point score." This measure could indicate the potential for an undesired fear response. For individual scores the calculation is simply the efficacy scale minus the threat scale. A positive critical point score indicates danger control (desired) while a negative value indicates fear control. For application to population samples it was originally recommended that the threat and efficacy scores be standardized before subtraction.

Measuring Risk Behaviors

In the original development of the RBD Scale, Witte et al. (1996) created the set of 12 measurement items based on the conceptual components of the EPPM (Table 1). To demonstrate the measure they evaluated it in a study of female undergraduate university students with respect to condom use in the prevention of genital warts. As part of a larger project, two data collections were used. The researchers conducted a mail survey to 300 participants, with 71 completions (23%). They also recruited experimental subjects on campus with 125 retained for the post-test survey. Experimental participants were randomly provided with one of three campaign packets, and controls received nothing. All participants in both studies completed the RBD Scale.

Table 1. Witte, Cameron, McKeon, and Berkowitz (1996) Scale to Measure the 4 Components of the Risk Behavior Diagnosis Scale.

(Response Efficacy)
1. [Recommended response] works in preventing [health threat].
2. [Doing/using recommended response] is effective in preventing [health threat].
3. If I [do/use recommended response], I am less likely to get [health threat].

(Self-Efficacy)

4. I am able to [do/use recommended response] to prevent getting [health threat].

5. [Recommended response] is easy to do/use to prevent [health threat].

6. [Doing/using recommended response] to prevent [health threat] is convenient.

(Severity)

7. I believe that [health threat] is severe.

8. I believe that [health threat] is serious.

9. I believe that [health threat] is significant.

(Susceptibility)

11. I am at risk for getting [health threat].

10. It is likely that I will contract [health threat].

12. It is possible that I will contract [health threat].

Confirmatory factor analysis indicated that each of the four scale components constituted a unique dimension, together accounting for 76% of variance and with a good model fit. A second-order confirmatory factor analysis supported the conceptualization of threat and efficacy as unique dimensions. Additive scales for threat and efficacy were computed (α = .73 and .71 respectively), critical point scores were determined, and participants were separated into high and low groups. ANOVA and discriminate analysis was used to assess validity against external measures of danger control and fear control responses. The critical point score was effective in differentiating the two response groups. The researchers concluded that the approach was reliable and held content, construct, and predictive validity. They also concluded that the tool would present an effective and easy clinical or field tool for individual or population assessment, and for message effect testing. The researchers published revised wording for many of the items in a 2001 guide to effective health communication (Table 2) (Witte, Meyer, & Martell, 2001). They also reported that standardization had not demonstrated sufficient utility to further recommend its use.

Table 2. Witte, Meyer, and Martell, D. (2001) Scale to Measure the 4 Components of the Risk Behavior Diagnosis Scale, Revised Wordings.

(Response Efficacy)

1. [Performing recommended response] prevents [health threat].

2. [Performing recommended response] works in deterring [health threat].

3. [Performing recommended response] is effective in getting rid of [health threat].

(Self-Efficacy)

4. I am able to [Perform recommended response] to prevent [health threat].

5. It is easy to [Perform recommended response] to prevent [health threat].

6. I can [Perform recommended response] to prevent [health threat].

(Severity)

7. [Health threat] is harmful.

8. [Health threat] is a serious threat.

9. [Health threat] is a severe threat.

(Susceptibility)

11. I am at risk for [Getting/experiencing health threat].

10. I am susceptible to [Getting/experiencing health threat].

12. It is possible that I will [Get/experience health threat].

The RBD Scale has been used in a number of studies since its inception. A cited reference search conducted in Web of Science indicates 73 published articles citing the original 1996 paper at the end of 2014. A complete list of citations is available from the first author of this chapter. The scale has been applied to a wide variety of health threats (e.g., radon exposure, farm safety, HIV/AIDS prevention, bulimia, dental hygiene, skin cancer, hearing loss, etc). Witte et al. provide a detailed account of the RBD Scale used in a clinical health counseling environment. An example of the development of an RBDS-based safety video on child booster car seats is available online at http://www.boosterseats4safety.org/research.aspx (Will, Sabo, & Porter, 2009).

Our examination of the body of work citing the original RBD Scale found that 14 cited the scale but did not employ it and 29 used partial instruments with only select components of the scale. Five articles used all four concepts with reduced items sets and 26 replicated the full scale. Here we provide an example of one of the full replications in which a dual-audience approach is also demonstrated. We then provide two examples in which a reduced item set is demonstrated.

Krieger and Sarge's (2013) study (full replication) was conducted with the purpose of examining the impact of disease prevention frames on female students' intentions to talk to a doctor about the human papillomavirus (HPV) vaccine and their mothers' intentions to encourage their daughters to talk to a doctor about the HPV vaccine. Two hundred and eighty-six female undergraduate students at a large, Midwestern university participated in a message design experiment. The authors removed 98 (34%) of the female students and their corresponding mothers from the data since the daughter had already received one or more doses of the vaccine. Therefore, this study utilized data from 188 female students and 115 corresponding mothers for the analyses. All these students and mothers completed the RBD scale.

To measure perceived effectiveness (i.e., response efficacy) of encouraging their daughter to talk with a physician about the HPV vaccine, mothers responded to three items (α = .89). Similarly, daughters answered a three-item scale (α = .76). Mothers further reported the degree to which they believed how easy it would be (i.e., self-efficacy) to encourage their daughter to speak to a doctor about the HPV vaccine by responding to three items. Daughters responded to the three similar items (α = .97). In order to operationalize susceptibility, mothers reported the degree to which they perceived their daughter was susceptible to getting HPV by responding to three items (α = .87). In a similar manner students used a scale to report the degree to which they perceived themselves susceptible to getting HPV by answering three items (α = .88). In measuring severity, mothers reported responded to three items (α = .86) to indicate the degree to which they believed HPV could be a serious threat to their daughter's life, health, and well-being. Daughters answered three similar items (α = .81). The final parallel question sets that were identified through this study appear in Table 3a and Table 3b.

Table 3a. Krieger and Sarge's Questionnaire Items (a: for mothers).

(Response Efficacy)
1. Encouraging my daughter is an effective way to get her to talk to her doctor about the HPV vaccine.
2. Encouraging my daughter would work in having her talk to her doctor about the HPV vaccine.
3. Encouraging my daughter would help my daughter talk to her doctor about the HPV vaccine.

(Self-Efficacy)

4. It would be easy for me to encourage my daughter to talk to her doctor about the HPV vaccine.

5. It would be simple for me to encourage my daughter to talk to her doctor about the HPV vaccine.

6. I would be comfortable encouraging my daughter to talk to her doctor about the HPV vaccine.

(Susceptibility)

7. My daughter is at high risk for getting HPV.

8. It is likely that my daughter will get HPV.

9. There is a high chance that my daughter will get HPV.

(Severity)

10. If my daughter were to get HPV it would be a very serious threat to her quality of life.

11. If my daughter were to get HPV it would be a very severe threat to her health.

12. If my daughter were to get HPV it would be harmful to her well-being.

Table 3b. Krieger and Sarge's Questionnaire Items (a: for daughters).

(Response Efficacy)

1. Talking to my health care provider would help me make a good decision about whether or not to get the HPV vaccine.

2. Talking to my health care provider would work in making a good decision about whether or not to get the HPV vaccine.

3. Talking to my health care provider would be an effective way to make a good decision about whether or not to get the HPV vaccine.

(Self-Efficacy)

4. It would be easy for me to talk to a parent/guardian about getting the HPV vaccine.

5. It would be simple for me to talk to a parent/guardian about getting the HPV vaccine.

6. I would be comfortable talking to a parent/guardian about getting the HPV vaccine.

(Susceptibility)

7. I am at high risk for getting HPV.

8. I am likely to get HPV.

9. My chances of getting HPV are high.

(Severity)
10. HPV is a serious threat to my quality of life.
11. HPV would be a severe threat to my health.
12. HPV would be harmful to my well-being.

In Popova's (2014) study (a partial replication), levels of threat and efficacy were measured on continuous scales and they were then used to predict the dependent variables–attitudes and behavioral intentions to use novel smokeless tobacco products. A nationally representative probability-based sample of 1,836 adult smokers participated in an online pretest-posttest experiment. All participants completed the reduced RBD scale via both a pretest and posttest.

To measure perceived threat, this study combined perceived severity and perceived susceptibility. Perceived severity was measured by two items (pretest α = .90, posttest α = .91). Similarly, perceived susceptibility was measured by two items (pretest α = .95, posttest α = .96). In order to operationalize perceived efficacy, the author combined individual items of response efficacy and self-efficacy. While perceived response efficacy was measured by two items (pretest α = .74, posttest α = .87), self-efficacy was measured with one item.

Table 4. Popova's (2014) 7 Item Instrument.

(Response Efficacy)
1. Staying away from snus is effective in preventing cancer.
2. If I do not use snus, I am less likely to develop health risks.
(Self-Efficacy)
3. It is easy for me to stay away from new smokeless tobacco products, such as snus.
(Susceptibility)
4. I am at risk of developing cancer from using snus.
5. It is likely that my health will suffer from using snus.
(Severity)
6. How harmful new smokeless tobacco products, such as snus, are for general health.
7. To what extent new smokeless tobacco products cause heart attack, cancer, and oral cancer.

Basil and colleagues conducted three consecutive studies with a reduced item set: 1) a content analysis examining the use of EPPM factors in actual workplace safety messages, 2) an experiment testing these messages with 212 construction trainees, 3) a replicated experiment with 1,802 men across four English-speaking countries (Basil, Basil, Deshpande, & Lavack, 2013). Their approach was unique in that its first study consisted of a content analysis of English-language safety communications materials from government departments and occupational health and safety organizations across North America. In their final study, a two-by-two repeated measures experiment was utilized to assess people's reactions to workplace safety messages in the form of safety posters. To operationalize threat, the authors combined severity and susceptibility. The perceived severity of the messages was assessed with two items (α = .88). In a similar manner susceptibility was assessed with two items (α = .81). In measuring efficacy, the authors combined individual items of response efficacy and self-efficacy (total four, two from each construct; α = .91). It is also interesting to note that the researchers did not include contextualization within the measurement items as is typically done. This was feasible due to the clear contextualization provided by the treatment materials.

Table 5. Basil et al. (2013) 8 Item Instrument.

(Response Efficacy)
1. Doing what the ad suggests will prevent the negative outcome.
2. The ad suggests an effective behavior in getting rid of serious consequences.

(Self-Efficacy)
3. I am able to do what the advertisement suggests.
4. I am capable of preventing the problem this advertisement shows.

(Susceptibility)
5. I am at risk for the negative outcome.
6. This problem could easily apply to me.

(Severity)
7. The negative outcome has serious consequences.
8. I believe this issue could be very severe.

Use of Existing Measures and Future Studies

In this review we have examined the creation and development of a single scale measure designed to serve three distinct but related purposes. The RBDS can be used to provide clinical insight into the orientation of a single patient toward a health threat and preventive measures. It may be used in the same way to estimate population (audience) orientations or it may be used experimentally to test and develop targeted health communications. Further, it has been designed in a manner to make it easily adaptable to a wide range of health threats and recommended responses. In this manner the RBDS is a remarkably flexible tool for health communication researchers and practitioners alike.

An ongoing challenge in both research and applied work lies in respondent burden. Survey questionnaires face logistical limitations on length and many clinical environments have strong limitations on time for client contact. It is no surprise then that the RBD Scale has been parsed into smaller discrete units to examine only select concepts and/or to employ fewer item measures per concept (even single items). The broad application of the scale in these modified approaches also provides the researcher or practitioner with ample guidance and demonstration of effective application in this circumstance. Future work might be undertaken to statistically analyze such studies in order to make specific recommendations on a reduced scale.

Recommended Readings

Choi, H. J., Krieger, J. L., & Hecht, M. L. (2013). Reconceptualizing efficacy in substance use prevention research: refusal response efficacy and drug resistance self-efficacy in adolescent substance use. *Health Communication, 28*(1), 40–52.

Krieger, J. L., & Sarge, M. A. (2013). A serial mediation model of message framing on intentions to receive the human papillomavirus (HPV) vaccine: Revisiting the role of threat and efficacy perceptions. *Health Communication, 28*(1), 5–19.

Napper, L. E., Harris, P. R., & Klein, W. M. P. (2014). Combining Self-Affirmation With the extended parallel process model: The consequences for motivation to eat more Fruit and Vegetables. *Health Communication, 29*(6), 610–618.

Roberto, A. J., Eden, J., Savage, M. W., Ramos-Salazar, L., & Deiss, D. M. (2014). Outcome evaluation results of school-based cybersafety promotion and cyberbullying prevention intervention for middle school students. *Health Communication, 29*(10), 1029–1042.

References

Basil, M., Basil, D., Deshpande, S., & Lavack, A. M. (2013). Applying the extended parallel process model to workplace safety messages. *Health Communication, 28*(1), 29–39.

Krieger, J. L., & Sarge, M. A. (2013). A serial mediation model of message framing on intentions to receive the human papillomavirus (HPV) vaccine: Revisiting the role of threat and efficacy perceptions. *Health Communication, 28*(1), 5–19.

Popova, L. (2014). Scaring the snus out of smokers: Testing effects of fear, threat, and efficacy on smokers' acceptance of novel smokeless tobacco products. *Health Communication, 29*(9), 924–936.

Will, K. E., Sabo, C. S., & Porter, B. E. (2009). Evaluation of the Boost'em in the Back Seat Program: Using fear and efficacy to increase booster seat use. *Accident Analysis and Prevention, 41*(1), 57–65.

Witte, K., & Allen, M. (2000). A meta-analysis of fear appeals: Implications for effective public health campaigns. *Health Education & Behavior, 27*(5), 591–615.

Witte, K., Cameron, K. A., McKeon, J. K., & Berkowitz, J. M. (1996). Predicting risk behaviors: Development and validation of a diagnostic scale. *Journal of Health Communication, 1*(4), 317–342.

Witte, K., Meyer, G., & Martell, D. (2001). The risk behavior diagnosis scale. In K. Witte, G. Meyer, & D. Martell, *Effective Health Risk Messages* (pp. 67–76). Thousand Oaks, CA: Sage.

19. Risk Perception Attitude (RPA) Framework

Computing the Four Attitudinal Groups

ERIN L. MEAD,
University of Maryland
RAJIV N. RIMAL,
George Washington University

In health communication, fear appeals constitute a popular persuasive approach for promoting behavior change. Several theories propose that fear can be used to motivate individuals to change behavior by increasing perceptions of the severity of and their susceptibility to diseases and risk factors (for a review see: Peters, Ruiter, & Kok, 2013; Witte & Allen, 2000). For example, in the health belief model (Janz & Becker, 1984) and protection motivation theory (Rogers, 1975) perceived risk is a significant predictor of an individual's likelihood of taking preventive action. However, fear appeals can backfire. When faced with a threat that increases fear and risk perceptions, individuals either attempt to control the perceived danger through the recommended behavior change (called "danger control response") or to reduce their fear through defensive avoidance or opposition (called "fear control response").

As part of the extended parallel process model, Witte (1992) showed that the nature of the response to a fear appeal is based on self-efficacy and response efficacy beliefs. First introduced by Bandura (1977), self-efficacy is defined as individuals' perceptions of their ability to successfully perform a behavior. Response efficacy is defined as individuals' perceptions of the effectiveness of a behavior in reducing their risk. Fear appeal messages lead to danger control processes when coupled with messages designed to increase self-efficacy and response efficacy beliefs; without an efficacy message, individuals are more likely to engage in fear control processes (Witte & Allen, 2000).

Derived from the extended parallel process model, the risk perception attitude (RPA) framework posits that the association between risk perceptions and behaviors is best understood in the context of individuals' efficacy beliefs (Rimal & Real, 2003). Whereas the extended parallel process model focuses on threat and efficacy as properties of messages, risk perceptions and efficacy beliefs are conceptualized as person-level variables in the RPA framework. Presence of threat and efficacy messages in the media can enhance individuals' risk perceptions and efficacy beliefs, and thereby motivate behavior change. However, risk perceptions and efficacy beliefs can be enhanced from sources in addition to the media, including discussions with other individuals, personal contemplation, and past experiences.

According to the RPA framework, individuals' responses toward behavior change communications can be classified according to their risk perceptions and efficacy beliefs. Risk perceptions have two dimensions: perceptions of the severity of harm from the disease or risk factor (called "perceived severity") and perceptions of susceptibility to that disease or risk factor (called "perceived susceptibility"). Efficacy beliefs also comprise two dimensions: confidence in one's ability to successfully perform a recommended behavioral action (called "self-efficacy belief") and perceived effectiveness of the recommended behavioral action to reduce or eliminate the risk (called "response efficacy belief"). A self-efficacy belief is not invariant across behaviors and contexts; rather, it fluctuates according to specific behaviors and situations (Maibach & Murphy, 1995). For example, a woman who is self-efficacious in her ability to use a condom with every sexual encounter to prevent sexually transmitted diseases might or might not be self-efficacious in her ability to quit smoking. Moreover, self-efficacy is tied to situations; the same woman is likely more confident in her ability to quit smoking when in a group of nonsmokers than when socializing with friends who are smoking. Individuals who perceive high risk and feel efficacious are likely to view the potential risks as challenges to overcome, whereas individuals who perceive high risk but have low efficacy are likely to hold fatalistic attitudes toward their vulnerability.

Based on risk perceptions and efficacy beliefs, the RPA framework categorizes individuals into four attitudinal groups. First, those who perceive high risk and hold high efficacy beliefs are characterized by a *responsive attitude*. Realizing the risks, believing they have the ability to avert the impending threat, and believing the recommended action will be effective, these individuals are the most motivated to engage in self-protective behavior. Second, those who perceive high risk but have low efficacy beliefs are characterized as having an *avoidance attitude*. Although motivated to take action through their awareness of the risks, they are less motivated than those with a responsive attitude to adopt the recommended action because of low confidence in their ability. They are more likely to try to remove their fear through denial of their risk or avoidance of the issue. Third, individuals who perceive low risk but hold strong efficacy beliefs are characterized by a *proactive attitude*. They are more motivated to take action by their desire for prevention rather than their perceived risk status. Fourth, those with low risk perceptions and low efficacy beliefs are characterized by an *indifference attitude* and are the least likely to take the recommended action. These individuals do not believe they are at risk and/or that the risk is severe and, even if they did believe in the risk, they do not believe they have the ability to avert the threat.

The formulation of the four attitudinal groups is useful for predicting individuals' motivations and self-protective behaviors as well as for audience segmentation purposes (Rimal & Real, 2003). Segmenting the audience based on key characteristics is useful for tailoring health communication campaigns and programs specific to the needs of the target audience. For example, a campaign aimed at promoting a behavior change among the avoidance group could emphasize efficacy information; similarly, a campaign directed at the proactive group may focus on enhancing risk perceptions.

The RPA framework has been tested across a variety of health behaviors, including climate change information seeking (Mead et al., 2012), HIV/AIDS prevention (Rimal et al., 2009), influenza vaccination (Real, Kim, & Conigliaro, 2013), breast cancer prevention (Rimal & Juon, 2010), breast cancer information seeking (Lee, Hwang, Hawkins, & Pingree, 2008), diabetes information seeking (Turner, Rimal, Morrison, & Kim, 2006), workplace safety (Real, 2008), food safety (Kennedy, Worosz, Todd, & Lapinski, 2008), skin cancer prevention (Turner et al., 2006), and nutrition promotion (Sullivan, Beckjord, Rutten, & Hesse, 2008). These studies illustrate different options for the measurement of risk perceptions, efficacy beliefs, and the four RPA attitudinal groups according to the needs of the study, which will be discussed in the next section.

Measuring Risk Perception Attitude

Measures of the RPA groups were first developed by Rimal and Real (2003) to study the influence of risk perceptions and efficacy beliefs on the salience of the issue of skin cancer, information seeking about skin cancer, and skin cancer-related behaviors. In the first phase of the study, the authors developed and tested the initial set of questions to capture individuals' risk perceptions and efficacy beliefs through an experimental manipulation of perceived risk and efficacy beliefs with regard to skin cancer. For the second phase, the authors finalized the questions through the results of the first phase and feed-back from the pilot test of the survey instrument. For risk perceptions, three questions asked participants about their vulnerability to skin cancer in the next year, two years, and five years on a 10-point Likert scale. For efficacy beliefs, three questions asked participants about their self-efficacy, or confidence to perform a preventive behavior, and three questions asked about the response efficacy of each behavior on a 5-point Likert scale. See Table 1 for the survey questions.

Table 1. Scales to Measure Risk Perceptions and Efficacy Beliefs, from Rimal & Real (2003) and Rimal & Juon (2010).

Survey Questions	Responses
Risk Perceptions: Perceived Susceptibility *"How likely are you to get [name of disease] in…"*	
1. the next year? 2. the next two years? 3. the next five years?	1–5 or 0–9 scale, ranging from "not at all likely" to "extremely likely"
Risk Perceptions: Perceived Severity *"If you got [name of disease],"*	
1. how deadly would it be?	1–7 scale, ranging from "not at all deadly" to "extremely deadly"
2. it would destroy both me and my family.	1–7 scale, ranging from strongly disagree to strongly agree
3. it would be impossible to recover from.	1–7 scale, ranging from strongly disagree to strongly agree
Self-Efficacy Beliefs (context of skin cancer prevention): *"How confident are you that you could…"*	
1. wear sunscreen each time you went out in the sun? 2. wear protective clothing each time you went out in the sun? 3. limit your time in the sun?	0–9 scale, ranging from not at all confident to extremely confident

Survey Questions	Responses
Response-Efficacy Beliefs (context of skin cancer prevention): *"If you performed each action, how effective would be it be preventing skin cancer?"*	
1. if you wore sunscreen each time you went out in the sun 2. if you wore protective clothing each time you went out in the sun 3. if you limited your time in the sun	0–9 scale, ranging from not at all effective to extremely effective

In the first step of the analysis, *perceived risk* was calculated by averaging the three responses to the perceived susceptibility questions (Rimal & Real, 2003). The Cronbach's alpha indicated high internal reliability ($\alpha = 0.96$). A high- and a low-risk group were calculated through a median split of the averaged score. In other words, the median value was calculated and used as the cut-off point to create the two groups. In the second step of the analysis, the self-efficacy and response efficacy scores were multiplied for each behavior separately, and then the three behaviors were averaged to create one *efficacy belief* score. The Cronbach's alpha indicated moderate internal reliability ($\alpha = 0.76$). A high- and a low-efficacy group were calculated through a median split of the averaged score. In the final step of the analysis, the four RPA groups were created from the risk perceptions and efficacy scores. Those who fell into both the low risk group and the low efficacy group were categorized as having an *indifference attitude*, while those who fell into both the low risk group and the high efficacy group were categorized as having a *proactive attitude*. Those who fell into both the high risk group and the high efficacy group were categorized as having a *responsive attitude*, while those who fell into both the high risk group and the low efficacy group were categorized as having an *avoidance attitude*.

In a subsequent study (Rimal & Juon, 2010), the perceived risk variable included both perceived severity and perceived susceptibility and the efficacy variable included both self-efficacy and response efficacy. These two variables were left as continuous variables in regression models. The four RPA framework groups were obtained through the interaction analysis method recommended by Aiken and West (1991). This method analyzes the relationship between risk perception and a behavioral variable at two levels of efficacy beliefs—one standard deviation above the mean (characterized as high efficacy) and one standard deviation below the mean (characterized as low efficacy) and allows the depiction of the four RPA framework groups (see Rimal & Juon, 2010, Figure 1).

Extending the above work, Mead et al. (2012) applied the RPA framework to adolescents' seeking of information about climate change by investigating: (a) the correlation between adolescents' and their parents' RPA attitudinal groups; (b) the association between adolescents' RPA attitudinal groups and their information seeking behaviors; and (c) the role of parents' RPA attitudinal groups in their adolescents' information seeking. Perceived risk was conceptualized as perceived severity, and a score was created from the mean of eight questions that asked respondents how much they thought global warming would harm different individuals or groups (e.g., themselves, their family, future generations) on a 4-point Likert scale. Efficacy beliefs were conceptualized as response efficacy, that is, the effectiveness of specific human activities to mitigate climate change, based on two questions. See Table 2 for the survey questions.

Table 2. Mead et al.'s Scale to Measure Risk Perceptions and Efficacy Beliefs.

Survey Questions	Responses
Risk Perceptions (Perceived Severity)	
How much do you think global warming will harm:	(1) Not at all, (2) Only a little, (3) A moderate amount, (4) A great deal
1. You personally?	
2. Your family?	
3. Your community?	
4. People in the United States?	
5. People in other modern industrialized countries?	
6. People in developing countries?	
7. Future generations of people?	
8. Plant and animal species?	
Response-Efficacy Beliefs	
1. Thinking about the energy-saving actions you're already taking and those you'd like to take over the next 12 months: If you did most of these things, how much do you think it would reduce your personal contribution to global warming?	(1) Not at all, (2) A little, (3) Some, (4) A lot

Survey Questions	Responses
2. If most people in the United States did these same actions, how much would it reduce global warming?	

In the first stage of the analysis, "don't know" and missing responses were mean imputed for each question. In the second stage of the analysis, the eight perceived severity questions were averaged into an index of *perceived risk* for parents and adolescents. The Cronbach's alpha indicated high internal reliability for both parents ($\alpha = 0.97$) and adolescents ($\alpha = 0.95$). In the third stage of the analysis, the two response efficacy questions were averaged into an index of *efficacy beliefs* for parents and adolescents. The Cronbach's alpha indicated moderate internal reliability for both parents ($\alpha = 0.79$) and adolescents ($\alpha = 0.75$). In the fourth stage of the analysis, the four RPA framework groups were formulated by conducting a cluster analysis of the risk and efficacy variables. The cluster analysis created four groups that maximized the differences in risk and efficacy among them.

Use of Existing Measures and Future Studies

Based on the description provided in this chapter, we can identify three methods for creating the four RPA framework groups (responsive, avoidance, proactive, and indifference) from people's risk perception and efficacy belief scores. In the first method, the two scores are simply subjected to median splits, thus creating high-risk and low-risk groups and high-efficacy and low-efficacy groups. Through cross-tabulations, the four groups are then identified. This method, while simple and intuitive, suffers from the limitation about threshold assumptions—the idea that a person right below the median is somehow qualitatively different from another person right above the median on one of the two variables. The second method uses one of the two variables (say, risk perception) as the independent variable and the other (efficacy belief) as the moderator in a regression equation. The "high" and "low" groups are then delineated by separating into values that are one standard deviation above the mean and one standard deviation below the mean. This method is considered superior on many counts (see Aiken & West, 1991), but it requires that the risk and efficacy variables first show an interaction effect; if not, we cannot create the four distinct RPA framework groups. A cluster analysis is the third method through which the four RPA framework groups can be delineated. This method is also superior to the median-split method, but it introduces an element of artificiality, in that it maximizes the difference in risk and efficacy values. So, which of these methods is preferable? We recommend the regression method, provided there is a significant risk perception x efficacy belief interaction. If not, the cluster method will also likely yield meaningful results. We recommend the use of the median split method for illustrative (not hypothesis-testing) purposes only.

This chapter reviewed scales that have been used across a variety of health domains to measure risk perceptions and efficacy beliefs following the RPA framework. Building upon the Rimal and Real (2003) study, researchers have adapted the measures to fit the needs of their studies. For example, Rimal and Real (2003) used one question to measure self-efficacy to prevent cancer and one question to measure perceived susceptibility of cancer, and created the RPA groups using a median split. Sullivan et al. (2008) averaged measures of perceived severity and susceptibility to create the risk perceptions score about diabetes and averaged measures of self-efficacy and response efficacy to create the efficacy beliefs score about diabetes prevention. The authors created the four RPA framework groups through a four-group cluster analysis. In their study of influenza vaccinations among health care personnel, Turner et al. (2006) measured self-efficacy to perform protective behaviors and perceived vulnerability to influenza, and created the four RPA framework groups using a k-means cluster analysis with perceived vulnerability and self-efficacy as the clustering variables.

As these examples illustrate, future studies can adapt existing measures of efficacy beliefs and risk perceptions to the needs of their study. Measures should be adapted to be specific to the disease, health risks, and related be-haviors of interest to the study. The number of questions asked to capture the constructs can be determined by the needs (and constraints) of the study. Moreover, researchers can determine which dimensions of efficacy beliefs (that is, self-efficacy and/or response efficacy) and risk perceptions (that is, perceived severity and/or perceived susceptibility) are most relevant to cap-ture for their study. In addition, RPA groups can be calculated in a variety of ways, including median splits, cluster analysis, and regression analysis.

Recommended Readings

Mead, E., Roser-Renouf, C., Rimal, R. N., Flora, J. A., Maibach, E. W., & Leiserowitz, A. (2012). Information seeking about global climate change among adolescents: The role of risk perceptions, efficacy beliefs and parental influences. *Atlantic Journal of Communication, 20*(1), 31–52.

Rimal, R. N., Brown, J., Mkandawire, G., Folda, L., Böse, K., & Creel, A. H. (2009). Audience segmentation as a social-marketing tool in health promotion: Use of the risk perception attitude framework in HIV prevention in Malawi. *American Journal of Public Health, 99*(12), 2224–2229.

Rimal, R. N., & Real, K. (2003). Perceived risk and efficacy beliefs as motivators of change. *Human Communication Research, 29*(3), 370–399.

Smith, R. A., Greenberg, M., & Parrott, R. L. (2014). Segmenting by risk perceptions: Predicting young adults' genetic-belief profiles with health and opinion-leader covariates. *Health Communication, 29*(5), 483–493.

Witte, K., & Allen, M. (2000). A meta-analysis of fear appeals: Implications for effective public health campaigns. *Health Education and Behavior, 27*(5), 591–615.

References

Aiken, L. S., & West, S. G. (1991). *Multiple regression: Testing and interpreting interactions.* Newbury Park, CA: Sage.

Bandura, A. (1977). Self-efficacy: Toward a unifying theory of behavioral change. *Psychological Review, 84*(2), 191–215. doi: 10.1037//0033-295x.84.2.191.

Janz, N. K., & Becker, M. H. (1984). The health belief model: A decade later. *Health Education and Behavior, 11*(1), 1–47. doi: 10.1177/109019818401100101.

Kennedy, J., Worosz, M., Todd, E. C., & Lapinski, M. K. (2008). Segmentation of US consumers based on food safety attitudes. *British Food Journal, 110*(7), 691–705. doi: doi:10.1108/00070700810887167.

Lee, S. Y., Hwang, H., Hawkins, R., & Pingree, S. (2008). Interplay of negative emotion and health self-efficacy on the use of health information and its outcomes. *Communication Research, 35*(3), 358–381. doi: 10.1177/0093650208315962.

Maibach, E., & Murphy, D. A. (1995). Self-efficacy in health promotion research and practice: Conceptualization and measurement. *Health Education Research, 10*(1), 37–50. doi: 10.1093/her/10.1.37.

Mead, E., Roser-Renouf, C., Rimal, R. N., Flora, J. A., Maibach, E. W., & Leiserowitz, A. (2012). Information seeking about global climate change among adolescents: The role of risk perceptions, efficacy beliefs and parental influences. *Atlantic Journal of Communication, 20*(1), 31–52. doi: 10.1080/15456870.2012.637027.

Peters, G. J. Y., Ruiter, R. A. C., & Kok, G. (2013). Threatening communication: A critical re-analysis and a revised meta-analytic test of fear appeal theory. *Health Psychology Review, 7*(SUPPL1), S8-S31. doi: 10.1080/17437199.2012.703527.

Real, K. (2008). Information seeking and workplace safety: A field application of the risk perception attitude framework. *Journal of Applied Communication Research, 36*(3), 339–359. doi: 10.1080/00909880802101763.

Real, K., Kim, S., & Conigliaro, J. (2013). Using a validated health promotion tool to improve patient safety and increase health care personnel influenza vaccination rates. *American Journal of Infection Control, 41*(8), 691–696. doi: 10.1016/j. ajic.2012.09.027.

Rimal, R. N., Brown, J., Mkandawire, G., Folda, L., Böse, K., & Creel, A. H. (2009). Audience segmentation as a social-marketing tool in health promotion: Use of the risk perception attitude framework in HIV prevention in Malawi. *American Journal of Public Health, 99*(12), 2224–2229. doi: 10.2105/ajph.2008.155234.

Rimal, R. N., & Juon, II. S. (2010). Use of the risk perception attitude framework for promoting breast cancer prevention. *Journal of Applied Social Psychology, 40*(2), 287–310. doi: 10.1111/j.1559-1816.2009.00574.x.

Rimal, R. N., & Real, K. (2003). Perceived risk and efficacy beliefs as motivators of change. *Human Communication Research, 29*(3), 370–399. doi: 10.1111/j.1468-2958.2003.tb00844.x.

Rogers, R. W. (1975). A protection motivation theory of fear appeals and attitude change. *The Journal of Psychology: Interdisciplinary and Applied, 91*(1), 93–114. doi: 10.1080/00223980.1975.9915803.

Sullivan, H. W., Beckjord, E. B., Rutten, L. J. F., & Hesse, B. W. (2008). Nutrition-related cancer prevention cognitions and behavioral intentions: Testing the risk perception attitude framework. *Health Education and Behavior, 35*(6), 866–879. doi: 10.1177/1090198108326164.

Turner, M. M., Rimal, R. N., Morrison, D., & Kim, H. (2006). The role of anxiety in seeking and retaining risk information: Testing the risk perception attitude framework in two studies. *Human Communication Research, 32*(2), 130–156. doi: 10.1111/j.1468-2958.2006.00006.x.

Witte, K. (1992). Putting the fear back into fear appeals: The extended parallel process model. *Communication Monographs, 59*(4), 329–349. doi: 10.1080/03637759209376276.

Witte, K., & Allen, M. (2000). A meta-analysis of fear appeals: Implications for effective public health campaigns. *Health Education and Behavior, 27*(5), 591–615. doi: 10.1177/109019810002700506.

20. Self-Efficacy

NICHOLE EGBERT,
Kent State University
& PHILLIP R. REED,
Kent State University

Albert Bandura (1977) pioneered the concept of self-efficacy as a "unifying theory of behavioral change" (p. 91) and based on the state of behavioral theory nearly 50 years later he did not overstate his case. Self-efficacy has become a key component of nearly every theory of behavior change used by social scientists, including the theory of planned behavior (Ajzen, 1991), protection motivation theory (Maddux & Rogers, 1983), the health belief model (Rosenstock, Strecher, & Becker, 1988), and the extended parallel process model (Witte, 1992). It might be said that no other single concept has had such an impact on predicting and promoting behavioral change through communication messages as self-efficacy. Self-efficacy is defined as a person's perceived ability to execute a specific behavior in a specific situation, and should not be misconstrued as a general trait or personality characteristic (Strecher, DeVellis, Becker, & Rosenstock, 1986).

Bandura argued that self-efficacy beliefs are highly context specific (1977); they depend not only upon the specific skill needed to complete a task, but also upon the perceived difficulty of that skill and the context in which the skill is carried out. Therefore, items in a self-efficacy measure must be tailored specifically to the skill relevant to the study outcomes. Whether adapting an existing measure or designing an entirely new one, there are several considerations that are key to effective measures of self-efficacy (beyond the usual psychometric concerns). In constructing items for a measure of self-efficacy, the designer must ensure that the items: 1) address the full spectrum of the domain of activity, 2) reflect the degree of task difficulty expected, and 3) avoid incorporating related constructs (Bandura, 2006).

Measuring Self-Efficacy

Multidimensionality of the Skill or Activity

As efficacy is domain specific, rather than a global concept (Bandura, 1977), efficacy measures must be similarly specific. The scale designer must ensure that the items are tailored to the domain of functioning. However, it is also important that the domain of activity is fully covered, rather than assuming the functional domain to be unidimensional (Bandura, 2006). To ensure a comprehensive assessment, the measure should address all relevant aspects of efficacy that pertain to the domain. For instance, Ryan et al. (2013) developed a measure to test the three types of efficacy perceptions of junior physicians in regard to prescribing medication: filling out prescriptions (e.g., "I can write the prescription legibly"), making decisions about appropriate medication (e.g., "I can decide on the most appropriate dose"), and requesting help when necessary (e.g., "I can ask for help with prescribing if necessary"). In addition to providing a comprehensive test of the functional domain of prescription writing, the multiple dimensions allow for more fine-grained analyses and specific recommendations.

Multi-dimensional self-efficacy scales have a number of benefits. In early phases of measure design, separate analysis of each dimension permits flaws in one dimension's measurement to be identified individually. Those specific items can be corrected or abandoned while retaining useful dimensions. Another benefit is that with appropriate pre-testing, researchers can determine relationships between the various dimensions. A longitudinal investigation may reveal that efficacy in one dimension relies on efficacy in another (to extend the Ryan et al., 2013, example, the decision-making dimension might rely on such other dimensions as recall of medication particulars or use of medication databases). Finally, multiple dimensions of self-efficacy can identify more specific relationships between variables. For example, although it is helpful to determine in general that efficacy in prescribing medication predicts errors in prescriptions, it is more useful to know if the greatest contributor to low prescribing efficacy is a physician's lack of confidence that he or she can ask for help.

Difficulty of Task

Specificity of task difficulty is equally as important as specificity of dimension. Items in a self-efficacy measure should specify standards of functional ability (Bandura, 2006). Without incorporating differences in the magnitude of difficulty, efficacy assessments may fail to differentiate the population under study (Bandura, 1977). Setting extremely high levels of function can result in persons with moderate perceptions of efficacy reporting very low efficacy scores. Conversely, low levels of function are considered achievable by most persons, greatly reducing the variance found in the population. However, incorporating extremes of difficulty still has value, particularly in longitudinal studies of intervention training or mastery development. Bandura (1977) noted that strong efficacy beliefs persist despite failure to perform the relevant function. Weak beliefs, however, are destroyed with far fewer disconfirming experiences. The strength of belief is tied inextricably to the magnitude of the task's difficulty. Even persons with a strong belief in their efficacy to drive a car are unlikely to have a similarly strong belief in their ability to execute a bootleg turn on ice with two flat tires. Thus, a study investigating emergency vehicle drivers may find such an item useful, whereas a more general study on driver preparedness would not.

Low difficulty items are of more general value. Failure in a low difficulty task is more likely to impact perceptions of self-efficacy negatively, particularly for persons with weak efficacy beliefs. Low efficacy beliefs for simple tasks suggest that confidence is needed for fundamental skills in the domain. This is particularly valuable information for the development and design of training or intervention exercises. Vishwanath (2007; see Figure 1) provided a good example of providing a specific level of task difficulty. In developing a unidimensional measure of efficacy in general information searches, Vishwanath specified precise conditions under which the function is enacted. All items begin with the stem phrase "You can search for information on _____," and then indicate a specific barrier to information searching (e.g., "without help"). This specificity of function difficulty reduces the impact of error related to differences in individual experiences with a functional domain. Thus, with specific obstacles included in the items, one person's memories of information searches with available help and another person's memories of searches with neither help nor computer access generate less unexplained variance in their self-efficacy scores.

Figure 1. Information Search Efficacy (Vishwanath, 2007).

You can search for information on _____ even if you know nothing about the topic.
You can search for information on _____ without help from anyone.
You can search for information on _____ if no one showed you how to search for the information.
You can search for information on _____ if you had no access to computing technology such as the Internet or personal computers.
You can search for information on _____ even if the information is not available online.

Conceptual Validity

In addition to ensuring that the measure is comprehensive in scope yet tailored to the skill under investigation, it is also important that items in a self-efficacy measure do not incorporate related constructs (Bandura, 2006). For instance, self-efficacy is often confused with outcome expectancy. Efficacy is strictly about one's perceived ability to perform a specific function. Outcome expectancy is instead a prediction about the consequences of performing, or failing to perform, that function. Both of these constructs are important determinants of goals and impact behavioral intention, but they are not predicted to do so in the same manner (Bandura, 1986). Behavioral intention is less likely to be confused with self-efficacy conceptually, however, imprecise wording of items can cause respondents to confuse the two constructs (Bandura, 2006). Efficacy measures should rely on statements of what the person "can do" rather than what he or she "will do." Efficacy and "can" refer to an individual's capability. Intention and "will" are predictions of expected behavior.

A study of self-efficacy beliefs regarding pelvic floor exercise following surgery illustrates the preceding distinctions (Burkert, Knoll, Scholz, Roigas, & Gralla, 2012). The various dimensions of efficacy in this domain are measured with specific items such as, "I am confident that I can return to regular pelvic floor exercise even if I have relapsed several times." These items are distinct from other measures that address outcome expectancies ("If I perform pelvic floor exercise regularly then I can do something about the incontinence"), behavioral intentions ("I intend to perform pelvic floor exercise several times a week"), and action planning ("I have made a detailed plan regarding how I will perform pelvic floor exercise"). Such specificity is not only necessary to measure self-efficacy accurately, but also indicates a number of related constructs that are useful in judging the validity of one's own efficacy measures.

These particular concerns of self-efficacy measures should guide a researcher in developing or adapting scales. The importance of incorporating the entirety of a function's domain, the function's difficulty, and avoiding related constructs, should support and strengthen standard tests of validity and reliability. In some cases, however, researchers wish to capture a slightly more general set of health behaviors, and for that reason, the following section highlights a measure of self-efficacy in health promotion, along with its relevant psychometrics.

Self-Rated Abilities for Health Practices Scale

The Self-Rated Abilities for Health Practices Scale (SRAHPS; Becker, Stuifbergen, Oh, & Hall, 1993) is designed to measure self-perceived ability in implementing health promotion behaviors. It provides an excellent example of a self-efficacy measure tailored to a specific functional domain and is psychometrically robust. The SRAHPS specifically addresses nutrition, exercise, psychological well-being, and health responsibility (acquiring information and assistance). Although the measure is designed specifically for health promotion, the general nature of each of the four areas makes this measure well-suited to adaptation across many health contexts.

The SRAHPS (Becker et al., 1993) was designed to measure consistent self-efficacy, rather than changes in efficacy following an intervention. The scale has been used with populations of adults with disabilities (Stuifbergen & Becker, 1994), older adults' self-care (Callaghan, 2003, 2005), and self-efficacy of family caregivers (Acton, 2002). Other researchers have used the SRAHPS to study self-efficacy following interventions in contexts ranging from adults with multiple sclerosis (Ennis, Thain, Boggild, Baker, & Young, 2006) to older adults living in Iranian villages (Hosseini, Torkani, & Tavakol, 2013).

The SRAHPS (Becker et al., 1993) consists of 28 items; four areas with 7 items in each area. Respondents rate each item on how well they are able to perform the behavior on a 5-point scale, anchored at 0 (Not at all) and 4 (Completely). To ensure that self-efficacy is the construct truly being measured, it is important that researchers make clear to the respondents that each item is understood to begin with "I am able to…" This can be accomplished through a note at the beginning of the measure, a note prior to each area, or by actually inserting the words before each item. The SRAHPS can be scored as a global index, summing the ratings of all items, or as an index of each area, summing only the 7 items for that area.

Figure 2. Self-Rated Abilities for Health Practices Scale Items and Subscales.

Nutrition: I am able to

Find healthy foods that are within my budget
Eat a balanced diet
Figure out how much I should weigh to be healthy
Tell which foods are high in fiber content
Figure out from labels which foods are good for me
Drink as much water as I need to drink every day
Brush my teeth regularly

Exercise: I am able to

Do exercises that are good for me
Fit exercise into my regular routine
Find ways to exercise that I enjoy

      Find accessible places for me to exercise in the community
      Know when to quit exercising
      Do stretching exercises
      Keep from getting hurt when I exercise
   Psychological Well-Being: I am able to
      Figure out things I can do to help me relax
      Keep myself from feeling lonely
      Do things that make me feel good about myself
      Avoid being bored
      Talk to friends and family about things that are bothering me
      Figure out how I respond to stress
      Change things in my life to reduce stress
  Health Practices: I am able to
      Figure out where to get information to take care of my health
      Watch for negative changes in my body's condition
      Recognize what symptoms should be reported to a doctor
      Use medication correctly
      Find a doctor who gives me good advice about how to stay healthy
      Know my rights and stand up for myself

      Get help from others when I need it

Overall, the index has demonstrated both validity and reliability across varied populations. A panel of expert reviewers (including health promotion nurses, tool development experts, and nurses in practice with disabled persons) vetted an early form of the SRAHPS (Stuifbergen & Becker, 1994). Content validity was further supported by a pilot test of disabled persons. These pilot tests reduced an initial set of 50 items to the 28 used currently. In its initial development, the SRAHPS (Becker et al., 1993) was tested at a county health fair with undergraduate students and with adults with disabilities recruited through a state advocacy group. Cronbach's alphas measuring reliability ranged from .91 to .94 for the index as a whole. Alphas for the various areas ranged from as low as .76 (for the exercise area among disabled adults) to as high as .92 (for the exercise area among health fair attendees).

Use of Existing Measures and Future Studies

It is not uncommon to hear researchers bemoan the splintered state of a body of literature in which each study employs a unique measure of a seemingly identical construct. This practice can make it difficult to compare results and conduct meta-analyses that move the state of knowledge forward. However, in the case of self-efficacy, it is understandable why so many unique measures exist. Adapting a measure of self-efficacy to the specific health-related behavior is imperative in the determination of the relationship between self-efficacy and the related health outcome. Even in the case of the SRAHPS, as reviewed above, the scope of the health behaviors in the self-efficacy measure should match those of the health outcome. For instance, when Jackson, Tucker, and Herman (2007) employed this measure in their sample of college students, they examined the relationship between self-efficacy in health promotion behaviors and the degree of health-promoting lifestyle. Their study found that health promotion self-efficacy was strongly related to engagement in six dimensions of a healthy lifestyle (spiritual growth, health responsibility, physical activity, nutrition, interpersonal relations, and stress management). Hence, one reason the measure worked was because its scope and specificity level was congruent with the outcome in question. On the other hand, as in the prescription example offered early in this chapter, breaking down a more specific behavior into smaller units is more appropriate when the outcome is the number of prescription errors.

We have provided some guidelines to assist researchers wishing to include self-efficacy measures in future research, as well as providing an example of an easily-adaptable measure that follows these guidelines. When developing new measures, researchers should take care to 1) address the full spectrum of the domain of activity, 2) reflect the degree of task difficulty expected, and 3) avoid incorporating related constructs (Bandura, 2006). As self-efficacy has been shown to be so valuable across domains of health behaviors, both general and specific, appropriate measurement techniques are imperative to capturing its full capacity.

Recommended Readings

Bandura, A. (1977). Self-efficacy: Toward a unifying theory of behavioral change. *Psychological Review, 84,* 191–215.

Bandura, A. (2006). Guide for constructing self-efficacy scales. In F. Pajares & T. Urdan (Eds.), *Self-efficacy beliefs of adolescents. Greenwich,* CT: Information Age Publishing.

Strecher, V. J., DeVellis, B. M., Becker, M. H., & Rosenstock, I. M. (1986). The role of self-efficacy in achieving health behavior change. *Health Education & Behavior, 13,* 73–92.

van der Bijl, J. J., & Shortridge-Baggett, L. M. (2001). The theory and measurement of the self-efficacy construct. *Research and Theory for Nursing Practice, 15*(3), 189–207.

Witte, K. (1992). Putting the fear back into fear appeals: The extended parallel process model. *Communication Monographs, 59,* 329–349.

References

Acton, G. J. (2002). Health-promoting self-care in family caregivers. *Western Journal of Nursing Research, 24,* 73–86.

Ajzen, I. (1991). The theory of planned behavior. *Organizational Behavior and Human Decision Processes, 50*(2), 179–211.

Bandura, A. (1977). Self-efficacy: Toward a unifying theory of behavioral change. *Psychological Review, 84,* 191–215.

Bandura, A. (1982). Self-efficacy mechanism in human agency. *American Psychologist, 37,* 122–147.

Bandura, A. (1986). *Social foundations of thought and action: A social cognitive theory.* Englewood Cliffs, NJ: Prentice-Hall.

Bandura, A. (2006). Guide for constructing self-efficacy scales. In F. Pajares & T. Urdan (Eds.), *Self-efficacy beliefs of adolescents.* Greenwich, CT: Information Age Publishing.

Becker, H., Stuifbergen, A., Oh, H. S., & Hall, S. (1993). Self-rated abilities for health practices: A health self-efficacy measure. *Health Values: The Journal of Health Behavior, Education & Promotion, 17*(5), 42–50.

Burkert, S., Knoll, N., Scholz, U., Roigas, J., & Gralla, O. (2012). Self-regulation following prostatectomy: Phase-specific self-efficacy beliefs for pelvic-floor exercise. *British Journal of Health Psychology, 17,* 273–293.

Callaghan, D. M. (2003). Health-promoting self-care behaviors, self-care self-efficacy, and self-care agency. *Nursing Science Quarterly, 16,* 247–254.

Callaghan, D. (2005). Healthy behaviors, self-efficacy, self-care, and basic conditioning factors in older adults. *Journal of Community Health Nursing, 22,* 169–178.

Ennis, M., Thain, J., Boggild, M., Baker, G. A., & Young, C. A. (2006). A randomized controlled trial of a health promotion education programme for people with multiple sclerosis. *Clinical Rehabilitation, 20,* 783–792.

Hosseini, H., Torkani, S., & Tavakol, K. (2013). The effect of community health nurse home visit self-care self-efficacy of the elderly living in selected Falavarjan villages in Iran in 2010. *Iranian Journal of Nursing and Midwifery Research, 18,* 47–53.

Jackson, E. S., Tucker, C. M., & Herman, K. C. (2007). Health value, perceived social support, and health self-efficacy as factors in a health-promoting lifestyle. *Journal of American College Health, 56*(1), 69–74.

Maddux, J. E., & Rogers, R. W. (1983). Protection motivation and self-efficacy: A revised theory of fear appeals and attitude change. *Journal of Experimental Social Psychology, 19,* 469–479.

Rosenstock, I. M., Strecher, V. J., & Becker, M. H. (1988). Social learning theory and the health belief model. *Health Education & Behavior, 15*(2), 175–183.

Ryan, C., Ross, S., Davey, P., Duncan, E. M., Fielding, S., Francis, J., Johnston, M., Ker, J., Lee, A. J., MacLeod, M. J., Maxwell, S., McKay, G., McLay, J., Webb, D., & Bond, C. (2013). Junior doctors' perceptions of their self-efficacy in prescribing, their prescribing errors and the possible causes of errors. *British Journal of Clinical Pharmacology, 76*, 980–987.

Strecher, V. J., DeVellis, B. M., Becker, M. H., & Rosenstock, I. M. (1986). The role of self-efficacy in achieving health behavior change. *Health Education & Behavior, 13*, 73–92.

Stuifbergen, A. K., & Becker, H. A. (1994). Predictors of health-promoting lifestyles in persons with disabilities. *Research in Nursing & Health, 17*, 3–13.

Vishwanath, A. (2007). Information search efficacy: A new measure and its initial tests. *Communication Research Reports, 24*, 195–203.

Witte, K. (1992). Putting the fear back into fear appeals: The extended parallel process model. *Communication Monographs, 59*, 329–349.

21. *Sensation Seeking*

Scales for Adolescents and Emerging Adults

CLAUDE H. MILLER,
University of Oklahoma

Sensation seeking (SS) (Zuckerman, 1979, 1994) is an arousal-based motivational state of interest to health communication researchers through its association with impulsivity, substance use, unsafe sex, and other forms of risky health behavior. A large research literature has characterized SS as a key personality trait predictive of risk-taking behaviors, particularly among young people (e.g., Arnett, 1998; 2005; Donohew, Lorch, & Palmgreen, 1991; Miller & Quick, 2010; Stephenson & Palmgreen, 2001), that peaks during adolescence (ages 10–18), and remains high throughout emerging adulthood (ages 19–25, Arnett, 2004, 2007). However, beyond emerging adulthood, Zuckerman (1974) reports a negative correlation between age and SS, and Galvan et al. (2007) report a significant negative correlation between chronological age and impulsivity, a construct closely related to SS. Similarly, Steinberg et al. (2008) assert age differences in sensation-seeking follow a curvilinear pattern, with sensation seeking increasing between ages 10 and 15, then remaining stable or declining thereafter.

Originally arising out of sensory deprivation research (Curtis & Zuckerman, 1968; Hocking & Robertson, 1969), SS has been associated with sensory arousal and the need for physical and mental stimulation (Zuckerman, 1979, 1994). Similar to stimulus seeking (Kish & Busse, 1968; Kish & Leahy, 1970), which is associated with exploration, curiosity, experience seeking, and sociability, SS has been measured—both as a set of personality constructs and as an array of risk preferences—using four subscales assessing thrill and adventure seeking, social and sexual disinhibition, experience seeking, and boredom susceptibility (Zuckerman, Eysenck, & Eysenck, 1978).

Zuckerman (1979) has characterized high SS individuals as having a greater sociobiological appetite for novelty and complexity relative to others; and also as more likely to approach novel, risky sources of sensory stimulation, while avoiding mundane, routine, and commonplace experiences. In short, SS is often characterized as the seeking of intense, novel stimuli, typically at the risk of potentially significant social, financial, legal, and physical costs (Zuckerman, 1994).

Within the field of health communication, researchers and policymakers have identified high sensation seekers as the primary targets for a variety of health risk campaigns (Palmgreen, Donohew, & Harrington, 2001). More specifically, Donohew, Lorch, & Palmgreen (1998) have developed the sensation-seeking targeting strategy (SENTAR) for designing risk prevention messages focusing on those features that are most likely to appeal to and resonate with high sensation seeking populations. The SENTAR approach calls for design elements employing vivid images, quick cuts, and fast pacing, along with dynamic movement, and vibrant sound effects to produce what Morgan et al. (2003) refer to as high message sensation value. Relative to low sensation value, messages seen as high in sensation value can prompt deeper processing and more favorable evaluations across an array of outcome variables (Stephenson, 2002, 2003).

Recent SS research has shown individuals' greater need for intensity of stimulation depends on their physiology (Norbury, Manohar, Rogers, & Husain, 2013) as well as the nature of their social environment (Arnett, 1994), with SS being associated with a host of social behaviors, including sexual risk-taking (Donohew et al., 2000; Sheer & Cline, 1995), drug use (Donohew et al., 1991; Stephenson & Palmgreen, 2001), tobacco use (Skara, Sussman, & Dent, 2001), and online gaming dependency (Mehroof & Griffiths, 2010). Research has also demonstrated how SS may interact with other factors and personality traits such as psychological reactance (Miller & Quick, 2010), affect lability and negative urgency (Karyadi, Coskunpinar, Dir, & Cyders, 2013), aggression (Zuckerman, 2007), impulsivity (Donohew et al., 2000; Zuckerman, 2007), and gender (Beck, Thombs, Mahoney, & Fingar, 1995; Stephenson, Hoyle, Palmgreen, & Slater, 2003; Zuckerman et al., 1978) among others (see Zuckerman, 2007).

Measuring Sensation Seeking

One of the most widely used scales for the measurement of SS has been Zuckerman and colleagues' Sensation Seeking Scale (SSS), originally comprised of four subscales developed from item factor analyses within a number of experimental studies. The SSS has gone through numerous revisions (in chronological order: Zuckerman, Kolin, Price, & Zoob, 1964; Zuckerman & Link, 1968; Zuckerman, 1971; Zuckerman, Eysenck and Eysenck, 1978; Zuckerman, 1994; Gray & Wilson, 2007), with a later version, Form V, consisting of a 40-item yes/no personality questionnaire used to assess the four SS factors—Experience Seeking (ES); Thrill/Adventure Seeking (TAS); Disinhibition (Dis); and Boredom Susceptibility (BS)—as well as a total SSS score. Gray and Wilson (2007) adapted the 40-item forced choice yes/no scale by separating and reordering it into an 80-item Likert-type scale measured along a 7-point disagree/agree continuum, and removed 19 items deemed dated and no longer reliable. Although these various versions and adaptations of the SSS have proved valid for assessing SS among adult populations, they were unsuitable for more contemporary populations of adolescent and emerging adults.

Sensation Seeking Scale for Adolescents

Based upon Zuckerman et al.'s SSS Form V, and Huba, Newcomb, and Bentler's (1981) Sensation Seeking Scale for Adolescents, Stephenson and colleagues developed their own Sensation Seeking Scale for Adolescents called the SSS-A, a 20-item scale demonstrating good internal consistency, measuring each of Zuckerman's four SS factors with 5-item subscales updated and adapted to resonate with a later generation of adolescents (Stephenson et al., 1999; Hoyle & Stephenson, 1999). So as not to confound the SSS-A as a predictor of substance use, Stephenson and colleagues removed all mention of alcohol and drugs from their measures, yet they were still able to demonstrate good predictive validity, showing moderate to strong correlations between SS and substance use (see Table 1).

Table 1. Stephenson et al.'s (1999) Sensation Seeking Scale for Adolescents (SSS-A).

Experience Seeking (ES)
1. I would like to explore strange places.
5. I like modern or abstract paintings.
9. I like to try new foods.
13. People should dress the way they want.
17. I would like to take off on a trip with no pre-planned routes or timetables.

Thrill and Adventure Seeking (TAS)

2. I would like to try rock climbing.

6. I like to do frightening things.

10. I would like to try parachute jumping.

14. I would like to ski down a steep mountain.

18. I would like to try bungee jumping.

Disinhibition (Dis)

3. I like wild parties.

7. I like to be around real partiers.

11. I would like to live in the fast lane.

15. I like watching sexy scenes in movies.

19. I would like to have new and exciting experiences, even if they are illegal.

Boredom Susceptibility (BS)

4. I hate watching a movie for the second time.

8. I get bored seeing the same kids all the time.

12. I get bored with people who always say the same things.

16. I get restless when I spend too much time at home.

20. I prefer friends who are excitingly unpredictable.

Note: Items measured on a 5-point, Likert-type "strongly disagree," "disagree," "neither disagree nor agree," "agree," "strongly agree" continuum. Alpha Reliabilities for each of the subscales above can be found in Hoyle and Stephenson (1999). Coefficient alpha for the entire scale was $\alpha = .82$ (Stephenson et al., 1999).

The SSS-A was further refined by Hoyle et al. (2002) into a shorter 8-item measure called the Brief Sensation Seeking Scale (BSSS) using two items for each of Zuckerman's original four factors. Hoyle and colleagues sought to avoid the use of terminology inappropriate for contemporary adolescents and emerging adults by excluding colloquialisms or references that were likely to appear dated and unfamiliar to them. With less than half the items of the SSS-A, and one fifth the items of the SSS Form V, the BSSS reduces test fatigue while reliably assessing SS across youth populations of varying age, sex, and ethnicity, with alpha reliabilities ranging between .68 and .85 (Hoyle et al., 2002).

Table 2. Hoyle et al.'s (2002) Brief Sensation-Seeking Scale (BSSS).

Experience Seeking (ES)
1.   I would like to explore strange places.
5.   I would like to take off on a trip with no pre-planned routes or timetables.

Thrill and Adventure Seeking (TAS)
3.   I like to do frightening things.
7.   I would like to try bungee jumping.

Disinhibition (Dis)
4.   I like wild parties.
8.   I would like to have new and exciting experiences, even if they are illegal.

Boredom Susceptibility (BS)
2.   I get restless when I spend too much time at home.
6.   I prefer friends who are excitingly unpredictable.

Note: Items measured on a 5-point, Likert-type "strongly disagree," "disagree," "neither disagree nor agree," "agree," "strongly agree" continuum. Coefficient alpha for the entire scale was α = .76.

Use of the BSSS Measure and Future Studies

Hoyle et al. (2002) provide evidence of the reliability and validity of the BSSS, and offer it as an effective self-report measure of the SS personality trait for use with adolescents and emerging adult populations. Despite its brevity—which is an important consideration when measuring multiple constructs as both predictor and criterion variables within health risk studies—the BSSS holds true to the four factors forming the original content domain of Zuckerman's full 40-item SSS Form V. Across populations varying in sex, age, and ethnic background, the BSSS provides scores that are significantly correlated with a range of risk-related outcomes including the use of tobacco, alcohol, marijuana, inhalants, hallucinogens, and cocaine.

Besides predicting tobacco, alcohol, and marijuana use, Miller and Quick (2010), using the CDC's Youth Risk Behavioral Surveillance System, found scores on the BSSS to be positively correlated with risky sex, and negatively correlated with student grade point average for an emerging adult population of college students. Examining an adolescent population, Hoyle et al. (2002) conducted over 6000 interviews with students in grades 5–12, and found higher sensation seeking to be significantly associated with less negative attitudes toward tobacco, alcohol, marijuana, inhalants, and hallucinogens, with the single largest positive correlation (.49) being between BSSS scores and intention to try marijuana at least once. This last finding, which essentially constitutes a susceptibility measure, is particularly important since it shows how the BSSS can be used as a predictor of substance initiation, act as a key targeting instrument, and policy makers to use in planning effective anti-substance campaigns.

The BSSS can be used as a critical predictor variable in a manner similar to the risk behavior diagnosis scale (RBD) developed for use with the extended parallel process model of fear appeals (EPPM; Witte, 1992; Witte, Cameron, McKeon, & Berkowitz, 1996), and the scales for measuring vested interest (Miller, Adame, & Moore, 2013; and see Chapter 26 this volume). Moreover, the four dimensions of SS can be used to direct the development of appropriate content for anti-risk messages.

As mentioned, Donohew et al.'s (1998) SENTAR, which focuses specifically on message features high in message sensation value, can be used to design anti-risk messages capable of eliciting greater message processing for more effective health campaign design strategies (Palmgreen, Donohew, Lorch, Hoyle, & Stephenson, 2001). The BSSS may be used in conjunction with SENTAR to identify susceptible populations. Because high sensation seeking is associated with less negative attitudes toward substance use and a greater propensity to engage in unsafe sex and other risky health behaviors, the BSSS offers a relatively quick and efficient means for targeting those high sensation seeking adolescents and emerging adults who are the most susceptible to negative health outcomes.

Recommended Readings

Donohew, L., Zimmerman, R., Cupp, P. S., Novak, S., Colon, S., & Abell, R. (2000). Sensation seeking, impulsive decision-making, and risky sex: Implications for risk-taking and design of interventions. *Personality and Individual Differences, 28,* 1079–1091.

Hoyle, R. H., Stephenson, M. T., Palmgreen, P., Lorch, E. P., & Donohew, R. L. (2002). Reliability and validity of a brief measure of sensation seeking. *Personal Individual Differences, 32,* 401–414.

Miller, C. H. & Quick, B. (2010). Sensation seeking and psychological reactance as health risk predictors for an emerging adult population. *Health Communication, 25,* 266–75.

Palmgreen, P., Donohew, L., Lorch, E. P., Hoyle, R. H., & Stephenson, M. T. (2001). Television campaigns and adolescent marijuana use: Tests of a sensation seeking targeting. *American Journal of Public Health, 91*, 292–296.

Stephenson, M. T., Hoyle, R. H., Palmgreen, P., & Slater, M. D. (2003). Brief measures of sensation seeking for screening and large-scale surveys. *Drug and Alcohol Dependence 72*, 279–286.

References

Arnett, J. J. (1994). Sensation seeking: A new conceptualization and a new scale. *Personality and Individual Differences, 16*, 289–296.

Arnett, J. J. (1998). Risk behavior and family role transitions during the twenties. *Journal of Youth and Adolescence, 27*, 301–320.

Arnett, J. J. (2004). *Adolescence and emerging adulthood: A cultural approach* (2nd ed.). Englewood Cliffs, NJ: Prentice Hall.

Arnett, J. J. (2005). The developmental context of substance use in emerging adulthood. *Journal of Drug Issues, 35*, 235–253.

Arnett, J. J. (2007). Emerging adulthood: What is it, and what is it good for? *Childhood Development Perspectives, 1*, 68–73.

Beck, K. H., Thombs, D. L., Mahoney, C. A., & Fingar, K. M. (1995). Social context and sensation seeking: Gender differences in college student drinking motivations. *International Journal of Addiction, 30*, 1101–1115.

Curtis, G. C. & Zuckerman, M. (1968). A psychopathological reaction precipitated by sensory deprivation, *American Journal of Psychiatry, 125*, 255–260.

Donohew, L., Lorch, E. P., & Palmgreen, P. (1991). Sensation seeking and targeting of televised anti-drug PSAs. In L. Donohew, H. E. Sypher, & W. J. Bukoski (Eds.), *Persuasive communication and drug abuse prevention* (pp. 209–226) Hillsdale, NJ: Lawrence Erlbaum Associates.

Donohew, L., Lorch, E. P. & Palmgreen, P. (1998). Application of a theoretic model of information exposure to health interventions. *Human Communication Research, 24*, 454–468.

Donohew, L., Zimmerman, R., Cupp, P. S., Novak, S., Colon, S., & Abell, R. (2000). Sensation seeking, impulsive decision-making, and risky sex: Implications for risk-taking and design of interventions. *Personality and Individual Differences, 28*, 1079–1091.

Galvan, A., Hare, T., Voss, H., Glover, G., & Casey, B. J. (2007). Risk-taking and the adolescent brain: Who is at risk? *Developmental Science, 10*, F8–F14.

Gray, J. M., & Wilson, M. A. (2007). A detailed analysis of the reliability and validity of the sensation seeking scale in a UK sample. *Personality and Individual Differences, 42*, 641–651.

Hocking, J. & Robertson, M. (1969). Sensation Seeking Scale as a predictor of need for stimulation during sensory restriction. *Journal of Consulting & Clinical Psychology, 33*, 367–369.

Hoyle, R. H., & Stephenson, M. T. (1999). *The sensation seeking scale for adolescents.* Unpublished manuscript.

Hoyle, R. H., Stephenson, M. T., Palmgreen, P., Lorch, E. P., & Donohew, R. L. (2002). Reliability and validity of a brief measure of sensation seeking. *Personal Individual Differences, 32,* 401–414.

Huba, G. J., Newcomb, M. D., & Bentler, P. M. (1981). Comparison of canonical correlation and interbattery factor analysis on sensation seeking and drug use domains. *Applied Psychological Measurement, 5,* 291–306.

Karyadi, K., Coskunpinar, A., Dir, A. L., & Cyders, M. A. (2013). The interactive effects of affect lability, negative urgency, and sensation seeking on young adult problematic drinking. *Journal of Addiction, 2013,* 7 pages. Retrieved January 8, 2015 from the National Center for Biotechnology Information website: http://dx.doi.org/10.1155/2013/636854

Kish, G. B., & Busse, W. (1968). Correlates of stimulus-seeking: Age, education, intelligence, and aptitudes. *Journal of Consulting and Clinical Psychology, 32,* 633–637.

Kish, G. B., & Leahy, L. (1970). Stimulus-seeking, age, interests, and aptitudes: An amplification. *Perceptual and Motor Skills, 30,* 670.

Mehroof, M., & Griffiths, B. D. (2010). Online gaming addiction: The role of sensation seeking, self-control, neuroticism, aggression, state anxiety, and trait anxiety. *Cyberpsychology, Behavior, and Social Networking, 13,* 313–316. doi:10.1089/cyber.2009.0229.

Miller, C. H., & Quick, B. (2010). Sensation seeking and psychological reactance as health risk predictors for an emerging adult population. *Health Communication, 25,* 266–75.

Morgan, S. E., Palmgreen, P., Stephenson, M. T., Hoyle, R. H., & Lorch, E. P. (2003). Associations between message features and subjective evaluations of the sensation value of anti-drug public service announcements. *Journal of Communication, 53,* 512–526.

Norbury, A., Manohar, S., Rogers, R. D., & Husain, M. (2013). Dopamine modulates risk-taking as a function of baseline sensation-seeking trait. *The Journal of Neuroscience, 33,* 12982–12986, doi: 10.1523/JNEUROSCI.5587–12.2013. Retrieved January 8, 2015 from the Society for Neuroscience website: http://www.jneurosci.org/content/33/32/12982.short ·

Palmgreen, P., Donohew, L. & Harrington, N. G. (2001). Sensation seeking in anti-drug campaign and message design. In R. E. Rice & C. K. Atkins (Eds.), *Public communication campaigns: Theory, practice and effects (pp. 300–304).* Thousand Oaks, CA: Sage.

Palmgreen, P., Donohew, L., Lorch, E. P., Hoyle, R. H., & Stephenson, M. T. (2001). Television campaigns and adolescent marijuana use: Tests of a sensation seeking targeting. *American Journal of Public Health, 91,* 292–296.

Sheer, V. C., & Cline, R. J. (1994). The development and validation of a model explaining sexual behavior among college students: Implications for AIDS communication campaigns. *Human Communication Research, 21,* 280–304.

Skara, S., Sussman S., & Dent, C. W. (2001). Predicting regular cigarette use among continuation high school students. *American Journal of Health Behavior, 25*, 147–156.

Steinberg, L., Albert, D., Cauffman, E., Banich, M., Graham, S., & Woolard J. (2008). Age differences in sensation seeking and impulsivity as indexed by behavior and self-report: Evidence for a dual systems model. *Developmental Psychology, 44*, 1764–1778. doi: 10.1037/a0012955.

Stephenson, M. T. (2002). Sensation seeking as a moderator of the processing of anti-heroin PSAs. *Communication Studies, 53*, 358–380.

Stephenson, M. T. (2003). Examining adolescents' responses to anti-marijuana PSAs. *Human Communication Research, 29*, 343–369.

Stephenson M. T., Hoyle, R. H., Palmgreen, P., & Slater, M. D. (2003). Brief measures of sensation seeking for screening and large-scale surveys. *Drug and Alcohol Dependence 72*, 279–286.

Stephenson, M. T., & Palmgreen, P. (2001). Sensation seeking, perceived message sensation value, personal involvement, and processing of anti-marijuana PSAs. *Communication Monographs, 68*, 49–71.

Stephenson, M. T., Palmgreen, P., Hoyle, R. H., Donohew, L., Lorch, E. P., & Colon, S. E., (1999). Short-term effects of an anti-marijuana media campaign targeting high sensation seeking adolescents. *Journal of Applied Communication Research, 27*, 175–195.

Stephenson, M. T., Velez, L. F., Chalela, P., Ramirez, A., & Hoyle, R. H. (2007). The reliability and validity of the Brief Sensation Seeking Scale (BSSS-8) with young adult Latino workers: Implications for tobacco and alcohol disparity research. *Addiction, 2*, 79–91.

Witte, K. (1992). Putting the fear back into fear appeals: The extended parallel process model. *Communication Monographs, 59*, 329–349.

Witte, K., Cameron, K. A., McKeon, J. K., & Berkowitz, J. M. (1996). Predicting risk behaviors: Development and validation of a diagnostic scale. *Journal of Health Communication, 1*, 317–342.

Zuckerman, M. (1971). Dimensions of sensation seeking. *Journal of Consulting and Clinical Psychology, 36*, 45–52.

Zuckerman, M. (1974). Sensation seeking. In H. London and J. Exner (Eds.), *Dimensions of personality*. New York: Wiley.

Zuckerman, M. (1979). *Sensation seeking: Beyond the optimal level of arousal*. Hillsdale, NJ: Erlbaum.

Zuckerman, M. (1994). *Behavioral expressions and biosocial bases of sensation seeking*. New York: Cambridge University Press.

Zuckerman, M. (2007). *Sensation seeking and risky behavior*. Washington, DC: American Psychological Association.

Zuckerman, M., Eysenck, S. B. J., & Eysenck, H. J. (1978). Sensation seeking in England and America: Cross-cultural, age, and sex comparisons. *Journal of Consulting and Clinical Psychology, 46*, 139–149.

Zuckerman, M., Kolin, E. A., Price, L., & Zoob, I. (1964). Development of a sensation-seeking scale. *Journal of consulting psychology, 28,* 477–482.

Zuckerman, M., & Link, K. (1968). Construct validity for the sensation seeking scale. *Journal of Consulting and Clinical Psychology, 32,* 420–426.

22. *Social Support*

STEPHEN A. RAINS,
University of Arizona

Social support plays a central role in health and well-being (Cohen & Syme, 1985; Uchino, 2004). Despite widespread agreement about the benefits of social support, the way(s) in which it produces salutatory effects are not fully understood (Lakey & Cohen, 2000; Thoits, 2011). Support processes have been examined by scholars representing a range of disciplines from the social sciences to medicine. In this body of research, social support has been conceptualized and studied in a myriad of ways. This chapter considers measures of social support developed from four traditions that are particularly relevant to health communication. Social support is examined as behaviors enacted by others to provide physical or emotional assistance, perceptions that others are available to serve as a support resource, a preference for support from particular types of people, and specific messages shared with others. Each tradition is briefly reviewed and representative measures considered.

Measuring Social Support

Received Support

Research on received support focuses on the degree to which one has been the recipient of specific acts of assistance during a given time period. Such assistance is defined broadly and can include advice and information, comforting and empathy, as well as physical acts such as providing transportation or help with housework. Received support is thought to improve health by bolstering one's coping efforts (Lakey & Cohen, 2000). The inventory of socially supportive behaviors (ISSB; Barrera, Sandler, & Ramsay, 1981) is one widely-used scale for evaluating received support.

Scale development. The ISSB was developed to evaluate the relative frequency with which individuals are the recipients of helping behaviors. This measure is noteworthy because it captures both tangible and intangible forms of assistance received by individuals during a given time period. The ISSB was designed to be a general measure of naturally occurring helping behaviors.

The ISSB begins with a stem asking participants to "Rate the frequency with which each of the 40 items occurred during the preceding month." Ratings are made on a 5-point scale with the intervals: 1= not at all; 2 = once or twice; 3 = about once a week; 4 = several times a week; 5 = about every day. The items in the ISSB are summed to formed a composite measure of support received during a given time period. The items in the ISSB are displayed in Table 1.

Table 1. The ISSB.

ISSB Items
Looked after a family member when you were away.
Was right there with you (physically) in a stressful situation.
Provided you with a place where you could get away for a while.
Watched after your possessions when you were away (pets, home, etc.).
Told you what s/he did in a situation that was similar to yours.
Did some activity together to help you get your mind off things.
Talked with you about some interests of yours.
Let you know that you did something well.
Went with you to someone who could take action.
Told you that you are OK just the way you are.
Told you that s/he would keep the things that you talk about private—just between the two of you.
Assisted you in setting a goal for yourself.
Made it clear what was expected of you.
Expressed esteem or respect for a competency or personal quality of yours.
Gave you some information on how to do something.
Suggested some action that you should take.
Gave you over $25.
Comforted you by showing you some physical affection.
Gave you some information to help you understand a situation you were in.
Provided you with some transportation.

ISSB Items

Checked back with you to see if you followed the advice you were given.

Gave you under $25.

Helped you understand why you didn't do something well.

Listened to you talk about your private feelings.

Loaned or gave you something (a physical object other than money) that you needed.

Agreed that what you wanted to do was right.

Said things that made your situation clearer and easier to understand.

Told you how s/he felt in a situation that was similar to yours.

Let you know that s/he will always be around if you need assistance.

Expressed interest and concern in your well-being.

Told you that s/he feels very close to you.

Told you who you should see for assistance.

Told you what to expect in a situation that was about to happen.

Loaned you over $25.

Taught you how to do something.

Gave you feedback on how you were doing without saying it was good or bad.

Joked and kidded to try to cheer you up.

Provided you with a place to stay.

Pitched in to help you do something that needed to get done.

Loaned you under $25.

In Barrera and colleagues' initial evaluation of the instrument, the test-retest correlation between individual items across a span of two days ranged between .44 and .94. Total ISSB scores were strongly correlated ($r = .88$) and the reliability coefficients were high ($\alpha = .93$ and .94) across the two measurement points. Barrera and colleagues reported statistically significant correlations between the ISSB and measures of support availability, network size, and perceived family cohesiveness. Additional tests of the ISSB offer evidence of its utility as a global measure of received support (Stokes & Wilson, 1984).

Support Availability

Whereas received support focuses on the reception of specific supportive acts during a given time period, support availability (also referred to as perceived support) considers individuals' perceptions that they have access to support resources. Support availability involves the general perception that, if necessary, one could acquire various types of support ranging from advice and empathy to physical assistance. Support availability is proposed to impact health and well-being by influencing individuals' appraisals of stressors (Lakey & Cohen, 2000). Individuals who feel greater levels of available support perceive situations as being less stressful and more manageable. As with received support, a number of measures of support availability exist. The multidimensional scale of perceived social support (MSPSS; Zimet, Dahlem, Zimet, & Farley, 1988) is one widely-used measure evaluating support availability.

Scale development. The MSPSS was created to evaluate individuals' perceptions of the availability and adequacy of support from members of their social network. The MSPSS is unique in that it considers evaluations of three support sources: friends, family members, and a significant other. The scale includes a total of 12 items that form three factors (one for each of the three support sources). The items included in the MSPSS are displayed in Table 2.

Table 2. The MSPSS.

MSPSS Items
There is a special person who is around when I am in need.[SO]
There is a special person with whom I can share my joys and sorrows.[SO]
My family really tries to help me.[FM]
I get the emotional help and support I need from my family.[FM]
I have a special person who is a real source of comfort to me.[SO]
My friends really try to help me.[FR]
I can count on my friends when thing go wrong.[FR]
I can talk about my problems with family.[FM]
I have friends with whom I can share my joys and sorrows.[FR]
There is a special person in my life who cares about my feelings.[SO]
My family is willing to help me make decisions.[FM]
I can talk about my problems with my friends.[FR]

Note: SO = significant other subscale; FM = family subscale; FR = Friends subscale

In Zimet and colleagues' initial evaluation of MSPSS, they conducted a principal components analysis that showed three distinct dimensions corresponding to support from family, friends, and a significant other. The reliability coefficients for all three dimensions exceed .84 and reliability for the total scale was .88. Test-retest reliability assessed over at least a three-month interval was .85 for the total scale, although the reliabilities for individual dimensions ranged between .72 and .85. The three subscales were negatively associated with depression and anxiety, with one minor exception. The factor structure, reliability, and validity of the MSPSS have been demonstrated in several other studies (Kazarian & McCabe, 1991; Zimet, Powell, Farley, Werkman, & Berkoff, 1990) and among specialized populations (Cecil, Stanley, Carrion, & Swann, 1995; Stanley, Beck, & Zebb, 1998).

Preference for Support from Weak Ties

Weak-tie support network preference is an individual-difference factor that involves the degree to which individuals have an enduring preference for support from particular types of social network members (Wright & Miller, 2010). This construct is rooted in Granovetter's (1973) basic distinction between strong ties such as family and friends with whom one communicates frequently and weak ties who are not interpersonally close but with whom one can acquire resources. In the context of health, weak ties may take the form of other individuals who are coping or have coped with a particular condition. Weak ties are argued to be a novel support resource in that, relative to strong ties, they have greater utility, more objectivity, reduced potential for social complications, and are less risky disclosure targets (Wright & Miller, 2010).

Scale development. The weak-tie support network preference scale (WTSNP; Wright & Miller, 2010) was developed to evaluate individuals' preference for social support from weak ties. The WTSNP consists of 19 total items representing four dimensions: utility, objectivity, risk, and comfort. The subscales may be combined into an aggregate measure or examined separately. The items in the WTSNP are displayed in Table 3.

Table 3. The WTSNP.

WTSNP Items
I feel comfortable discussing my problems with close friends and family (reverse coded).[C]
I know that I can count on my close friends and family members to help me when I have personal problems (reverse coded).[C]
My close friends and family get too emotional when I discuss my problems with them.[R]
It is less risky to discuss my problems with people who are not as intimate with me as close friends and family members.[R]

WTSNP Items
I discuss my problems with people who are not close to me so I don't have to worry about my family and close friends finding out.[R]
People who don't know me very well are less likely to pass judgment on me.[R]
My close friends and family tend to have viewpoints too similar to my own to help much.[R]
I can get help discussing my problems with people who don't know me very well without feeling obligated to help them in return.[R]
People I'm not intimate with tend to judge me less harshly than my close friends and family members.[R]
My family and close friends often tend to judge me when I discuss my problems with them.[R]
I find people who don't know me very well see things more objectively than my family and close friends.[O]
People who are not involved with me emotionally can offer me better advice about my problems.[O]
Often times I can get a more objective perspective discussing my problems with relative strangers who are different from me than I can from family or close friends.[O]
I can discuss personal problems in greater depth with people I don't know very well than with my family and close friends.[O]
I feel as though my close friends and family provide me with better advice about personal problems than people who don't know me very well (reverse-coded).[O]
I find that I can get more objective information about my problems from people who are not close friends or family members.[O]
I get more understanding from people who don't know me very well than from close friends and family.[O]
People who don't know me very well offer the most objective viewpoints about my problems.[O]
My close friends and family are able to offer objective advice despite their strong feelings about me (reverse-coded).[O]

Note: C = comfort subscale; R = risk subscale; U = utility subscale; O = objectivity subscale

Wright and Miller (2010) conducted two studies to evaluate the WTSNP. Confirmatory factor analyses showed that 19 items representing the four factors adequately fit the sample data in both studies. Tests of three and five-factor models offered evidence to justify the four-factor model. The reliability coefficients for the four factors ranged from .73 to .91. Wright and Miller reported statistically significant correlations between the dimensions of the WTSNP and relationship closeness, stressor-related anxiety, and coping efficacy.

Support Message Dimensions

Measures of social support have also been developed to help identify supportive messages during interaction. The goal of such frameworks is to offer an approach for examining the content of supportive exchanges. Unlike the previous self-report measures, these frameworks involve using human coders to evaluate support message content. One widely used coding scheme is the social support behavior code (SSBC; Cutrona & Suhr, 1992).

Scale development. The SSBC is rooted in the assumption that social support is a multidimensional construct. Social support messages may address qualitatively different issues. A total of 23 supportive messages are grouped into five macro categories in the SSBC, including: informational, emotional, esteem, network, and tangible support. This framework is applied in two steps by two or more raters. Coders first determine the unit of analysis, which could consist of an entire speaking turn, individual sentences, or thought units. Coders then attempt to classify each message into one of the 23 categories. Fairly extensive training may be required for coders to achieve an acceptable level of inter-coder agreement in applying the coding framework. The SSBC is presented in Table 4.

Table 4. The SSBC.

SSBC Support Type	Purpose of Message
Informational support	
Advice	Offers ideas and suggests actions
Referral	Refers the recipient to some other source of help
Situation appraisal	Reassesses or redefines the situation
Teaching	Provides detailed information, facts, or news about the situation or about skills needed to deal with the situation
Tangible Assistance	
Loan	Offers to lend the recipient something
Direct task	Offers to perform a task directly related to the stress

SSBC Support Type	Purpose of Message
Indirect task	Offers to take over one or more of the recipient's other responsibilities while the recipient is under stress
Active participation	Offers to join the recipient in action that reduces the stress
Willingness	Expresses willingness to help
Esteem Support	
Compliment	Says positive things about the recipient or emphasizes the recipient's abilities
Validation	Expresses agreement with the recipient's perspective on the situation
Relief of blame	Tries to alleviate the recipient's feelings of guilt about the situation
Network Support	
Access	Offers to provide the recipient with access to new companions
Presence	Offers to spend time with the person
Companions	Reminds the recipient of availability of companions such as others who are similar in interests or experiences
Emotional Support	
Relationship	Stresses the importance of closeness and love in relationship with the recipient
Physical affection	Offers physical contact, including hugs, kisses, hand-holding, shoulder patting
Confidentiality	Promises to keep the recipient's problem in confidence
Sympathy	Expresses sorrow or regret for the recipient's situation or distress
Listening	Makes attentive comments as the recipient speaks
Empathy	Expresses understanding of the situation or discloses a personal situation that communicates understanding
Encouragement	Provides the recipient with hope and confidence
Prayer	Prays with the recipient

The SSBC has been applied to evaluate support messages in numerous health communication studies such as among disability communities online (Braithwaite, Waldron, & Finn, 1999) and health bloggers coping with anorexia (Tong, Heinmann-LaFave, Jeon, Kolodziej-Smith, & Warshay, 2013). In these studies, the authors were able to achieve acceptable levels of intercoder agreement for the five macro categories in the SSBC.

Use of Existing Scales and Future Studies

The myriad of ways in which social support is conceptualized and thought to function is reflected in the diversity of measures that have been developed to assess this phenomenon. Four traditions of social support measures that are particularly relevant to health communication were considered in this chapter: received support, perceived support availability, preference for weak-tie support, and support message dimensions. Efforts to identify the measure most appropriate for a given study should begin by considering the broader perspective from which one wishes to investigate social support. Understanding the way which social support is being conceptualized will offer guidance about the specific tradition of support measure that is most appropriate for one's investigation.

Recommended Readings

Rains, S. A., Peterson, E., & Wright, K. B. (2015). Communicating social support in computer-mediated contexts: A meta-analytic review of content analyses examining support messages shared online among individuals coping with illness. *Communication Monographs*. Advanced online publication.

Segrin, C., & Passalacqua, S. A. (2010). Functions of loneliness, social support, health behaviors, and stress in association with poor health. *Health Communication, 25*, 312–322.

Weiner, A. S., & Hannum, J. W. (2013). Differences in the quantity of social support between geographically close and long-distance friendships. *Journal of Social and Personal Relationships, 30*, 662–672.

Wright, K. B., & Rains, S. A. (2013). Weak-tie support network preference, stigma, and health outcomes in computer-mediated support groups. *Journal of Applied Communication Research, 41*, 309–324.

References

Barrera, M., Sandler, I. N., & Ramsay, T. B. (1981). Preliminary development of a scale of social support: Studies on college students. *American Journal of Community Psychology, 9*, 435–447.

Braithwaite, D. O., Waldron, V. R., & Finn, J. (1999). Communication of social support in computer-mediated groups for people with disabilities. *Health Communication, 11*, 123–151.

Cecil, H., Stanley, M. A., Carrion, P. G., & Swann, A. (1995). Psychometric properties of the MSPSS and NOS in psychiatric outpatients. *Journal of Clinical Psychology, 51*, 593–602.

Cohen, S., & Syme, S. L. (1985). *Social support and health.* New York: Academic Press.

Cutrona, C. E., & Suhr, J. A. (1992). Controllability of stressful events and satisfaction with spouse support behaviors. *Communication Research, 19*, 154–174.

Granovetter, M. (1973). The strength of weak ties. *American Journal of Sociology 78*, 1360–1380.

Kazarian, S. S., & McCabe, S. B. (1991). Dimensions of social support in the MSPSS: Factorial structure, reliability, and theoretical implications. *Journal of Community Psychology, 19*, 150–160.

Lakey, B., & Cohen, S. (2000). Social support theory and measurement. In S. Cohen, L. Underwood, & B. Gottlieb (Eds.), *Measuring and intervening in social support* (pp. 29–52). New York: Oxford University Press.

Stanley, M. A., Beck, J. G., & Zebb, B. J. (1998). Psychometric properties of the MSPSS in older adults. *Aging and Mental Health, 2*, 186–193.

Stokes, J. P., & Wilson, D. G.(1984). The inventory of socially supportive behaviors: Dimensionality, prediction, and gender differences. *American Journal of Community Psychology, 12*, 53–69.

Thoits, P. A. (2011). Mechanisms linking social ties and support to physical and mental health. *Journal of Health and Social Behavior, 52*, 145–161.

Tong, S. T., Heinmann-LaFave, D., Jeon, J., Kolodziej-Smith, R., & Warshay, N. (2013). The use of pro-ana blogs for online social support. *Eating Disorders, 21*, 408–422.

Uchino, B. N. (2004). *Social support and physical health: Understanding the health consequences of relationships.* New Haven, CT: Yale University Press.

Wright, K. B., & Miller, C. H. (2010). A measure of weak-tie/strong-tie support network preference. *Communication Monographs, 77*, 502–520.

Zimet, G. D., Dahlem, N. W., Zimet, S. G., & Farley, G. K. (1988). The multidimensional scale of perceived social support. *Journal of Personality Assessment, 52*, 30–41.

Zimet, G. D., Powell, S. S., Farley, G. K., Werkman, S., & Berkoff, K. A. (1990). Psychometric characteristics of the multidimensional scale of perceived social support. *Journal of Personality Assessment, 55*, 610–617.

23. Stigma

MARY J. BRESNAHAN,
Michigan State University
& JIE ZHUANG,
Michigan State University

Goffman (1963) presented a conceptual guidebook for understanding stigma, but offered no plan for studying stigma systematically. Measuring stigma has continued to be elusive because stigmatizers often cloak stigma in self-report and experimental research (Earnshaw & Chaudoir, 2009). It is relatively easy to document the experience of recipients of stigma but more difficult to get stigmatizers to reveal their stigma. Smith (2007) explained that "stigma communication is the messages spread through communities to teach their members to recognize the disgraced and to react accordingly" (p. 464). The goal of this chapter is to provide a comprehensive overview of existing stigma theories and measures.

Three classes of stigma theories study perception and enactment of stigma: 1) attribution theories of stigma, 2) stigma as power disparity, and 3) stigma as a communicative event. Link and Phelan's (2001) 5-factor model typifies the attribution approach defining 5 stigma behaviors including labeling, negative attribution, separation, status loss, and discrimination. Subsequent research has developed scales to measure these stigma behaviors (Bresnahan & Zhuang, 2011). The idea of stigma as power disparity focuses on structural and social imbalances in the creation, maintenance, and experience of stigma (Parker & Aggleton, 2003; Scambler, 2004). Positional, relational, informational, and social power inequality enables stigmatizers to enforce negative evaluation downgrading others who are afflicted with an undesirable condition. Earnshaw and Chaudoir (2009) observe that "stigma serves to keep some people in a relative position of power because they do not possess the devalued attribute and others in a relative position of subordination because they possess the devalued attribute" (p. 1161). The communication of stigma model considers how stigma is enacted between stigmatizers and the stigmatized both verbally and nonverbally (Smith, 2007).

There is some consensus about the dimensions of stigma and less consensus about how to measure stigma. The majority of measures have focused on the experience of being stigmatized rather than stigmatizers.

Measuring Stigma: Recent Studies of Stigma

Indicative of this increasing scholarly interest in stigma, journals in three disciplines have recently devoted an entire issue to studies of stigma (*Basic and Applied Social Psychology*, 2013, vol. 35, 1; *Communication Studies*, 2014, vol. 65, 2; *Social Science & Medicine*, 2014, vol. 103, 1). We summarize how stigma measurement has been advanced in each of these volumes.

Basic and Applied Social Psychology

In 2013, *Basic and Applied Social Psychology* published 14 articles covering a broad range of stigma topics. We focus on 4 of these studies that involved measurement. DePierre, Puhl, and Luedicke conducted two studies examining whether the food addict label was less stigmatized compared to 7 other stigma labels including 3 obesity labels. Participants ranked each of the 8 stigmatized conditions for social distance, sympathy/concern, anger/disgust, and responsibility concluding that the food addict label was less stigmatized compared to other obesity labels. Ilic et al. measured consequences of stigma for people with mental illness. They conducted a validation study of the Multifaceted Stigma Experience Scale demonstrating four dimensions including hostile discrimination (6 Likert items), benevolent discrimination (3 items), taboo (3 items), and denial (3 items).

While they did not provide actual items to measure stigma, Chaudoir, Earnshaw, and Andel (2013) discussed anticipated stigma, which they defined as "the degree to which individuals anticipate or expect to be the target of discrimination or social rejection because of their situation" (p. 76). Finally, Herek, Saha, and Burack (2013) measured three dimensions of stigma—felt stigma, enacted stigma, and stigma management. Deriving from the Perceived Stigma of HIV/AIDS scale (Westbrook & Bauman, 1996) and the HIV Stigma Scale (Berger, Ferrans, & Lashley, 2001), Herek, Saha, and Burack developed a 7-item Likert scale of felt stigma. They measured enacted stigma asking for the frequency of occurrence for 22 stigmatizing incidents. Stigma management was measured with 15 items asking participants how frequently they used these coping strategies. There were 3 indicators of stigma management each with 5 items including avoidance, interaction seeking, and concealment of HIV status. They also measured 3 psychosocial correlates of stigma including dispositional optimism, self-esteem, and psychological distress.

Communication Studies

The special issue of *Communication Studies* included 7 studies mostly based on content analysis; however, the categories measured could easily be converted into scaled items. For example, Salek compared downplaying a stigmatized condition with trying to educate in the case of how religion affected the Romney presidential bid. Stearns suggested measuring 3 stigmatizing behaviors—silencing, incivility, and bullying and the consequences of these behaviors such as loss of self-esteem, stress, embarrassment, fear of retaliation, and life dissatisfaction. Striley investigated the stigma of excellence with open-ended surveys conducted with 169 gifted adolescents. Her analysis showed there is merit in measuring labeling, the amount of value placed on conformity, how a condition poses a relational threat and causes uncertainty, problems in self-esteem, loneliness, and social alienation for the victims of stigma. Holton, Farrell, and Fudge analyzed messages for 4 kinds of social stigma cues: labeling, description of psychiatric symptoms, social skill deficits, and physical symptoms. Finally, the only psychometric article included in this issue was the study by Smith that providing an empirical test for her model of interpersonal stigma communication. She measured 9 variables to probe stigma including danger (4 Likert items), responsibility (3 items), sympathy (3 items), frustration (3 items), severity (3 items), risk (3 items), intervention support (6 items), likelihood of telling others (1 item), and disgust sensitivity (7 items).

Social Science & Medicine

A special issue of *Social Science & Medicine* included 16 articles investigating *social power* in a range of stigmatized conditions including mental illness, homosexuality, obesity, HIV/AIDS, and depression. Researchers in this issue termed social power as structural stigma (Reid, Dovidio, Ballester, & Johnson, 2014), structural discrimination (Yang et al., 2007), and structural racism (Lukachko, Hatzenbuehler, & Keyes, 2014). The goal was to explore the effect of structural stigma and the interaction between structural and individual stigma. The issue included reviews of stigma research, meta-analyses, theory building pieces, and qualitative studies utilizing in-depth interviewing. The current discussion focuses on five empirical studies measuring structural stigma.

Angermeyer and colleagues (2014) measured individual and structural discrimination from the perspective of the stigmatizer at both individual and societal levels. They operationalized individual discrimination by asking respondents to rate the extent to which they were willing to engage in relationships with an individual with a major depressive disorder including (a) rent a room, (b) work together, (c) live as a neighbor, (d) take care of a child, (e) marry into a family, (f) introduce to friends, and (g) recommend for a job. Respondents were presented with nine medical conditions and were asked to select three diseases for which they believed available social resources should be reduced.

Hatzenbuehler et al. (2014) analyzed data from the General Social Survey (GSS) to investigate stigmatizers' attitudes toward homosexuality. Four Likert items measured attitudes toward homosexuality including (a) If some people in your community suggested that a book in favor of homosexuality should be taken out of your public library, would you favor removing this book, or not?; (2) Should a man who admits that he is a homosexual be allowed to teach in a college or university, or not?; (3) Suppose a man who admits that he is a homosexual wanted to make a speech in your community. Should he be allowed to speak, or not?; (4) Do you think that sexual relations between two adults of the same sex is always wrong, almost always wrong, wrong only sometimes, or not wrong at all?

Lukachko and colleagues conducted an archival study measuring structural racism with four indicators, including political participation, employment and job status, education attainment, and judicial treatment. The dimension of political participation consisted of three items, including registered to vote, voted, and state elected officials; employment and job status consisted of (a) civilian labor, (b) employed, (c) executive/managerial position, and (d) professional specialty; receiving bachelor's degree or higher was used to measure educational attainment, and judicial treatment was measured by (a) incarcerated, (b) disenfranchised, and (c) death row.

Link and Phelan (2014) measured stigma-power with three processes: (a) cultural designation of value, (b) concern with staying in, and (c) being kept away. Cultural assessment of values was operationalized as two dimensions: devaluation-discrimination and daily indignities. Perception of devaluation and discrimination was measured by a 12-item version of Perceived Devaluation-Discrimination Scale (Link, 1987). Daily indignities were measured with an 8-item scale assessing how frequently participants were taken advantage of, had hurt feelings, or had people act uncomfortably around them.

Concern with staying in was measured with a 6-item scale drawing on the concept of "rejection sensitivity" developed by Downey et al. (2004). Respondents were given scenarios describing situations in which they might be identified as having a mental illness or losing control and asked how concerned they would be in this situation. Stigma consciousness was assessed by a 5-item scale asking participants the extent to which they were aware of their stigmatized status and their monitoring of status. Secrecy was measured by a 5-item scale estimating the frequency of concealing their history of psychiatric hospitalization in the past three months.

Being kept away was assessed by a 5-item scale measuring the extent to which respondents avoided rejecting interactions or engaged in interactions with others who also have mental illness. Finally, being kept down (i.e., losing self-esteem) was measured using an 8-item self-esteem scale developed by Rosenberg (1989) asking respondents' agreement with questions about whether they think they can do things as well as most people.

Lastly, Pachankis et al.'s stigma measure toward gay men was constituted by (a) policies affecting sexual minorities and (b) attitudinal indicators toward policies affecting homosexuals. The researchers coded the presence or absence of (a) amendments banning same-sex marriage, (b) sexual nondiscrimination employment laws, (c) a category recognizing sexual orientation as a protected category in hate crimes reporting, (d) nondiscrimination laws toward homosexual students and anti-bullying laws based on sexual orientation, and (e) statutes restricting same-sex or non-married couples from adopting. Using these categories, public opinion toward protection policies for gay/lesbian couples were collected from 41 national polls from 1999 to 2008.

The three issues devoted to stigma covered a wide range of stigma-related topics and employed a variety of methodologies to study stigma. Besides summarizing the three special issues, this chapter also presents a matrix of additional measures of stigma in Table 1. There are 4 inclusion criteria: 1) innovative dimensions of stigma, 2) frequently cited and used measures, 3) multiple items in a measure, and 4) attention to the validity of the measure.

Table 1. Ten Measures of Stigma.

Source	Source/ year	S stigma-tizer R recipient B both	Theory	Method	Measures
Brown, Macintyre, & Trujillo (649 citations)	*AIDS Education and Prevention,* 2003	B	PLWHIV/ AIDS	Review of 22 studies that measure attitude toward HIV/ AIDS	CDC Health Risk Survey, AIDS Social Anxiety Scale, Attitude toward AIDS & PLHA Scale, State/trait anxiety inventories, Fear of AIDS scale

Source	Source/ year	S stigma- tizer R recipient B both	Theory	Method	Measures
Clement, Brohan, Henderson, Hatch, & Thornicort	*BMC Psychiatry*, 2012	R	Mental illness stigma theory	Scale Validation study Measures can be adapted to other stigmatized conditions	**BACE** 30 Likert items measure knowledge, accessibility, social sanctioning, guilt and shame, and reluctance to admit there is a problem
Corrigan, Watson, & Miller (**295 citations**)	*Journal of Family Psychology*, 2006	S	Mental illness stigma theory	**S1** phone survey **S2** content analysis of focus group discussions	7 items measure attributions about person with condition and 7 items measuring attributions about family members
DISC-12 Thorncroft et al., 2009	*The Lancet,* 2009	R	Mental illness stigma theory	Scale Validation study Measures can be adapted to other stigmatized conditions	21 items measure unfair treatment; 4 items measure exclusion; 2 items measure overcoming stigma; 5 items for positive treatment
Earnshaw & Chaudoir (Review Stigma Measures)	*AIDS & Behavior,* 2009	B	New HIV Stigma Framework	Review of 25 stigma measures	Measures: **S**—prejudice, stereotype, discrimination; **R**—enacted, anticipated, internalized stigma, outcomes: psychological & behavioral health
Gabbidon et al. **QUAD** scale	*BMC Psychiatry,* 2013	R	Mental illness stigma theory	Questionnaire on Anticipated Discrimination	QUAD consists of 14 Likert items measuring felt stigma in multiple contexts.

Source	Source/ year	S stigma- tizer R recipient B both	Theory	Method	Measures
Interian et al. study (in- cludes multiple stigma mea- sures)	*Psychi- atric Services,* 2010	B	5 measures of men- tal illness stigma	220 pri- mary care Hispanic patients were surveyed in waves 5 times over 3 years	12-item perceived discrimination; 3-item mental health treatment stigma; 6-item social distance; 7-item use of anti- depressants; health questionnaire
ISMI Scale (Ritsher et al., 2003)	*Psychia- try Re- search,* 2003	R	Mental Ill- ness Stigma Theory	29 item Internal- ized stigma of mental illness scale	6 items measure stereotype en- dorsement; 7 items for discrimination experience; 5 items for social withdraw- al, and 5 items for stigma resistance
Myers & Rosen (**320 ci- tations**)	*Inter- national Journal of Obesi- ty,* 1999	R	Obesity stigma	Measures for obesi- ty can be adapted to other stigmatized conditions	2 measures: wheth- er /how often this happened to you 11 item inventory of stigmatizing situations 21 10-point ordinal items for coping
Steward et al., (**144 ci- tations**)	*Social Science & Med- icine,* 2008	R	Herek's (2002) HIV Stigma framework	**S1** an- alyzed interviews for 4 types of stigma **S2** sur- veyed PLWHIV for dis- closure/ avoidance impact on depression	Enacted stigma: 21-item index of stigma events Vicarious stigma: 20 items for experi- ence of stigma Felt normative stigma: 15 items prevalence stigma Internalized stigma: 15 items belief that PLWHIV should be stigmatized

Measuring Stigma

Bresnahan & Zhuang's Stigma Scale

Based on the heavily cited (3093 citations) 2001 Link and Phelan conceptualizing of stigma study that identified 5 dimensions, Bresnahan and Zhuang (2011) developed items to operationalize these dimensions and conducted a validation study for this measure that can be adapted to any form of stigma. The 5 dimensional stigma scale shows acceptable validity and reliability. To this point the newly introduced measure has been used in 11 other studies. The 5 stigma dimensions include items measuring labeling, negative attribution, controllability, separation, and status loss. The scale could not validate items to measure discrimination as the magnitude of agreement with such items was low. These are the items included in this measure.

Labeling Items:
Label 1 HIV/AIDS is a loaded gun.
Label 2 HIV/AIDS is a death sentence.
Label 3 HIV/AIDS is a ticking time bomb.
Label 4 HIV/AIDS is a vessel of disease.
Label 5 HIV/AIDS is a thief stealing people's life.
Label 6 HIV/AIDS is a disaster.

Negative Attribution:
1. A person who has HIV/AIDS has no will power.
2. A person who has HIV/AIDS likes instant gratification.
3. A person who has HIV/AIDS took the path of least resistance.
4. A person who has HIV/AIDS is weak in character.
5. A person who has HIV/AIDS is self-indulgent.
6. People who have HIV/AIDS bring the disease on themselves.
7. People who have HIV/AIDS take high health risk.

Distancing:
1. I would stay away from a person with HIV/AIDS.
2. I would not want contact with any body fluid from someone with HIV/AIDS.
3. I would not want contact with saliva from someone with HIV/AIDS.
4. I would not want to share food with someone who has HIV/AIDS.
5. I would not want contact with the blood of someone with HIV/AIDS.

Status Loss:
1. Other people look down on people who have HIV/AIDS.
2. People who have HIV/AIDS are judged negatively.

3. People who have HIV/AIDS often suffer status loss.
4. HIV/AIDS makes a person disempowered.

Controllability:
1. I can control HIV/AIDS by refusing to have unsafe sex.
2. I know what needs to be done to prevent HIV/AIDS.
3. HIV/AIDS is controllable.
4. I can control HIV/AIDS by not engaging in risky behaviors.

The Revised Berger HIV Stigma Scale

Berger, Ferrans, and Lashley (2001) developed an instrument to assess the stigma perceived by people living with HIV. With a total of 41 items, the instrument consists of four sub-dimensions measuring personalized stigma, disclosure communication, negative self-image, and public attitudes. Since its development, this scale has been widely cited and heavily used. Subsequently, Bunn, Solomon, Miller, and Forehand (2007) revised the Berger et al. scale by shortening it to 32 items and renaming personalized stigma to enacted stigma and retaining the rest three dimensions. In Bunn et al.'s (2007) study, the revised scale was administered to 157 individuals living with HIV. The revised measure consists of four subscales only including unique items, with adequate sub-scale reliabilities.

Enacted stigma (named personalized stigma in the original scale)
(1) Some people who know I have HIV have grown more distant.
(2) I am hurt by how people reacted to learning I have HIV.
(3) People avoid touching me if they know I have HIV/AIDS.
(4) I have stopped socializing with some people due to their reactions to learning I have HIV/AIDS.
(5) I have lost friends by telling them I have HIV.
(6) People I care about stopped calling me after learning that I have HIV/AIDS.
(7) People seem afraid of me because I have HIV/AIDS.
(8) People have physically backed away from me because I have HIV/AIDS.
(9) People who know that I have HIV/AIDS ignore my good points.
(10) People do not want me around their children once they know that I have HIV/AIDS.
(11) I regret having told some people that I have HIV/AIDS.

Disclosure communication
(1) For many years of my life, no one has known that I have HIV.
(2) I am very careful who I tell that I have HIV.
(3) I never feel the need to hide the fact that I have HIV. (RC)
(4) I worry that people who know I have HIV will tell others.
(5) I work hard to keep my HIV/AIDS a secret.
(6) Telling someone I have HIV/AIDS is risky.
(7) I worry that people may judge me when they learn that I have HIV/ AIDS.

Negative self-image
(1) I feel guilty because I have HIV.
(2) I feel ashamed of having HIV/AIDS.
(3) People's attitudes about HIV make me feel worse about myself.
(4) I feel I am not as good a person as others because I have HIV.
(5) I never feel ashamed of having HIV. (RC)
(6) Having HIV makes me feel unclean.
(7) Having HIV in my body is disgusting to me.
(8) Having HIV makes me feel that I am a bad person.

Public attitudes
(1) People with HIV lose their jobs when their employers learn that they have HIV/AIDS.
(2) People with HIV are treated as outcasts.
(3) Most people with HIV/AIDS are rejected when others learn that they have HIV/AIDS.
(4) Most people believe that a person who has HIV is dirty.
(5) Most people think that a person with HIV is disgusting.
(6) Most people are uncomfortable around someone with HIV.

Use of Existing Measures and Future Studies

Studies of stigma analyze cognitive, affective, behavioral, and communicative components. There is an emergent consensus for some behaviors important in the creation, maintenance, and experience of stigma as shown in the Bresnahan and Zhuang (2011) operationalization of Link and Phelan and the revised Berger et al. scale (Bunn et al., 2007). Five themes emerge from analysis of stigma studies including 1) responses to stigma such as negative attribution, discrimination, bullying, and hate crimes, 2) denial of access to opportunity, 3) the choice whether to reveal or conceal the stigmatized condition, 4) coping strategies, and 5) the negative outcomes of stigma on recipients including depression, shame, and embarrassment. Van Brakel (2005) insightfully suggests: "The similarity in the consequences of stigma in many different cultural settings and the crosscutting applicability of many items from stigma instruments suggest that it would be possible to develop a generic set of stigma assessment instruments" (p. 11). So far, this has not happened.

Recommended Readings

Beaulieu, M., Adrien, A., Potvin, L., & Dassa, C. (2014). Stigmatizing attitudes towards people living with HIV/AIDS: Validation of a measurement scale. *BMC Public Health, 14,* 1246–1259. http://www.biomedcentral.com/1471-2458/14/1246

Foster, L. R., & Byers, E. S. (2013). Stigmatization of individuals with sexually transmitted infections: Effects of illness and observer characteristics. *Journal of Applied Social Psychology, 43,* E141–E152. 10.1111/jasp.12036.

Holzemer, W. L., Human, S., Arudo, J., Rosa, M. E., Hamilton, M. J., Corless, I.,...& Maryland, M. (2009). Exploring HIV stigma and quality of life for persons living with HIV infection. *Journal of the Association of Nurses in AIDS Care, 20*(3), 161–168. doi: 0.1016/j.jana.2009.02.002. doi: 10.1080/09540120802032627.

Kalichman, S. C., Simbayi, L. C., Cloete, A., Mthembu, P. P., Mkhonta, R. N., & Ginindza, T. (2009). Measuring AIDS stigmas in people living with HIV/AIDS: The internalized AIDS-related stigma scale. *AIDS Care, 21*(1), 87–93. doi: 10.1080/09540120802032627.

Kheswa, G. (2014). Exploring HIV and AIDS Stigmatisation: Children's perspectives. *Mediterranean Journal of Social Sciences, 5,* 529—541. doi: 10.5901/mjss. 2014. v5n15p529.

Mahajan, A. P., Sayles, J. N., Patel, V. A., Remien, R. H., Ortiz, D., Szekeres, G., & Coates, T. J. (2008). Stigma in the HIV/AIDS epidemic: A review of the literature and recommendations for the way forward. *AIDS (London, England), 22*(Suppl 2), S67. Doi: 0.1097/01.aids.0000327438.13291.62.

References

Angermeyer, M. C., Matschinger, H., Link, B. G., & Schomerus, G. (2014). Public attitudes regarding individual and structural discrimination: Two sides of the same coin? *Social Science & Medicine, 103,* 60–66. doi: 10.1016/j.socscimed.2013.11.014.

Berger, B. E., Ferrans, C. E., & Lashley, F. R. (2001). Measuring stigma in people with HIV: Psychometric assessment of the HIV stigma scale. *Research in Nursing & Health, 24,* 518–529. doi:10.1002/nur.10011.

Bresnahan, M. I., & Zhuang, J. (2011). Towards a theory of stigma. *Journal of Health Psychology, 15,* 231–243. doi:10.1348/135910709X457946.

Brown, L., Macintyre, K., & Trujillo, L. (2003). Interventions to reduce HIV/AIDS stigma: What have we learned? *AIDS Education and Prevention, 15*, 49–69. doi: 10.1521/aeap.15.1.49.23844.

Bunner, J. Y., Solomon, S. E., Miller, C., & Forehand, R. (2007). Measurement of stigma in people with HIV: A reexamination of the HIV stigma scale. *AIDS Education and Prevention, 19*, 198–209. doi:10.1521/aeap.2007.19.3.198.

Chaudoir, S. R., Earnshaw, V. A., & Andel, S. (2013). "Discredited" versus "discreditable": Understanding how shared and unique stigma mechanisms affect psychological and physical health disparities. *Basic and Applied Social Psychology, 35*, 75–87. doi:10 .1080/01973533.2012.746612.

Clement, S., Brohan, E., Jeffery, D., Henderson, C., Hatch, S. L., Thornicroft, G. (2012). Development and psychometric properties the Barriers to Access to Care Evaluation scale (BACE) related to people with mental ill health. *BMC Psychiatry, 12*, 36–47. doi:10.1186/1471-224X-12-36.

Corrigan, P. W., Watson, A. C., & Miller, F. E. (2006). Blame, shame, and contamination: The impact of mental illness and drug dependence stigma on family members. *Journal of Family Psychology, 20*, 239. doi: 10.1037/0893-3200.20.2.239.

DePierre, J. A., Puhl, R. M., & Luedicke, J. (2013). A new stigmatized identity? Comparisons of a "food addict" label with other stigmatized health conditions. *Basic and Applied Social Psychology, 35*, 10–21. doi: 10.1080/01973533.2012.746148.

Downey, G., Mougios, V., Ayduk, O., London, B. E., & Shoda, Y. (2004). Rejection sensitivity and the defensive motivational system: Insights from the startle response to rejection cues. *Psychological Science, 15*, 668–673. doi: 10.1111/j.0956-7976.2004.00738.x.

Earnshaw, V. A., & Chaudoir, S. R. (2009). From conceptualizing to measuring HIV stigma: A review of HIV stigma mechanism measures. *AIDS and Behavior, 13*, 1160–1177. doi:10.1007/s10461-009-9593-3

Gabbidon, J., Brohan, E., Clement, S., Henderson, R. C., & Thornicroft, G. (2013). The development and validation of the Questionnaire on Anticipated Discrimination (QUAD). *BMC Psychiatry, 13*, 297–309. doi: 10.1186/1471-244X-13-297.

Goffman, E. (1963). *Stigma: Notes on the management of spoiled identity.* New York: Simon and Schuster.

Hatzenbuehler, M. L., Bellatorre, A., Lee, Y., Finch, B. K., Muennig, P., & Fiscella, K. (2014). Structural stigma and all-cause mortality in sexual minority populations. *Social Science & Medicine, 103*, 33–41. doi: 10.1016/j.socscimed.2013.06.005.

Herek, G. M., Saha, S., & Burack, J. (2013). Stigma and psychological distress in people with HIV/AIDS. *Basic and Applied Social Psychology, 35*, 41–54. doi:10.1080/0197 3533.2012.746606.

Holton, A. E., Farrell, L. C., & Fudge, J. L. (2014). A threatening space? Stigmatization and the framing of autism in the news. *Communication Studies, 65*, 189–207. doi: 10.1080/10510974.2013.855642.

Ilic, M., Reinecke, J., Bohner, G., Röttgers, H. O., Beblo, T., Driessen, M.,...& Corrigan, P. W. (2013). Belittled, avoided, ignored, denied: Assessing forms and consequences of stigma experiences of people with mental illness. *Basic and Applied Social Psychology*, *35*(1), 31–40. doi: 10.1080/01973533.2012.746619.

Interian, A., Ang, A., Gara, M., Link, B., Rodriguez, M., & Vega, W. (2010). Stigma and depression treatment utilization among Latinos: Utility of four stigma measures. *Psychiatric Services*, *61*, 373–379. doi:10.1176/appi.ps.61.4.373.

Link, B. G., & Phelan, J. C. (2001). Conceptualizing stigma. *Annual Review of Sociology*, *27*, 363–385. doi:10.1146/annurev.soc.27.1.363.

Link, B. G., & Phelan, J. (2014). Stigma power. *Social Science & Medicine*, *103*, 24–32. doi: 10.1016/j.socscimed.2013.07.035.

Luhtanen, R., & Crocker, J. (1992). A collective self-esteem scale: Self-evaluation of one's social identity. *Personality and Social Psychology Bulletin*, *18*, 302–318 doi: 10.1177/0146167292183006.

Lukachko, A., Hatzenbuehler, M. L., & Keyes, M. K. (2014). Structural racism and myocardial infarction in the United States. *Social Science & Medicine*, *103*, 42–50. doi:10.1016/j.socscimed.2013.07.021.

Myers, A., & Rosen, J. C. (1999). Obesity stigmatization and coping: Relation to mental health symptoms, body image, and self-esteem. *International Journal of Obesity and Related Metabolic Disorders: Journal of the International Association for the Study of Obesity*, *23*, 221–230. doi: 10.1038/sj.ijo.0800765.

Pachankis, J. E., Hatzenbuehler, M. L., & Starks, T. J. (2014). The influence of structural stigma and rejection sensitivity on young sexual minority men's daily tobacco and alcohol use. *Social Science & Medicine*, *103*, 67–75. doi: 10.1016/j.socscimed.2013.10.005.

Parker, R., & Aggleton, P. (2003). HIV and AIDS-related stigma and discrimination: a conceptual framework and implications for action. *Social Science & Medicine*, *57*, 13–24. doi: 10.1016/S0277-9536(02)00304-0.

Reid, A. E., Dovidio, J. F., Ballester, E., & Johnson, B. T. (2014). HIV prevention interventions to reduce sexual risk for African Americans: The influence of community-level stigma and psychological processes. *Social Science & Medicine*, *103*, 118–125. doi:10.1016/j.socscimed.2013.06.028.

Ritsher, J., Otilingam, P. G., & Grajales, M. (2003). Internalized stigma of mental illness: Psychometric properties of a new measure. *Psychiatry Research*, *121*, 31–49. doi: 10.1016/j.psychres.2003.08.008.

Rosenberg, M. (1989). *Society and the adolescent self-image*. Middletown, CT: Wesleyan University Press.

Salek, T. A. (2014). Faith turns political on the 2012 campaign trail: Mitt Romney, Franklin Graham, and the stigma of nontraditional religions in American politics. *Communication Studies*, *65*, 174–188. doi: 10.1080/10510974.2013.851097.

Scambler, G. (2004). Re-framing stigma: Felt and enacted stigma and challenges to the sociology of chronic and disabling conditions. *Social Theory & Health*, *2*, 29–46. doi: 10.1057/palgrave.sth.8700012.

Smith, R. A. (2007). Language of the lost: An explication of stigma communication. *Communication Theory, 17,* 462–485. doi: 10.1111/j.1468-2885.2007.00307.x.

Smith, R. A. (2014). Testing the model of stigma communication with a factorial experiment in an interpersonal context. *Communication Studies, 65,* 154–173. doi: 10.1080/10510974.2013.851095.

Stearns, S. A. (2014). This Goffmanian conundrum: Supporting the status quo or forced to manage societal ramifications? *Communication Studies, 65,* 208–222. doi: 10.1080/10510974.2013.851098.

Steward, W. T., Herek, G. M., Ramakrishna, J., Bharat, S., Chandy, S., Wrubel, J., & Ekstrand, M. L. (2008). HIV-related stigma: Adapting a theoretical framework for use in India. *Social Science & Medicine, 67,* 1225–1235. doi: 10.1016/j.socscimed.2008.05.032.

Striley, K. M. (2014). The stigma of excellence and the dialectic of (perceived) superiority and inferiority: Exploring intellectually gifted adolescents' experiences of stigma. *Communication Studies, 65*(2), 139–153. doi: 10.1080/10510974.2013.85172.

Thorncroft, G., Brohan, E., Rose, D., Sartorius, N., & Leese, M. (2009). Global pattern of experience and anticipated discrimination against people with schizophrenia: A cross-sectional survey. *The Lancet, 373,* 408–415. doi: 10.1016/S0140-6736(08)61817-6.

Van Brakel, W. H. (2006). Measuring health-related stigma—a literature review. *Psychology, Health & Medicine, 11,* 307–334. doi: 10.1080/13548500600595160.

Westbrook, L. E., & Bauman, L. J. (1996). *Perceived stigma of HIV/AIDS scale.* Bronx, NY: Albert Einstein College of Medicine.

24. Subjective Numeracy

KERK F. KEE,
Chapman University
& YUHUA (JAKE) LIANG,
Chapman University

Numeracy is the ability to understand numerical information. This specific ability is critical to comprehending health information as well as weighing the risks and benefits of medical treatment options. Numerical information is often used in decision aids designed to empower patients in shared decision-making, especially when they are asked to consent to a medical procedure that involves calculated risks and benefits. Patients may evaluate quantitative data such as survival likelihood, treatment success rates, complication rates, and comparative procedural statistics, among others.

However, difficulty in understanding numerical risk information can lead to treatment decisions that do not align with patients' goals. Such a misalignment can possibly lead to a lower level of perceived provider satisfaction. Physicians and patients both succeed in sharing the decision-making process only when patients can fully comprehend the medical information they receive, and then apply it to choose the treatment option that is most compatible with their personal goals and/or values.

Numeracy presents a systemic challenge for effective health communication, especially for many Americans with low numeracy. About "22% of Americans scored in the lowest 2 levels for quantitative literacy, a performance level that corresponds to having the ability to solve only single-operation arithmetic problems (e.g., what is the difference in cost between 2 items?)" (Fagerlin et al., 2007, p. 672). Furthermore, Lipkus and colleagues (2001) informed us that even populations with more formal education reported low numeracy.

Numeracy has received much research attention in health communication, medical decision-making, and public health research over the last couple of decades. Prior studies found that individuals with low numeracy are less likely to recall risk information presented in pictographs or text (Zikmund-Fisher, Smith, Ubel, & Fagerlin, 2007), misinterpret risk information in the health context (Sheridan, Pignone, & Lewis, 2003), perceive inaccurately the risk of developing cancer (Donelle, Arocha, & Hoffman-Goetz, 2008), underutilize cancer screening for early detection (Ciampa, Osborn, Peterson, & Rothman, 2010), overestimate mammography's reduction of the risk of developing breast cancer (Schwartz, Woloshin, Black, & Welch, 1997), adhere to recommended health behaviors among patients living with chronic disease (Ciampa et al., 2010), seek health information online to a lesser degree (Rakovski et al., 2012), and report lower patient-provider satisfaction (Ciampa et al., 2010). This body of literature clearly documents the detrimental effects of low numeracy on health decisions, although these studies conceptualize numeracy differently.

Previous researchers have advanced conceptual definitions for numeracy, including a person's *ability* to understand risks expressed in numbers, such as frequencies, probabilities, and percentages (Lipkus et al., 2001); *aptitude* with ratios, probabilities, and fractions (Fagerlin et al., 2007); and *difficulty* in using numbers in daily life (Ciampa et al., 2010). Framing numeracy as a difficulty may be attributed to the observation that ratio and probability concepts are often not intuitive for many individuals (Nelson, Moser, & Han, 2013). Golbeck and colleagues (2005) define numeracy as "the degree to which individuals have the capacity to access, process, interpret, communicate, and act on numerical, quantitative, graphical, biostatistical, and probabilistic health information needed to make effective health decisions" (p. 375). Morris and colleagues (2013) conceptualize numeracy as a dimension of health literacy, while Rakovski and colleagues (2012) suggest that numeracy and health literacy are empirically two distinct constructs. Based on existing research, we summarize numeracy as *the ability to understand numeric or quantitative information*. For readers interested in a more exhaustive review of numeracy, we refer them to Reyna and colleagues (2009).

Measuring Subjective Numeracy

The measurement of numeracy has followed objective and subjective approaches. These approaches both measure the underlying construct of numeracy. The objective measure relies on actual mathematical tests, tapping into individuals' abilities to reason with numbers. The objective measure has been validated and well received (see Lipkus et al., 2001). However, the current chapter focuses solely on the *Subjective Numeracy Scale* (SNS) due to certain advantages over the objective measure. We compare and contrast these advantages in the following sections. Moreover, one should note that the 8-item SNS measure (Fagerlin et al., 2007) differs from a number of past studies that have ostensibly used subjective numeracy. Some previous studies used two items from the Health Information National Trends Survey (e.g., Ciampa et al., 2010; Nelson et al., 2013; Smith, Wolf, & Wagner, 2010) to measure subjective numeracy. However, 2-item measures prevent tests for structural properties using factor analytic approaches; therefore, we limit our discussion to the 8-item SNS measure from Fagerlin et al.

The SNS measure has specific advantages to overcome certain challenges for practitioners, making it more efficient to administer across populations. First, research participants generally do not enjoy taking an aptitude test. Validated measures of objective numeracy require actual mathematical calculations. This requirement may induce a negative reaction to the research study and/or decrease study completion rates. For longitudinal studies, this reaction may also lower the retention rate of voluntary participants. Second, when administered through an online survey, researchers have little assurance that participants are performing the mathematical calculations without assistance, such as using a computing device, or asking a friend for help. Third, when administered through the telephone, the simultaneous tasks of remembering all the components of the question and performing the calculations can stimulate cognitive overload, social desirability effects, and perceived demand characteristics, resulting in an inaccurate assessment of telephone participants' numeracy. In response to these challenges, Fagerlin and colleagues (2007) developed the SNS to measure numeracy in a more efficient and less aversive fashion.

The SNS consists of two dimensions. The first four items are designed to measure individuals' beliefs about cognitive abilities and skill in performing different mathematical operations, such as fraction and percentage calculations. The last four items measure individuals' general preferences for the presentation of numerical and probabilistic information, such as graphs.

Table 1. Fagerlin et al.'s Subjective Numeracy Scale.

Cognitive Abilities (1=*not at all good*, 6–*extremely good*)
1. How good are you at working with fractions?
2. How good are you at working with percentages?
3. How good are you at calculating at 15% tip?
4. How good are you at figuring out how much a shirt will cost if it is 25% off?

Preference for Display of Numeric Information

1. When reading the newspaper, how helpful do you find tables and graphs that are parts of a story? (1=*not at all*, 6=*extremely*)

2. When people tell you about the chance of something happening, do you prefer that they use *words* ("it rarely happens") or *numbers* ("there's a 1% chance"?) (1=*always prefer words*, 6=*always prefer numbers*)

3. When you hear a weather forecast, do you prefer predictions using *percentages* (e.g., "there will be a 20% chance of rain today") or predictions using only *words* (e.g., "there is a small chance of rain today")? (1=*always prefer percentages*, 6=*always prefer words*, reverse coded)

4. How *often* do you find numerical information to be useful? (1=*never*, 6=*very often*)

SNS's development and validity may be examined in light of the objective measure. The objective measure tested participants' actual ability to make decisions based on numeric assessment (e.g., what is the best risk of getting a disease: 1 in 100, 1 in 1000, or 1 in 10?). The SNS measure paralleled the objective measures without using a numeric assessment. Fagerlin and colleagues (2007) found that the SNS correlated significantly with the objective measure developed by Lipkus and colleagues (2001) ($r = 0.63$–0.68). Furthermore, the SNS was completed in less time (24 seconds per item v. 31 seconds per item, $p < 0.05$), less stressful (1.62 v. 2.69, $p < 0.01$) and less frustrating (1.92 v. 2.88, $p < 0.01$). More participants (50%) who completed the SNS versus 8% who completed the objective scale volunteered to participate in another study (Odds Ratio = 11.00, 95% CI = 2.14–56.65).

In terms of validity, SNS has not received a full range of efforts to validate. Specifically, the scale validation and follow up studies appeared to aim to establish the SNS's criterion validity rather than assessing the overall construct validity. Although the SNS has received empirical support in terms of its correlation with the objective measure, and it has several distinct advantages for data collection as discussed in the previous paragraph, we briefly review SNS's content, criterion-related, and construct validity (Kerlinger & Lee, 1999) in the following paragraphs.

Content validity refers to the extent to which a measure covers the full range of the subject matter. The SNS began with 42 items. The final scale was reduced to 8-items. Content validity decreases with the number of items; still, the final 8 item measure includes questions related to fractions, percentages, hypothetical applications of numeracy (e.g., tipping and discount), and preference for numeric information (e.g., "how often do you find numeric informational to be useful"). This wide range generally supports SNS's content validity, although multiple items per content area would further strengthen content validity.

Criterion-related validity is the extent to which a measure compares to other variables that assess the same construct. Two subtypes of this validity include *predictive validity* and *concurrent validity*. Predictive validity refers to the ability of the measure to predict an intended outcome. Predictive validity is often established by deploying longitudinal designs, which has not been used with the SNS at the writing of this chapter. In terms of concurrent validity, there is evidence in the original validation efforts because of the measure's correlation with the objective measure ($r = .68$). However, data from national representative samples in the United States and Germany (Galesic & Garcia-Retamero, 2010) did not yield relevant statistics to demonstrate isomorphism between the objective and subjective measures.

Construct validity refers to the extent to which a measure solely assesses the underlying construct. The SNS was developed out of criterion-related validity to approximate objective numeracy; validation efforts have not followed traditional rigors of establishing construct validity. Traditional approaches to establish construct validity involve (1) confirmatory factor analyses to establish the structural validity and dimensionality (such as parallelism), (2) test of convergence and discrimination with the use of nomothetic networks, (3) or multi-trait multi-method approaches. The SNS has limited empirical support in construct validity. The original validation study did not provide evidence to identify whether the 8-item measure conformed to the internal structure of a unidimensional measurement model. At the time of this writing, we are unaware of any such analysis that has been conducted. Researchers who apply SNS should keep the discussed aspects of validity in mind.

Use of Existing Measures and Future Studies

A number of studies have utilized the SNS since original development, often as an individual difference measure for statistical control or as a moderator for other variables. One encouraging area of work involved validating the numeracy construct using a Rasch Analysis (Weller et al., 2013). This approach to measurement follows Item Response Theory, which involves developing question items of varying difficulty, presenting these items to test respondents sequentially, and calculating their numeracy based on the difficulty of the final test items and their performance. Weller et al.'s (2013) approach resulted in a measure that correlated substantially with the objective measure ($r = .55$), and equally with SNS ($r = .55$). This correlation provides some indirect evidence that SNS may be as useful as objective measures in assessing numeracy, assuming that the Rasch Analysis resulted in more valid measure of numeracy.

Practically, health care providers should not assume that patients can understand the statistics and numerical information given to them. In fact, based on patients' numeracy level, providers would be well advised to take additional time to explain the quantitative information related to prescriptions and treatments in order to reduce the likelihood of unnecessary future visits due to preventable misunderstandings. Furthermore, providers can use different versions of a health message with individuals, depending on numeracy levels. For example, with low numeracy patients, a provider can use graphical displays and/or analogies (Galesic & Garcia-Retamero, 2010). By helping patients of all numeracy levels to make fully informed decisions, effective health communication can close the gap in medical interventions that are intended to improve the quality of care for patients.

Recommended Readings

Fagerlin, A., Zikmund-Fisher, B. J., Ubel, P. A., Jankovic, A., Derry, H. A., & Smith, D. M. (2007). Measuring numeracy without a math test: Development of the subjective numeracy scale. *Medical Decision-making, 27*, 672–680.

Galesic, M., & Garcia-Retamero, R. (2010). Statistical numeracy for health: A cross-cultural comparison with probabilistic national samples. *Archives of Internal Medicine, 170*, 462–468.

Golbeck, A. L., Ahlers-Schmidt, C. R., Paschal, A. M., & Dismuke, S. E. (2005). A definition and operational framework for health numeracy. *American Journal of Preventive Medicine, 29*, 375–376.

Nelson, W. L., Moser, R. P., & Han, P. K. (2013). Exploring objective and subjective numeracy at a population level: Findings from the 2007 Health Information National Trends Survey (HINTS). *Journal of Health Communication, 18*, 192–205.

Zikmund-Fisher, B. J., Smith, D. M., Ubel, P. A., & Fagerlin, A. (2007). Validation of the subjective numeracy scale: Effects of low numeracy on comprehension of risk communications and utility elicitations. *Medical Decision-making, 27*, 663–671.

References

Ciampa, P. J., Osborn, C. Y., Peterson, N. B., & Rothman, R. L. (2010). Patient numeracy, perceptions of provider communication, and colorectal cancer screening utilization. *Journal of Health Communication, 15*, 157–168. doi: 10.1080/10810730.2010.522699.

Donelle, L., Arocha, J., & Hoffman-Goetz, L. (2008). Health literacy and numeracy: Key factors in cancer risk comprehension. *Chronic Diseases in Canada, 29*, 1–8.

Fagerlin, A., Zikmund-Fisher, B. J., Ubel, P. A., Jankovic, A., Derry, H. A., & Smith, D. M. (2007). Measuring numeracy without a math test: Development of the subjective numeracy scale. *Medical Decision-making, 27,* 672–680. doi: 10.1177/0272989X07304449.

Galesic, M., & Garcia-Retamero, R. (2010). Statistical numeracy for health: A cross-cultural comparison with probabilistic national samples. *Archives of Internal Medicine, 170,* 462–468. doi: 10.1001/archinternmed.2009.481.

Golbeck, A. L., Ahlers-Schmidt, C. R., Paschal, A. M., & Dismuke, S. E. (2005). A definition and operational framework for health numeracy. *American Journal of Preventive Medicine, 29,* 375–376. http://dx.doi.org/10.1016/j.amepre.2005.06.012

Kerlinger, F. N., & Lee, H. B. (1999). *Foundations of behavioral research.* New York: Wadsworth.

Lipkus, I. M., Samsa, G., & Rimer, B. K. (2001). General performance on a numeracy scale among highly educated samples. *Medical Decision-making, 21,* 37–44. doi: 10.1177/0272989X0102100105.

Morris, N. S., Field, T. S., Wagner, J. L., Cutrona, S. L., Roblin, D. W., Gaglio, B., Mazor, K. M. (2013). The association between health literacy and cancer-related attitudes, behaviors, and knowledge. *Journal of Health Communication, 18*(sup1), 223–241. doi: 10.1080/10810730.2013.825667.

Nelson, W. L., Moser, R. P., & Han, P. K. (2013). Exploring objective and subjective numeracy at a population level: Findings from the 2007 Health Information National Trends Survey (HINTS). *Journal of Health Communication, 18,* 192–205. doi: 10.1080/10810730.2012.688450.

Rakovski, C., Sparks, L., Robinson, J. D., Kee, K. F., Bevan, J. L., & Agne, R. (2012). A regression-based study using jackknife replicates of HINTS III data: Predictors of the efficacy of health information seeking. *Journal of Communication in Healthcare, 5,* 163–170. http://dx.doi.org/10.1179/1753807612Y.0000000014

Reyna, V. F., Nelson, W. L., Han, P. K., & Dieckmann, N. F. (2009). How numeracy influences risk comprehension and medical decision-making. *Psychological Bulletin, 135,* 943–973. http://dx.doi.org/10.1037/a0017327

Schwartz, L. M., Woloshin, S., Black, W. C., & Welch, H. G. (1997). The role of numeracy in understanding the benefit of screening mammography. *Annals of Internal Medicine, 127,* 966–972. doi: 10.7326/0003-4819-127-11-199712010-00003.

Sheridan, S. L., Pignone, M. P., & Lewis, C. L. (2003). A randomized comparison of patients' understanding of number needed to treat and other common risk reduction formats. *Journal of General Internal Medicine, 18,* 884–892. doi: 10.1046/j.1525-1497.2003.21102.x.

Smith, S. G., Wolf, M. S., & von Wagner, C. (2010). Socioeconomic status, statistical confidence, and patient–provider communication: An analysis of the Health Information National Trends Survey (HINTS 2007). *Journal of Health Communication, 15,* 169–185. doi: 10.1080/10810730.2010.522690.

Weller, J. A., Dieckmann, N. F., Tusler, M., Mertz, C. K., Burns, W. J., & Peters, E. (2013). Development and testing of an abbreviated numeracy scale: A Rasch analysis approach. *Journal of Behavioral Decision-making, 26*, 198–212. doi: 10.1002/bdm.1751.

Zikmund-Fisher, B. J., Smith, D. M., Ubel, P. A., & Fagerlin, A. (2007). Validation of the subjective numeracy scale: Effects of low numeracy on comprehension of risk communications and utility elicitations. *Medical Decision-making, 27*, 663–671. doi: 10.1177/0272989X07303824.

25. *Uncertainty and Uncertainty Management*

ROXANNE PARROTT,
The Pennsylvania State University
RACHEL A. SMITH,
The Pennsylvania State University
& AMY E. CHADWICK,
Ohio University

Derived from uncertainty in illness theory (Mishel, 1981), uncertainty management theory (UMT; Brashers, 2001) addresses how individuals understand and
experience uncertainty, which encompasses the inability to determine meaning
associated with ambiguity about one's state of health, complexity associated
with treatment and care, a lack of information about diagnosis, and a lack of
predictability for prognosis (Brashers, 2001). Uncertainty management includes appraisals of the situation, appraisals of uncertainty, emotional responses
to uncertainty, and psychological and behavioral responses to uncertainty that
include information seeking, information avoidance, and advocacy (Brashers,
Goldsmith, & Hsieh, 2002; Brashers, Haas, Neidig, & Rintamaki, 2002).

According to UMT, uncertainty may be appraised as a danger, such that
not knowing might lead to harm, or uncertainty can be appraised as a benefit,
in which case, not knowing may help a person to maintain hope or optimism
(Brashers, 2001). When uncertainty is appraised as a danger, people have a
negative emotional response, feeling fear, anxiety, or worry. When uncertainty is appraised as a benefit, people have a positive emotional response, feeling
hope or happiness. Uncertainty can also be appraised as *neither* good nor bad
(neutral response), or *both* good and bad (combined response). Positive and
negative emotional responses to uncertainty can co-occur for different aspects
of the same health condition. For example, when treatment options for spinal
cord injuries are perceived to be few and to have minimal positive effects, this

uncertainty is appraised as a danger and leads to negative emotions, whereas uncertainty about the degree of functional impairment associated with the spinal cord injury itself may be evaluated more positively and produce hope (Parrott, Stuart, & Cairns, 2000).

Uncertainty appraised as a danger leads people to attempt to reduce uncertainty, whereas uncertainty appraised as a benefit may lead people to maintain or even increase their uncertainty (Brashers et al., 2000; Brashers & Babrow, 1996). The uncertainty management process involves seeking and/ or avoiding information; adapting to chronic uncertainty; and/or obtaining assistance with uncertainty management through social support (Brashers, 2001). Appraisals of uncertainty, emotional responses, and management strategies can vary and shift as new information is obtained or as uncertainty is reappraised, often through communication. The appraisal process and responses themselves affect the experience of uncertainty, uncertainty appraisal, and selection of uncertainty management behavior (Brashers, Neidig, & Goldsmith, 2000).

In asserting the significance of appraisals about the current situation and about uncertainty, as well as the significance of the emotions resulting from these appraisals, UMT has many parallels to appraisal theories. According to appraisal theories, emotions arise from assessments of environmental stimuli in relation to goals, motives, wants, and needs (Lazarus, 1991). Different patterns of appraisals about stimuli in the environment result in different emotions (Roseman & Smith, 2001). Thus, different appraisals are associated with the hope, happiness, fear, or anxiety individuals feel in response to uncertainty (Chadwick, 2015; Roseman, 2001).

An appraisal theory that is particularly relevant to UMT is Lazarus's cognitive-mediation theory (Lazarus, 1991, 2001). Cognitive-mediation theory posits two categories of appraisals, *primary appraisal*, in which individuals determine the meaning of the stimulus for them, and *secondary appraisal*, in which individuals assess their ability to cope with the consequences of the stimulus. The primary appraisal assesses whether an environmental stimulus has implications for the individual's well-being (e.g., *importance*), whether conditions are favorable or unfavorable to achieving relevant goals (e.g., *goal congruence*), and what is at risk in the situation (e.g., self- and social esteem, moral values, ego ideals, meanings and ideas, other persons and their well-being, or life goals). The secondary appraisal assesses who has control over the environmental stimulus, whether the individual can successfully achieve a reward or avoid harm in response to the stimulus, and whether the individual thinks the environmental situation will become better or worse (e.g., *future expectation*). The primary and secondary appraisals are rapid assessments, influence each other, have no inherent temporal ordering, and fully mediate emotions (Lazarus & Folkman, 1987). These appraisals are a more detailed and explicit description of the kinds of appraisals that may go into the broad assessment of whether uncertainty is a danger or a benefit, and the resulting emotion evoked than is usually provided in UMT.

Measuring Uncertainty and Uncertainty Management

When measuring uncertainty and uncertainty management, researchers should fully assess cognitive reactions, including primary and secondary appraisals, as well as emotional reactions. Typically, studies that have examined uncertainty in health contexts focus on documenting whether or not people are feeling uncertainty, as well as identifying what causes people to feel uncertain, such as the diagnosis and prognosis (e.g., Mishel, 1981; Lin, Acquaye, Vera-Bolanos, Cahill, Gilbert, & Armstrong, 2012). These types of studies measure the causes and consequences of uncertainty, but do not assess the key mediating mechanisms of appraisals and emotional responses to uncertainty comprising the uncertainty management process, and how these lead to different ways to increase or reduce uncertainty.

Illness uncertainty has received extensive focus in efforts to derive valid instruments, but the focus has largely remained on cognitive elements rather than emphasizing appraisals and emotions, particularly the positive emotion of hope. Mishel (1981) administered a survey to 259 hospitalized patients and, through exploratory factor analysis, developed a scale consisting of two dimensions to operationalize uncertainty management, with follow-up administration to 100 patients to further validate the instrument (see Table 1). The first, labeled multi-attributed ambiguity, includes 20 items (Cronbach α = .89) associated with all categories of illness events, while the second, labeled, unpredictability, has 8 items (Cronbach α = .72) that focus on whether a patient is confident in predicting the symptomatology and outcomes linked to the illness. Construct validity was assessed via assessing levels of stress, which should directly relate to a patient's inability to cope with uncertainty, finding an r = .35 to support the scale's validity, and r = .25 relating to unpredictability. Further, uncertainty should impair comprehension with a measure of comprehension found to negatively relate to ambiguity, r = -.63 and unpredictability, r = -.56 (Mishel, 1981).

Table 1. Mishel's (1981) Scale to Measure 2 Dimensions of Illness Uncertainty (MUIS—Mishel's Uncertainty in Illness Scale).

(Multi-attributed ambiguity)

1. I don't know what is wrong with me.
2. I have a lot of questions without answers.
3. I am unsure if my illness is getting better or worse.
4. It is unclear how bad my pain will be.
5. The explanations they give seem hazy to me.
6. I do not know when to expect things will be done to me.
7. My symptoms continue to change unpredictably.
8. The doctors say things to me that could have many meanings.
9. My treatment is too complex to figure out.
10. It is difficult to know if the treatments or medications I am getting are helping me.
11. There are so many different types of staff, it's unclear who is responsible for what.
12. Because of the unpredictability of my illness, I cannot plan for the future.
13. The course of my illness keeps changing; I have my good and bad days.
14. It's vague to me how I will manage after I leave the hospital.
15. I have been given many differing opinions about what is wrong with me.
16. It is not clear what is going to happen to me.
17. They have not told me how they will treat my illness.
18. It is difficult to determine how long it will be before I can care for myself.
19. They give me so much information that I cannot tell what is most important.
20. They have not given me a specific diagnosis.

(Unpredictability)

1. The purpose of each treatment is clear to me.
2. When I have pain, I know what it means about my condition.
3. I usually know if I am going to have a good or bad day.
4. It is clear to me when I am getting better or worse.
5. I understand everything explained to me.
6. I can predict how long my illness will last.
7. I can generally predict the course of my illness.
8. My physical distress is predictable; I know when it is going to get better or worse.

Mishel's scale has been used extensively and adapted to varying disease contexts, as well as different cultures (e.g., Giammanco et al., 2014). Sometimes, the adaptations include additional scale items, as with the version used with patients who have been diagnosed with primary brain tumors (Lin et al., 2012). Several items were added for use of the scale in this context (see Table 2).

Table 2. Items Added to MUIS for Use with Patients with Brain Tumors (Lin et al., 2012).

1.	The results of the tests are inconsistent or unclear.
2.	I do not know when to expect things (e.g., treatment, tests, etc.) will be done to me.
3.	When I have symptoms, I know what these mean about my condition.
4.	It is unclear how bad my symptoms will be.
5.	I can depend on the medical team to be there when I need them.

Other studies have extended the theoretical foundation of the MUIS to assess behaviors linked to uncertainty management in clinical trials, positing that knowledge, problem-solving skills, and patient-provider communication reflect avenues to address the meaning of uncertainty (e.g., a lack of knowledge), how to address uncertainty (e.g., utilize problem-solving skills), and outcomes associated with the skills gained (e.g., through physician-provider communication; Mishel et al., 2009). Select items associated with such an approach focused on decision-making for early state prostate cancer patients appear in Table 3.

Table 3. Sample Items Used in Mishel et al. (2009).

(Knowledge; 3 of 20 items)	
1.	Prostate cancer can recur even after prostatectomy.
2.	Rising PSA levels mean that a man has prostate cancer.
3.	Untreated prostate cancer can spread to the bones.
(Problem-solving; 3 of 10 items)	
1.	When I have to do something that makes me worry, I try to think about how I can handle my worry.
2.	When I have a lot of things to do, I try to plan my work more carefully.
3.	When I am short of money, I try to plan more carefully in the future.

(Patient-provider Communication; 3 of 5 items)
1. During the visit, how much did the doctor tell you about your illness and what he/she is doing to treat it?
2. During the visit, how much did you help with the planning of your treatment?
3. During the visit, how much did you tell the nurses and treatment staff about concerns you might be having about the treatment program?

Some studies have begun to assess appraisals of and emotional responses to uncertainty (e.g., Parrott, Peters, & Traeder, 2012). Other studies have examined behaviors in response to uncertainty, including information seeking (see Yang chapter in this volume), information avoidance, adaptation to chronic uncertainty, and seeking social support (see Rains chapter in this volume), and how these may vary by the source of uncertainty. For example, the uncertainty of experiencing stigmatization because of a health diagnosis may be appraised as a danger, evoking fear (Brashers, 2001) and resulting in an overall withdraw from interactions (Smith, 2011; also see Bresnahan & Zhuang's chapter in this volume), which directly addresses the social nature of the source of the uncertainty. Outside the clinical setting, UMT has guided efforts to explain outcomes associated with genetic conditions, leading to assessments (see Table 4) of illness uncertainty (Cronbach α = .81), uncertainty management (Cronbach α = .85), negative emotions associated with a diagnosis (Cronbach α = .85), and communication preferences (Cronbach α = .80) to more fully capture the theoretical scope of UMT (Parrott, Peters, & Traeder, 2012).

Table 4. Parrott et al.'s (2012) Scales to Assess UMT Constructs.

(Illness Uncertainty)
1. The symptoms of the condition are puzzling to me.
2. The condition doesn't make sense to me.
3. I understand the condition.
(Uncertainty Management)
1. I want to feel hopeful about the condition.
2. I want peace of mind with respect to the condition.
3. I want to feel like I am more in control with respect to the condition.
4. I want to feel that eventually everything will be OK.

(Negative feelings relating to the diagnosis)

1.   The condition makes me angry.

2.   The condition makes me sad.

3.   The condition makes me feel afraid.

(Communication preferences)

1.   I want to talk about how to manage my thoughts and feelings about (condition).

2.   I want to talk about how to use information about (condition) to make future decisions.

3.   I want to talk about how to test for (condition).

4.   I want to talk about how to treat (condition).

5.   I want to talk about what (condition) is.

The direction that Parrott et al. (2012) took with scales to assess uncertainty and uncertainty management emphasizes the significance of emotions and appraisals associated with the process of uncertainty management. Several of the appraisals relevant to uncertainty have been assessed in the context of climate change (Chadwick, 2010, 2015) and should be considered to further scale development linked to UMT. The measures in Table 5 have been modified from the original measures to focus on feelings of certainty/uncertainty rather than climate change.

Table 5. Measures of appraisals related to UMT adapted from Chadwick (2015).

(Appraisal of Importance)

Being certain about [target, e.g., my diagnosis]...

1.   Does not matter at all to me/Matters very much to me

2.   Is very important/Is very unimportant **R**

3.   Is very nonessential/Is very essential

4.   Is very significant/Is very insignificant **R**

5.   Is of no concern/Is of very much concern

6.   Is very relevant/Is very irrelevant **R**

7.   Is not needed at all/Is needed very much

(Note. **R** = reverse-coded item.)

(Appraisal of Goal Congruence)
Being certain about [Target, e.g., my diagnosis]…

1. is one of my goals.

2. relates to my personal goals.

3. would help me achieve other important goals.

4. helps me meet my personal goals.

5. fits with my personal values.

6. is consistent with my ideals.

7. is important to meeting my personal goals.

(Appraisal of Future Expectation)

1. Being certain about [Target, e.g., my diagnosis] will make the future wonderful.

2. Not being certain about [Target, e.g., my diagnosis] will make the future awful.

3. Failing to learn [Target, e.g., my diagnosis] will create a bleak future.

4. Learning [Target, e.g., my diagnosis] will create a bright future.

5. A more certain [Target, e.g., my diagnosis] equals a much better future.

6. An uncertain [Target, e.g., my diagnosis] equals a much worse future.

Use of Existing Measures and Future Studies

To continue progress in understanding the role of uncertainty in health communication, researchers need to fully assess *all* aspects of uncertainty: causes, mediating mechanisms, and consequences. This includes measuring whether people are feeling uncertain, what they are feeling uncertain about, their appraisals of the situation, their appraisals of uncertainty, the emotions that they are feeling, and the behaviors they intend to perform (or not perform) to manage their uncertainty. In addition, as uncertainty management often occurs through communication, attending to who is (and is not) selected for conversations or as sources of information, and how the causes and mediating mechanisms predict these communication patterns will capture critical aspects of how uncertainty management unfolds. Finally, because uncertainty management is a process, longitudinal studies are needed to capture appraisals and emotions before uncertainty management behaviors have occurred, through the management experience, and afterward to determine how the processes of appraisal and reappraisal of both emotions and uncertainty unfolds dynamically, and ultimately affects the uncertainty management process.

Additional Readings

Brashers, D. E. (2001). Communication and uncertainty management. *Journal of Communication, 51,* 477–497.

Brashers, D. F., Neidig, J. L., & Goldsmith, D. J. (2004). Social support and the management of uncertainty for people living with HIV and AIDS. *Health Communication, 16,* 305–331.

Lin, L., Acquaye, A. A., Vera-Bolanos, E., Cahill, J., Gilbert, M. R., & Armstrong, T. S. (2012). Validation of the Mishel's uncertainty in illness scale—brain tumor form (MUIS-BT). *Journal of Neuro-Oncology, 110,* 293–300.

Mishel, M. H. (1981). The measurement of uncertainty in illness. *Nursing Research, 30,* 258–263.

Parrott, R., Peters, K., & Traeder, T. (2012). Uncertainty management and communication preferences related to genetic relativism among families affected by Down Syndrome, Marfan Syndrome, and Neurofibromatosis. *Health Communication, 27,* 663–671.

References

Brashers, D. E. (2001). Communication and uncertainty management. *Journal of Communication, 51,* 477–497.

Brashers, D. E., Goldsmith, D. J., & Hsieh, E. (2002). Information seeking and avoiding in health contexts. *Health Communication Research, 28,* 258–271.

Brashers, D. E., Haas, S. M., Neidig, J. L., & Rintamaki, L. S. (2002). Social activism, self-advocacy, and coping with HIV illness. *Journal of Social and Personal Relationships, 19,* 113–133.

Brashers, D. E., Neidig, J. L., & Goldsmith, D. J. (2004). Social support and the management of uncertainty for people living with HIV and AIDS. *Health Communication, 16,* 305–331.

Chadwick, A. E. (2010). *Persuasive hope theory and hope appeals in messages about climate change mitigation and seasonal influenza prevention.* (PhD Dissertation), The Pennsylvania State University, State College, PA.

Chadwick, A. E. (2015). Toward a theory of persuasive hope: Effects of cognitive appraisals, hope appeals, and hope in the context of climate change. Health Communication, 30, 598 611. doi: 10.1080/10410236.2014.916777. Published online October 2014.

Lazarus, R. S. (1991). *Emotion and adaptation.* New York: Oxford University Press.

Lazarus, R. S. (2001). Relational meaning and discrete emotions. In K. R. Scherer, A. Schorr, & T. Johnstone (Eds.), *Appraisal processes in emotion: Theory, methods, research* (pp. 37–67). New York: Oxford University Press.

Lazarus, R. S., & Folkman, S. (1987). Transactional theory and research on emotions and coping. *European Journal of Personality, 1,* 141–169.

Lin, L., Acquaye, A. A., Vera-Bolanos, E., Cahill, J., Gilbert, M. R., & Armstrong, T. S. (2012). Validation of the Mishel's uncertainty in illness scale—brain tumor form (MUIS-BT). *Journal of Neuro-Oncology, 110,* 293–300.

Mishel, M.H. (1981). The measurement of uncertainty in illness. *Nursing Research, 30,* 258–263.

Mishel, M. H., Germino, B. B., Lin, L., Pruthi, R. S., Wallen, E. M., Crandell, J., & Blyler, D. (2009). Managing uncertainty about treatment decision-making in early stage prostate cancer: A randomized clinical trial, *Patient Education and Counseling, 77,* 349–359.

Parrott, R., Peters, K., & Traeder, T. (2012). Uncertainty management and communication preferences related to genetic relativism among families affected by Down Syndrome, Marfan Syndrome, and Neurofibromatosis. *Health Communication, 27,* 663–671.

Roseman, I. J. (2001). A model of appraisal in the emotion system: Integrating theory, research, and applications. In K. R. Scherer, A. Schorr, & T. Johnstone (Eds.), *Appraisal processes in emotion: Theory, methods, research* (pp. 68–91). New York: Oxford University Press.

Roseman, I. J., & Smith, C. A. (2001). Appraisal theory: Overview, assumptions, varieties, controversies. In K. R. Scherer, A. Schorr, & T. Johnstone (Eds.), *Appraisal processes in emotion: Theory, methods, research* (pp. 3–19). New York: Oxford University Press.

Smith, R. A. (2011). Stigma communication and health. In T. L. Thompson, R. Parrott, & J. Nussbaum (Eds.), *Handbook of health communication* (2nd ed., pp. 455–468). New York: Taylor & Francis.

Way, B. M., & Masters, R. D. (1996). Emotion and cognition in political information-processing. *Journal of Communication, 46,* 48–65.

26. *Vested Interest*

CLAUDE H. MILLER,
University of Oklahoma
& BRADLEY J. ADAME,
Arizona State University

One fundamental assumption of social science is that attitudes are linked to behaviors such that holding a particular attitude tends to engender a correspondingly relevant behavior (Allport, 1935; Glasman & Albarracan, 2006). Although the attitude-behavior association may not always be reliable, a significant body of research has identified a number of variables which, to varying degrees, moderate attitude-behavior consistency (Glasman & Albarracan, 2006; Johnson & Eagly, 1989). Focusing on the most hedonically relevant qualities of such moderators (Miller & Averbeck, 2013; and see Chapter 10 this volume). Crano and colleagues have developed Vested Interest Theory (VI), and demonstrated its reliability in predicting attitude-behavior consistency (Crano, 1983, 1997; Crano & Prislin, 1995; Lehman & Crano, 2002; Sivacek & Crano, 1982). Across a number of health, risk, and crisis-related contexts, VI can be useful for identifying and targeting those attitudes that are most consistently predictive of attitude-relevant behavior.

Because many attitudes are not reliably linked to relevant behaviors, accurate targeting is critical if time, money, and effort are to be spent on social influence attempts designed to modify or reinforce important behaviors. For example, although people may report having positive attitudes about the importance of voting, their actual voting behavior may be predicted better by their attitudes about the weather on election day. In this regard, attitudes that appear to be relevant in a given context may in fact bear little or no relationship with their respectively expected behaviors.

Vested interest theory posits the attitude-behavior relationship is a function of five dimensions of vestedness: stake, salience, certainty, immediacy, and self-efficacy. Drawing from the extended parallel process model of fear appeals (EPPM; Witte, 1992), Miller, Adame, and Moore (2013) have added a sixth variable, response-efficacy, to the VI framework. Within the context of disaster preparedness, Miller et al. (2013) expanded the VI model and developed reliable metrics to evaluate perceptions of each VI element in relation to specific disaster relevant (i.e., tornado and earthquake) attitude-objects. Although Crano and colleagues considered stake to be one of the five dimensions of vested interest, Miller et al. (2013) suggested it may be more useful to consider stake as the primary foundation with which the other components interact to create higher levels of vestedness. In brief, the essential elements of vested interest can be characterized as follows:

Stake. The first and most essential constituent of any attitude predictive of behavior is stake. An attitude holder's stake in a given attitude object (e.g., cancer screening) is represented by his or her basic subjective perception of the personal gain/loss consequence associated with that object. According to Sivacek and Crano (1982), the greater the number, magnitude, and duration of personal consequences, the greater the stake, the stronger the attitude, and the higher the likelihood of attitude-consistent actions (e.g., taking the time and making the effort to actually get screened for cancer). Research has described stake as a global proxy for VI, and more recently as a demographic variable distinguishing individuals as stakeholders within a particular crisis context, based upon their geographical location, and the prevailing climate and hazard attributes associated with that location (Miller et al., 2013). For example, people living along the West Coast have a stake in earthquake and wildfire preparedness, whereas people living in the Southeastern United States have more of a stake in tornado and hurricane preparedness.

Salience. A second component of VI involves how pronounced, noticeable, or intrusive an attitude object is. Crano's research has shown vestedness can be increased by accessibility priming, which tends to enhance the salience of the hedonic consequences of an attitude object (Crano & Prislin, 1995). For example, the more people are talking about an issue (e.g., the value of vitamin D), and the more it appears in the news, the more salient it will be, and thus, the more likely it will figure into attitude consistent behaviors (e.g., spending time in the sun, and/or taking a supplement each day).

Certainty. A third component of vested interest is certainty, or the confidence and conviction an individual attaches to the likelihood of gain/loss consequences of an attitude object occurring. If the hedonic consequences are uncertain, a relevant attitude is not likely to be of high vested interest. The probability of consequences associated with a decision to behave in an attitude consistent fashion refers to the certainty associated with that attitude. Consequences perceived to be certain (e.g., increasing the odds of contracting type 2 diabetes through excessive sugar consumption) significantly increase the likelihood of attitude-consistent behavior (controlling and reducing sugar intake), whereas uncertainty attenuates the motivation to act.

Immediacy. A fourth component of vested interest involves the immediacy of attitude relevant consequences. Crano (1995) asserts that the hedonic relevance of an object whose consequences are immediate will be perceived as more substantial relative to one whose consequences are perceived as removed in time. Thus, immediacy is a temporal component related to the perceived consequences of proximal versus distal attitude-consistent behavior. Proximal consequences, perceived as more immediate (e.g., catching the flu via annual exposure to a flu virus), reliably influence behavior (getting immunized) in contrast to distal consequences perceived as less immediate (e.g., developing lung cancer from years of smoking), which weaken the motivation to act in an attitude-consistent manner (quitting smoking).

Self-efficacy. A fifth component of vested interest involves perceptions about one's ability to perform actions consistent with affecting the gain/loss consequences associated with an attitude object. Obviously, if the relevant actions are perceived to be beyond the capability of an actor, efficacy will be perceived as low, attenuating vested interest and attitude-behavior-consistency. There is a large body of research indicating that one's self-perceived ability to enact an attitude relevant behavior directly impacts one's motivation to act, in lieu of or beyond one's actual ability (Bandura, 1977; 1982; 1994). Vested interest posits that when presented with a series of potential behavioral choices, the perception of ones' ability to cope effectively with challenges (e.g., quitting smoking) will moderate the decision to act such that high perceived self-efficacy (e.g., getting a nicotine patch) positively influences attitude-consistent behavior, whereas low perceived self-efficacy (e.g., quitting cold turkey) diminishes the incentive to act, or eliminates it as a viable choice option.

Response Efficacy. Finally, drawn from the EPPM, response efficacy is one's perception of the potential effectiveness of a recommended behavioral response. Research has demonstrated response efficacy (e.g. whether water conservation is an effective means of protecting a scarce resource) is distinct from self-efficacy (e.g. whether one thinks one's self capable of conserving water); although the concepts are closely related, effective measurement requires accounting for their key distinctions (Miller et al., 2013). For example, individual smokers might perceive themselves as entirely capable of wearing nicotine patches as directed (i.e., high perceived self-efficacy), but lack confidence in their effectiveness (i.e., low perceived response efficacy), and thus not be motivated to use them.

Each of the above components of VI influences attitude-behavior consistency, and together they interact to predict specific behavioral outcomes. For example, in their study on disaster preparedness, Miller et al. (2013) found perceived susceptibility to tornado and earthquake hazards decreased sharply as perceptions of certainty about their occurrence decreased and perceptions of self-efficacy increased. From a VI perspective, if one's goals involve initiating preventative behaviors and/or promoting preparedness activities, the first steps for initiating action would involve identifying stakeholders and assessing their perceptions of vestedness along each of the six dimensions outlined above. Determining the vested interest of context-specific stakeholders would then suggest ways to more effectively develop the types of appeals best suited to resonate with the sensibilities of those stakeholders (Andreasen, 2006) and motivate them to the greatest effect. Moreover, VI can provide the framework for targeting the key attitudes, beliefs, and expectations of people from various agencies, levels of involvement, and geographic regions to address the pertinent issues and threats presented by health, risk, and disaster relevant challenges. Along these lines, VI and related constructs have been applied to assess, target, and formulate influence strategies for a range of risk-related attitudes and behaviors, including such topics as earthquake and tornado preparedness (Mulilis & Lippa, 1990; Miller et al., 2013), food safety (Houghton, Kleef, Rowe, & Frewer, 2006), water consumption (Lam, 2006), and general pro-environmental attitudes (Meinhold & Malkus, 2005).

Measuring Vested Interest

The dimensions of VI can be used as predictor or criterion variables. The manipulation or measurement of VI in previous research by Crano and colleagues has focused primarily on assessing stake, which has generally been operationalized in terms of self-interest, or perceived costs, threats, and/or risks, such that the greater the self-interest, or the higher the costs and risks, the more vested participants are assumed to be. For example, concerning health insurance policy, Lehman and Crano (2002) used stake as a grouping variable, setting four levels of VI by designating those who were uninsured to be the most vested, followed by those who were underinsured with excessively costly insurance, followed by those with inadequate coverage for serious health problems, and finally, those who had insurance that was not excessively expensive designated as the least vested individuals.

Some studies have simply noted whether participants were in high or low self-interest categories (e.g., Johnson, Siegel, & Crano, 2014), or included a subset of the five dimensions of VI. For example, to predict participants' intentions to become organ donors, Siegel et al. (2008) used three 2-item scales to assess stake, immediacy, and salience (Table 1). Other studies have used a combination grouping/factorial approach, designating one or more dimensions of VI as grouping variables and manipulating others within a factorial message design (Adame & Miller, 2015). For example, Adame and Miller (2015) used region of the country (Oklahoma's tornado alley) to hold stake and salience as constants within their study of tornado disaster preparedness, while manipulating certainty, immediacy, response efficacy, and self-efficacy within high and low vestedness PSA TV spots using a factorial message design. Adame and Miller then used Miller et al.'s (2013) VI subscales (see below) as manipulation checks prior to assessing tornado disaster preparedness outcomes.

Table 1. Siegel et al.'s (2008) Vested Interest subscales.

Stake
1. By being [a live organ donor/an organ donor], I could save the life of a loved one.
2. By donating [an organ/my organs], I can help save a life.

Immediacy
1. My signing up to be [a live organ donor/an organ donor] would have an immediate impact on my life.
2. My signing up to be [a live organ donor/an organ donor] would have an immediate impact on my community.

Salience
1. I see lots of information about [live organ donation/organ donation] in the media.
2. [Live organ donation/organ donation] is a common conversation topic among people I know.

Note: Items measured on a 7-point, Likert-type strongly disagree/strongly agree continuum. Reliability correlations are as follows: Stake, $r = .53$; Immediacy, $r = .49$; Salience, $r = .44$.

Miller, Adame, and Moore's (2013) Vested Interest Subscales

Based on Witte's (1992; Witte et al., 1996) EPPM, which was designed to explain and predict individuals' reactions to fear appeal messages using several concepts similar to those articulated by VI, Miller et al. (2013) adopted a similar methodological framework for constructing VI scales to measure components of vested interest associated with those attitudes that best explain and predict individuals' disaster preparedness. Vested interest theory and the EPPM highlight similar elements within overlapping frameworks that can be useful for designing, constructing, and assessing social action campaigns specifically focused upon variables linking attitudes with relevant behaviors. Both models account for threat severity, or stake; and both account for an individual's perceived self-efficacy. However, in prior research, only the EPPM has provided a direct method for measuring these key variables via an audience analysis survey method.

On the other hand, as Miller et al. (2013) have noted, the EPPM does not address two important VI components—salience and immediacy—nor does it adequately assess certainty. Whereas the EPPM includes susceptibility, which is a similar construct, it does not assess the more encompassing concept of certainty. That is to say, even if one considers one's self susceptible to a given threat, crucial relevant outcomes may not necessarily be perceived as certain. On the other hand, if an outcome is considered certain, susceptibility becomes a foregone conclusion.

Just as the EPPM may be augmented by aspects of VI, so also may VI be enhanced by taking into consideration the EPPM's notion of response efficacy. Moreover, combining all of these elements—stake/severity, salience, certainty/susceptibility, immediacy, self-efficacy, and response efficacy—into a single more broadly defined construct of vestedness should have the potential to provide richer data, and lead to more practical applied research useful in designing, developing, and deploying the most effective health and social action campaigns.

Witte and colleagues developed a set of instruments called the risk behavior diagnosis scale (RBD; Witte, Cameron, McKeon, & Berkowitz, 1996) comprised of four subscales measuring perceived severity, susceptibility, response efficacy, and self-efficacy, that can be customized to fit various threat scenarios, and used to assess the central components of the EPPM. Using the same format as the RBD, Miller et al. (2013) developed three additional subscales to measure the perceived certainty, immediacy, and saliency of threatening outcomes associated with disaster preparedness. The three subscales derived from vested interest were added to three of the four EPPM subscales (perceived severity was not assessed, although it can be used to assess stake; see below).

Thus, a total of seven subscales, comprised of four to eight 7-point Likert-type items, may be customized as appropriate to assess VI relevant perceptions pertinent to health risk and disaster-related preparedness behaviors. Using polling data from an adult sample of Oklahoma residents, self-report responses from a convenience sample of University of Oklahoma college students, and a modified snowball sample of adult residents living in Southern California, Miller et al. (2013) collected data using six of the seven expanded

VI model subscales (severity/stake was held as a constant). Based on EFA results, a multi-group confirmatory factor analysis (CFA) using Maximum Likelihood estimation was performed to confirm the higher order structure of the three VI subscales across the three studies. The CFA model was refined and simplified based on fit, parsimony, and unity (i.e., the desire to specify a single model that could fit the data from all three studies. This procedure further reduced the 20 original VI items to 12, forming three factors defined by four items each. These three subscales along with three from the EPPM, and a seventh for assessing severity/stake are presented in Table 2, along with their alpha reliability statistics across all three data sets (as well as from Witte et al., 1996, for their 3-item severity subscale).

The following subscales provide participants with a brief definition of the relevant VI dimensional construct, followed by an introductory statement prompting them to think about the threat/risk within the appropriate context of interest. The versions presented below have been customized for general disaster preparedness, although they may be adapted for health risks as well, or for any social influence topic for which there is a concern for assessing the attitude-behavior consistency of a targeted construct.

Table 2. Miller et al.'s (2013) Vested Interest subscales.

Outcome Certainty (4-item α = .88)
Certainty is defined as the perceived probability of an event or outcome occurring.

Please answer the following questions regarding your perceptions of the certainty of [relevant local threat].

1. How likely is [relevant threat] to occur in your community?

Not Likely	1	2	3	4	5	6	7	Highly Likely

2. What is the chance of you being affected by [relevant threat]?

Small Chance	1	2	3	4	5	6	7	Large Chance

3. What are the odds you will be injured in [relevant threat]?

Not Likely	1	2	3	4	5	6	7	Highly Likely

4. What are the odds your property will be damaged in [relevant threat]?

Not Likely	1	2	3	4	5	6	7	Highly Likely

Immediacy of Outcomes (4-item α = .79)

Immediacy is defined as the perceived amount of time before the consequences of an event may come about.

Please answer the following questions regarding how immediately you think the consequences of [relevant local threat] will occur.

1. How far in the future might [relevant threat] affect you?

Not Far	1	2	3	4	5	6	7	Very Far

2. How long do you think it will be before [relevant threat] occurs in your area?

Not Long	1	2	3	4	5	6	7	Very Long

3. How long do you think it will be before your belongings or property are damaged by [relevant threat]?

Not Long	1	2	3	4	5	6	7	Very Long

4. How much time do you expect before [relevant threat] happens in your area?

Short Time	1	2	3	4	5	6	7	Long Time

Threat Salience (4-item α = .91)

Salience is defined as your awareness of the presence or prominence of a potentially threatening event.

Please answer the following questions regarding how salient [relevant local threat] is for you.

1. How often do you think about potential [relevant threat]?

Not Often	1	2	3	4	5	6	7	Very Often

2. How concerned are you about potential [relevant threat]?

Not Concerned	1	2	3	4	5	6	7	Very Concerned

3. How often do you think about the threat of [relevant threat]?

Not Often	1	2	3	4	5	6	7	Very Often

4. How often do you think about preparing for the possibility of [relevant threat]?

Not Often	1	2	3	4	5	6	7	Very Often

Susceptibility (5-item α = .85)

Susceptibility is defined as being vulnerable to harm or at risk for a particular threat.
Please answer the following questions regarding how susceptible and vulnerable you feel toward [living in (location)], a region of the country know to have frequent [relevant local threat].

1. How susceptible are you to getting injured [from relevant threat]?

Not Susceptible	1	2	3	4	5	6	7	Highly Susceptible

2. How susceptible is your property to getting damaged [from relevant threat]?

Not Susceptible	1	2	3	4	5	6	7	Highly Susceptible

3. What is the possibility your property will get damaged [from relevant threat]?

Not Possible	1	2	3	4	5	6	7	Highly Possible

4. How at risk is your community [from relevant threat]?

Not at Risk	1	2	3	4	5	6	7	Highly at Risk

5. Given that you live in [location], what is your risk [from relevant threat]?

Low Risk	1	2	3	4	5	6	7	High Risk

Response Efficacy (7-item α = .77)

Response efficacy is defined as the ability of a tool or procedure to produce a desired result.

The [relevant federal/state/local authority] recommends the use of [advocated response], which commonly includes such things as [list of three or four response methods]. Please answer the following questions regarding how effective various related responses may be to [relevant local threat].

1. How effective is [advocated response] at minimizing the negative consequences of [relevant threat]?

Not Effective	1	2	3	4	5	6	7	Highly Effective

2. How effective would [advocated response] be to reduce the damage caused by [relevant threat]?

Not Effective	1	2	3	4	5	6	7	Highly Effective

3. How effective do you think [advocated response] will be at lowering distress following [relevant threat]?

Not Effective	1	2	3	4	5	6	7	Highly Effective

4. How effective is [advocated response] at minimizing damage from [relevant threat] to your property or belongings?

Not Effective	1	2	3	4	5	6	7	Highly Effective

5. How effective is [advocated response] at reducing the impact of [relevant threat]?

Not Effective	1	2	3	4	5	6	7	Highly Effective

6. How effective is [advocated response] at reducing the potential harm caused by [relevant threat]?

Not Effective	1	2	3	4	5	6	7	Highly Effective

7. How effective are [list advocated response methods] at helping respond to [relevant threat]?

Not Effective	1	2	3	4	5	6	7	Highly Effective

Self-Efficacy (6-item α = .84)

Self-efficacy is defined as your ability to effectively produce a desired result.

Please answer the following questions regarding how effective you think you can be at preparing for and responding to [relevant local threat].

1. How capable are you at effectively preparing [recommended response] to help respond to [relevant threat]?

Not Capable	1	2	3	4	5	6	7	Highly Capable

2. How able are you to take the time to prepare [recommended response] for use in the event of [relevant threat]?

Not Able	1	2	3	4	5	6	7	Very Able

3. Can you afford to buy the items needed for [recommended response] in case of [relevant threat]?

Cannot Afford	1	2	3	4	5	6	7	Can Easily Afford

4. How easy would it be for you to prepare [recommended response] for use in [relevant threat]?

Not Easy	1	2	3	4	5	6	7	Very Easy

5. How much knowledge do you have about using [recommended response] in response to [relevant threat]?

No Knowledge	1	2	3	4	5	6	7	Great Knowledge

6. How effective are you at using [recommended response] in case of [relevant threat]?

Not Effective	1	2	3	4	5	6	7	Highly Effective

Threat Severity (3-item α = .90 for items 1–3; Witte et al., 1996)

Severity is defined as how high the stakes are, and how serious the consequences of a threatening event are perceived to be.

Please answer to the following questions regarding how serious you believe [relevant local threat] would be for you.

1. I believe [relevant threat] is severe.

| Strongly Disagree | 1 | 2 | 3 | 4 | 5 | 6 | 7 | Strongly Agree |

2. I believe [relevant threat] is serious.

| Strongly Disagree | 1 | 2 | 3 | 4 | 5 | 6 | 7 | Strongly Agree |

3. I believe [relevant threat] is significant.

| Strongly Disagree | 1 | 2 | 3 | 4 | 5 | 6 | 7 | Strongly Agree |

4. [Relevant threat] has serious financial consequences.

| Strongly Disagree | 1 | 2 | 3 | 4 | 5 | 6 | 7 | Strongly Agree |

5. [Relevant threat] leads to grave personal outcomes.

| Strongly Disagree | 1 | 2 | 3 | 4 | 5 | 6 | 7 | Strongly Agree |

6. [Relevant threat] is of great magnitude.

| Strongly Disagree | 1 | 2 | 3 | 4 | 5 | 6 | 7 | Strongly Agree |

Use of the VI Subscales and Future Studies

Recent research has applied Witte et al.'s (2001) EPPM for both formative campaign development, and the construction of more effective fear appeal messages. While this approach has proven heuristic value, further assessing key aspects of vestedness can be even more useful in predicting the likelihood of targeted populations' actual attitude consistent behaviors. When the purpose is to get people to act, rather than merely think or talk about acting, measuring the broader construct of VI can provide researchers and policy makers with a valuable indication of their intended audiences' psychological profile useful in outlining and identifying those aspects most critical for optimizing effective campaign message designs.

Vested interest theory suggests the most effective health campaigns should be strategically focused on stressing the immediacy, salience, and certainty of threat-relevant personal consequences for targeted audiences, and should identify effective responses useful in meeting health risk challenges and boosting perceived self-efficacy. Understanding the vested interest of a target audience can provide a foundation for identifying, assessing, and strengthening the key components necessary for optimizing the most effective campaigns prior to or in conjunction with addressing specific efficacy needs. Furthermore, the assessment of VI can be applied across a number of content areas where researchers seek to quantify the vestedness of specific targeted attitudes predicting behaviors relevant to such behaviors as smoking cessation, cancer screening, preventative medicine, obesity, substance use, organ donation, and safe sex.

Recent VI research has also begun to broaden the VI construct by expanding it to include circumstances in which individuals are both directly and indirectly affected by significant threats and concerns, and how such considerations may be related to attitude-behavior consistency (Johnson et al., 2014). This expansion was stimulated by research on interpersonal relationships suggesting that attitude-congruent action is not simply a self-centered phenomenon, but rather it may be more accurately assessed by taking into account the significant influences of intimate others in shaping one's opinions and actions. Research on interpersonal closeness suggests people in close relationships perceive their intimates to be extensions of themselves; taking this into account, Johnson et al. (2014) have demonstrated how the consideration of the concerns of close interpersonal relations can be critical in understanding the circumstances in which attitudes predict behaviors. Indirectly vested individuals—that is, those who have no direct vested interest, but who are associated with intimate others who do—may have less-extreme attitudes, and engage in fewer attitude-relevant actions than those who are directly vested, yet their attitude-relevant behaviors may nonetheless be reliably predicted by the indirect vestedness instilled by their consideration of close others. Moreover, Johnson et al. have shown that as closeness to a vested other increases, so too does the concomitant indirect vestedness influence attitude–behavior consistency.

Along with assessing direct vestedness, future research into attitude behavior consistency should assess and measure instances of indirect vestedness, particularly within personal health-risk contexts, where the interests of intimate others are bound to be of significant importance.

Recommended Readings

Adame, B. J. & Miller, C. H. (2015). Vested interest & disaster preparedness: Strategic campaign message design. *Health Communication, 30,* 271–281.

Crano, W. D. (1995). *Attitude strength: Antecedents and consequences.* Mahwah, NJ: Erlbaum.

Crano, W. D., & Prislin, R. (1995). Components of vested interest and attitude-behavior consistency. *Basic and Applied Social Psychology, 17,* 1–21.

Miller, C. H., Adame, B. J., & Moore, S. D. (2013). Vested interest theory and disaster preparedness. *Disasters, 37,* 1–27.

References

Adame, B. J. & Miller, C. H. (2015). Vested interest & disaster preparedness: Strategic campaign message design. *Health Communication, 30,* 271–281. doi: 10.1080 / 10410236.2013.842527.

Allport, G. W. (1935). Attitudes. In C. Murchinson (Ed.), *Handbook of social psychology.* Worcester, MA: Clark University Press.

Andreasen, A. R. (2006). *Social marketing in the 21st century.* Thousand Oaks, CA: Sage.

Bandura, A. (1977). Toward a unifying theory of behavioral change. *Psychological Review, 84,* 191–215.

Bandura, A. (1982). Self-efficacy mechanism in human agency. *American Psychologist, 37,* 122 147.

Bandura, A. (1994). Social cognitive theory of mass communication. In J. Bryant & D. Zillman (Eds.), *Media effects: Advances in theory and research* (pp. 61–90). Hillsdale, NJ: Erlbaum.

Crano, W. D. (1983). Assumed consensus of attitudes: The effect of vested interest. *Personality and Social Psychology Bulletin, 9*(4), 597–608. doi: 10.1177/0146167283094009.

Crano, W. D. (1995). Attitude strength and vested interest. In R. E. Petty & J. A. Krosnick (Eds.), *Attitude strength: Antecedents and consequences* (pp. 131–158). Mahwah, NJ: Erlbaum.

Crano, W. D., & Prislin, R. (1995). Components of vested interest and attitude-behavior consistency. *Basic and Applied Social Psychology, 17*(1 & 2), 1–21.

Glasman, L. R., & Albarracan, D. (2006). Forming attitudes that predict future behavior: A meta-analysis of the attitude-behavior relation. *Psychological Bulletin, 132,* 778–822. doi: 10.1037/0033–2909.132.5.778.

Houghton, J. R., van Kleef, E., Rowe, G., & Frewer, L. J. (2006). Consumer perceptions of the effectiveness of food risk management practices: A cross-cultural study. *Health, Risk & Society, 8,* 165–183.

Johnson, B. T., & Eagly, A. H. (1989). Effects of involvement on persuasion: A meta-analysis. *Psychological Bulletin, 106,* 290–314.

Johnson, I., Siegel, J. T., & Crano, W. D. (2014). Expanding the reach of vested interest in predicting attitude-behavior consistency. *Social Influence, 9,* 20–36. doi: 10.1080/15534510 .2012.738243.

Lam, S. P. (2006). Predicting intention to save water: Theory of planned behavior, response efficacy, vulnerability, and perceived efficiency of alternative solutions. *Journal of Applied Social Psychology, 36,* 2803–2824.

Lehman, B. J., & Crano, W. D. (2002). The persuasive effects of vested interest on attitude-criterion consistency in political judgment. *Journal of Experimental Social Psychology, 38,* 101–112. doi: 10.1006/jesp.2001.1489.

Meinhold, J. L., & Malkus, A. J. (2005). Adolescent environmental behaviors: Can knowledge, attitude, and self-efficacy make a difference? *Environment and Behavior, 37,* 511–532.

Miller, C. H., Adame, B. J., & Moore, S. D. (2013). Vested interest theory and disaster preparedness. *Disasters, 37,* 1–27.

Miller, C. H., & Averbeck, J. M., (2013). Hedonic relevance and outcome relevant involvement. *Electronic Journal of Communication, 23*(3). Retrieved January 2, 2015, from, http://www.cios.org/www/ejc/v23n34toc.htm#millerfr 2013

Mullis, J.-P., & Lippa, R. (1990). Behavioral change in earthquake preparedness due to negative threat appeals: A test of protection motivation theory. *Journal of Applied Social Psychology, 20,* 619–638.

Siegel, J. T., Alvaro, E., Lac, A., Crano, W. D., & Alexander, S. (2008). Intentions of becoming a living organ donor among Hispanics: A theoretical approach exploring differences between living and non-living organ donation. *Journal of Health Communication, 13,* 80–99.

Sivacek, J., & Crano, W. D. (1982). Vested interest as a moderator of attitude-behavior consistency. *Journal of Personality and Social Psychology, 43,* 210–221.

Witte, K. (1992). Putting the fear back into fear appeals: The extended parallel process model. *Communication Monographs, 59,* 329–349.

Witte, K., Cameron, K. A., McKeon, J. K., & Berkowitz, J. M. (1996). Predicting risk behaviors: Development and validation of a diagnostic scale. *Journal of Health Communication, 1,* 317–342.

27. *Willingness to Communicate about Health*

Kevin B. Wright,
George Mason University

Health communication scholars have long been interested in interpersonal communication issues in a variety of contexts, such as patient-provider interaction, communication within social support groups, and everyday conversations about health between individuals and their family members and friends (Street, Makoul, Arora, & Epstein, 2009; Wright & Rains, 2013).

For example, within the area of patient-provider communication, researchers have had a growing interest in the benefits of collaborative communication, which involves open discussion between patients and providers about health concerns as well as mutual problem solving and decision-making when discussing patient cases and treatment options (Dutta-Bergman, 2005). Collaborative communication has been linked to a variety of important outcomes for patients, including greater satisfaction with medical encounters, better adherence to treatments, and improved physical health outcomes (Naik, Kallen, Walder, & Street, 2008; Zolnierek & DiMatteo, 2009).

However, collaborative communication rests on the assumption that patients are willing to communicate with providers and others in their social network. This includes disclosing sensitive information about their lifestyle behaviors that may put them at risk for disease, such as smoking, overindulgence of alcohol and/or unhealthy food, and lack of exercise. Such topics may increase a patient's communication apprehension when interacting with providers. Moreover, individuals must be willing to communicate with providers in an assertive manner in situations where they feel the need to be advocates for their rights or specific preferences as patients (Brashers, Haas, & Neidig, 1999; Ruggiano, Whiteman, and Shtompel, 2014; Wright, Frey, & Sopory, 2007). For example, when patients feel that a certain procedure or course of treatment is incompatible with their lifestyle or long-term wishes, such as a surgery that may correct a physical problem but inhibit one's ability to engage in activities such as sports or a patient's preference for palliative care options over chemotherapy or other curative approaches to cancer treatment, they must be willing to communicate their concerns and wishes to providers. These situations can be daunting for patients who feel apprehensive toward having such conversations with their physician due to status differences or if patients have a more paternalistic view of provider-patient relationships. In such cases, it may be difficult for a patient to express his or her health concerns or preferences let alone challenge a physician or other provider such as a nurse.

Moreover, other areas of health communication beyond patient-provider interaction may be affected by a person's willingness to communicate about their health situation. For instance, social support has been linked to a variety of positive health outcomes in numerous studies. However, in order for social support to occur, individuals need to be willing to communicate about their specific problems or stressful situations they face as well as the type of support they would like to receive from members of their social network(s). When people face stigmatized health concerns, they are often less willing to communicate with close ties, such as friends and family members, about their health concerns, although there is some evidence that they may be willing to communicate with weak ties, such as with members of an online support group (Wright & Rains, 2013).

Given these issues, a number of researchers have become interested in the construct of willingness to communicate about health as a variable that may impact patient health outcomes in a variety of health communication contexts. In an effort to measure this construct, Wright, Frey, and Sopory (2007) developed the Willingness to Communicate about Health (WTCH) scale. Since that time, researchers have utilized this measure in a variety of health communication studies, and the scale has recently been adapted to measure more specific willingness to communicate about health topics, such as sexual health (Canzona, 2015). The purpose of this chapter is to discuss the theoretical influences on the development of the WTCH scale, recent applications of the WTCH scale, the limitations of the WTCH scale, and ways in which this scale could potentially be refined and applied in future health communication research.

Measuring Willingness to Communicate about Health

Willingness to communicate has been identified as an important predisposition that has important implications for interpersonal communication and relationships in a variety of contexts (McCroskey & Richmond, 1987; 1998).

Willingness to communicate was defined by McCroskey and Richmond (1998) as "an individual's predisposition to initiate communication with others" (p. 120). McCroskey and Richmond (1987) developed and tested the willingness to communicate scale and found that it had good reliability and good convergent, discriminant, and predictive validity. Although McCroskey and Richmond (1987) viewed willingness to communicate as a more general predisposition, they also argued that it was "probably to a major degree situationally dependent" (p. 129). With the growth of the health communication area, health communication scholars have becoming increasingly interested in the idea that (un)willingness to communicate can influence a number of important health behaviors and outcomes.

Prior to the development of the WTCH scale, a number of researchers had investigated willingness to communicate about specific health issues as opposed to developing a scale to measure this concept more generally across multiple contexts. For example, several researchers examined health communication topics that are often interpersonally difficult to discuss, such as willingness to communicate about organ donation to family members (McDonald et al., 2007; Smith, Kopfman, Lindsey, Yoo, & Morrison, 2004), or Crowell's (2004) study that investigated willingness to communicate about condom usage.

Based on the overall concept of willingness to communicate and this previous work within health contexts, Wright et al. (2007) sought to develop a generalized measure of willingness to communicate about health that would be potentially useful for both health communication researchers and health care practitioners. Wright et al. (2007) tested the scale with two samples (cancer patients and college students) and found that it exhibited good convergent and discriminant validity, and good predictive validity in terms of predicting patient advocacy on Brashers et al.'s (1999) Patient Self-Advocacy Scale (PSAS) across both samples. The factor loadings ranged from 0.35 to 0.83 and the Cronbach's alpha of the two subscales (by factors) were also acceptable (alpha = .71 for each subscale across both the cancer patient and student samples). The 10 items for the WTCH scale appear in Table 1.

Table 1. Willingness to Communicate about Health (WTCH) Scale (Wright et al., 2007).

Strongly Disagree = 1
Disagree = 2
Neutral = 3

Agree = 4

Strongly Agree = 5

1. I feel comfortable talking about health with health care providers.
2. I experience difficulties communicating successfully with health care providers.
3. I am quick to make an appointment to talk with a physician when I am not feeling well.
4. I am a competent communicator when talking about health issues.
5. When I don't feel well, I don't want to talk to others.
6. I am comfortable talking about my health with a wide variety of people not counting physicians.
7. I am comfortable talking with a variety of people about their health (not counting physicians).
8. I actively seek out information about health.
9. I frequently talk about health issues.
10. I only talk about health issues when I have to.

Since its development in 2007, several studies have utilized or been influenced by the WTCH construct/scale in a variety of health contexts. These studies provide examples of how the WTCH construct/scale can be applied to different contexts and questions/hypotheses regarding the relationship between WTCH and other variables.

Wright and Frey (2008) examined the role of WTCH among older patients in an environmentally restructured (i.e. pleasant 5-star hotel-like surroundings as opposed to a traditional hospital setting) cancer center. Specifically, these researchers examined relationships between patients' WTCH scores and their information seeking, perceptions of coping activities the center offered, and satisfaction with the center. The results indicated that WTCH appeared to play an important role in predicting patient information-seeking behaviors and the overall satisfaction with the care they received at the center. The study also found that perceptions of the health-care environment (the degree to which patients perceived the cancer center surroundings to be pleasant) mediated cancer patients' WTCH.

Canzona (2015) modified the Wright et al. (2007) WTCH scale and created a Willingness to Communicate about Sexual Health scale and used it to measure cancer survivors' willingness to communicate about sexual health (as well as their partners' willingness to communicate about sexual health) following chemotherapy, surgery (i.e. mastectomy), and other procedures that affect sexual activity. The results indicated that willingness to communicate about sexual health was predictive of conversations about sexual health between cancer survivors, their partners, and providers, as well as relational satisfaction.

Other studies that have cited Wright et al. (2007) have drawn upon the concept of WTCH theoretically without using the measure. These studies demonstrate promising areas of research where the WTCH scale could potentially be applied in future work.

For example, Ciletti's (2009) study assessed an intervention tool for improving patient-provider communication, which included items similar to the Wright et al. (2007) WTCH scale, such as "How comfortable are you when talking about your health with health care providers such as a doctor, nurse, nurse practitioner, etc.?" and "How well do you believe you communicate with your doctor(s)?" The results of the study found that individuals who indicated higher willingness to communicate with their health care providers were more likely to engage in self-advocacy and were more satisfied with their medical visit.

Ruggiano et al. (2014) drew upon Wright et al. (2007) in the theoretical framework for their study of older patient self-advocacy. One major theme that emerged from the interviews in this study was "deciding to self advocate," which the authors defined as patients' confidence in presenting knowledge, assessments, and opinions to their provider. This included behaviors such as "asking questions, making alternative requests to providers, acquiring second opinions, and disagreeing with providers" (p. 10). Although this was a qualitative study, the authors found that willingness to communicate about health issues was reported by participants to be an important factor in deciding to engage in self-advocacy with physicians.

Use of Existing Measures and Future Studies

Willingness to communicate about health will likely be a variable of interest for health communication scholars in the future given the long-standing interest in willingness to communicate and communication apprehension within the communication discipline, as well as widespread interest in interpersonal communication issues such as patient-provider interaction and collaborative communication, social support, and communication about health issues among family members and friends.

The WTCH scale represents an initial step in terms of measuring this concept. The scale can certainly be improved through future application and refinement. This measure would benefit from being used to measure not only general willingness to communicate about health, but also specific health issues (especially highly stigmatized health issues). Conceptually, as health stigma increases, willingness to communicate should decrease within most contexts. This may lead patients to disclose less about their health conditions, seek less information, and be less likely to engage in self-advocacy in their interactions with providers. Finding ways to increase the precision of the WTCH scale or the development of a similar measure may help researchers and clinicians identify patients and other individuals coping with health concerns who are less willing to discuss their health issues. This could be useful in terms of developing intervention strategies to help such people communicate more easily about their health issues as well as advocate for their specific needs.

More generally, the WTCH (or similar measure) could be used to assess a more general tendency to communicate about health concerns, which may be helpful for identifying individuals who may benefit from interventions such as referral to a support group or individual counseling, versus individuals who may need more attention in terms of helping them to develop their communication skills in health-related settings.

Recommended Readings

Canzona, M. R. (2015). *Breast cancer survivors' sexual health after oncology: Capturing patient, partner, and clinician narratives to enhance biopsychosocial care.* Unpublished doctoral dissertation, George Mason University.

Ciletti, A. (2009). *Combating the ticking clock: An analysis of using an intervention material as a tool for effective patient communication* Unpublished doctoral dissertation, Hawaii Pacific University.

Ruggiano, N., Whiteman, K., & Shtompel, N. (2014). "If I don't like the way I feel with a certain drug, I'll tell them." Older adults' experiences with self-determination and health self-advocacy. *Journal of Applied Gerontology,* Published online before print April 21, 2014, doi: 10.1177/0733464814527513.

Wright, K. B., & Frey, L. R. (2008). Communication and care in an acute cancer center: The effects of patients' willingness to communicate about health, health-care environment perceptions, and health status on information seeking, participation in care practices, and satisfaction. *Health Communication, 23(4),* 369–379.

References

Brashers, D. E., Haas, S. M., & Neidig, J. L. (1999). The Patient Self-Advocacy Scale: Measuring patient involvement in health care decision-making interactions. *Health Communication, 11,* 97–121.

Canzona, M. R. (2015). *Breast cancer survivors' sexual health after oncology: Capturing patient, partner, and clinician narratives to enhance biopsychosocial care.* Unpublished doctoral dissertation, George Mason University.

Ciletti, A. (2009). *Combating the ticking clock: An analysis of using an intervention material as a tool for effective patient communication.* Unpublished doctoral dissertation, Hawaii Pacific University.

Crowell, T. L. (2004). Seropositive individuals' willingness to communicate, self-efficacy, and assertiveness prior to HIV infection. *Journal of Health Communication, 9,* 345–424.

Dutta-Bergman, M. J. (2005). The relation between health-orientation, provider-patient communication, and satisfaction: An individual-difference approach. *Health Communication, 18,* 291–303.

McCroskey, J. C., & Richmond, V. P. (1987). Willingness to communicate. In J. C. McCroskey & J. A. Daly (Eds.), *Personality: interpersonal communication* (pp. 189–156). Newbury Park, CA: Sage.

McCroskey, J. C., & Richmond, V. P. (1998). Willingness to communicate. In J. C. McCroskey, J. A. Daly, M. M. Martin, & M. J. Beatty (Eds.), *Communication and personality: Trait perspectives* (pp. 118–131). Cresskill, NJ: Hampton Press.

McDonald, D., Ferreri, R., Jin, C., Mendez, A., Smail, J., Balcom, B. et al. (2007). Willingness to communicate about organ donation intention. *Public Health Nursing, 24,* 151–159.

Naik, A. D., Kallen, M. A., Walder, A., & Street, R. L. (2008). Improving hypertension control in diabetes mellitus the effects of collaborative and proactive health communication. *Circulation, 117,* 1361–1368.

Ruggiano, N., Whiteman, K., & Shtompel, N. (2014). "If I don't like the way I fee with a certain drug, I'll tell them." Older adults' experiences with self-determination and health self-advocacy. *Journal of Applied Gerontology,* Published online before print April 21, 2014, doi: 10.1177/0733464814527513.

Smith, S. W., Kopfman, J. E., Lindsey, L. L. M., Yoo, J., & Morrison, K. (2004). Encouraging family discussion on the decision to donate organs: The role of the willingness to communicate scale. *Health Communication, 16,* 333–346.

Street Jr., R. L., Makoul, G., Arora, N. K., & Epstein, R. M. (2009). How does communication heal? Pathways linking clinician–patient communication to health outcomes. *Patient Education and Counseling, 74,* 295–301.

Wright, K. B., & Frey, L. R. (2008). Communication and care in an acute cancer center: The effects of patients' willingness to communicate about health, health-care environment perceptions, and health status on information seeking, participation in care practices, and satisfaction. *Health communication, 23*(4), 369–379.

Wright, K. B., Frey, L., & Sopory, P. (2007). Willingness to communicate about health as an underlying trait of patient self-advocacy: The development of the Willingness to Communicate about Health (WTCH) measure. *Communication Studies, 58,* 35–51.

Wright, K. B., & Rains, S. A. (2013). Weak-tie support network preference, health related stigma, and health outcomes in computer-mediated support groups. *Journal of Applied Communication Research, 41,* 309–324.

Zolnierek, K. B. H., & DiMatteo, M. R. (2009). Physician communication and patient adherence to treatment: A meta-analysis. *Medical Care, 47,* 826–834.

Author Biographies

Editors

Do Kyun Kim (PhD, Ohio University) is an associate professor and Richard D'Aquin / BORSF Professor of Communication at the University of Louisiana at Lafayette. His main areas of expertise include diffusion of information and innovations, social network analysis, communication campaign and intervention, and communicative social change. He has also been involved in climate change communication research projects as an affiliate researcher of the Center for Climate Change Communication. In addition to a PhD degree in Communication, he has several academic degrees in different fields of social science, such as political science and economics. Dr. Kim has been involved in many domestic and international projects for health promotion and social change, dealing with cases in the United States, Botswana, South Africa, India, and South Korea. He has also applied this knowledge to several community, state, and national projects on health promotion and organizational/community change. He is the founder and executive director of Acadiana Community Education Center, which provides educationally marginalized people with diverse educational opportunities, such as computer skills and literacy education.

James W. Dearing (PhD, University of Southern California) is Professor and Chairperson of the Department of Communication at Michigan State University. Dr. Dearing was Principal Investigator of the Cancer Communication Research Center, a U.S. National Cancer Institute Center of Excellence in Cancer Communication Research, and Senior Scientist with Kaiser Permanente. Jim specializes in the diffusion of innovations, and the use of diffusion principles to disseminate and effectively implement and sustain worthy innovations. He works and speaks frequently with research and policy groups to accelerate the spread of evidence-based practices, programs, policies, and technologies, and to measure diffusion. He studied under and worked closely with Everett M. Rogers for 20 years. Dearing has led projects funded by the Bill & Melinda Gates Foundation, the John D. and Catherine T. McArthur Foundation, the Robert Wood Johnson Foundation, the W. K. Kellogg

Foundation, and U.S. federal agencies including the Agency for Healthcare Research and Quality, the National Science Foundation, and the Centers for Disease Control and Prevention. He has worked on studies about health care delivery improvement, cancer care coordination and communication, lifestyle/physical activity, science teaching and learning, alcohol and substance abuse innovations, and the scale-up strategies of inter-organizational teams on behalf of social innovations.

Chapter Contributors

Chapter 1

John Banas (PhD, University of Texas at Austin) is an associate professor in the Department of Communication at the University of Oklahoma, where he began working in 2006. Professor Banas primarily studies persuasion theory and interpersonal communication, which led to a research interest in the effects of communication competence in the context of health communication that resulted in, among other projects, this book chapter. Primarily a quantitative social scientist, his research has appeared in such journals as *Human Communication Research, Communication Monographs, Journal of Computer-Mediated Communication*, and *Health Communication.* professor Banas resides in Norman, Oklahoma with his wonderful wife (also a Professor in the Department of Communication at the University of Oklahoma), and their two daughters, ages 4 and 9 months. When he is not performing in an official professor capacity, Professor Banas enjoys playing tennis and skiing. His other hobby/obsession, due to his upbringing in Michigan and earning his undergraduate degree at Michigan State University, is watching Spartan football and basketball.

    Daniel R. Bernard (PhD, University of Oklahoma) is the executive director of the Veterans Education Program at California State University, Fresno. This program provides opportunity and access to resources at Fresno State and connects veterans to support organizations in the Central Valley. In addition, this program offers unique educational, vocational, and workforce development opportunities to veterans. Dr. Bernard's research focuses on persuasion and interpersonal theories often at the intersection of health communication. Other areas of research interest include deceptive communication, nonverbal communication, and risk communication. In addition to several book chapters, his research has appeared in the *Journal of Health Communication, Communication Research, Health Communication,* and the *Journal of Applied Social Psychology.*

Chapter 2

Kathryn Greene (PhD, The University of Georgia) is a professor in the Department of Communication at Rutgers University. She received her doctorate in Speech Communication from the University of Georgia in 1992. She has published in the area of health communication where her research foci explore the role of communication in health decision-making both from interpersonal and prevention perspectives. Her research received awards such as the National Communication Association's Outstanding Dissertation Award, top national and regional paper awards, article of the year awards, and the Southern States Communication Association's Early Career Research Award. She has also received several outstanding teaching awards and teaches courses in interpersonal communication, health communication, research methods, and persuasion. Professor Greene has published numerous manuscripts on privacy and disclosure of HIV information including a brief health disclosure intervention. This research has appeared in a book, book chapters, and journals such as the *Journal of Communication, Communication Monographs, Health Communication,* and *Journal of Health Communication.*

    Amanda Carpenter is a doctoral candidate in the Department of Communication at Rutgers University. Prior to Rutgers, she attended Michigan State University where she earned her BA and MA in health communication. She is interested in how individuals manage health information in relationships. Her research has been published in outlets such as the *Journal of Communication, Journal of Applied Communication Research,* and *Qualitative Health Research.*

Chapter 3

Hye-Jin Paek (PhD, University of Wisconsin–Madison) is an associate professor in the Department of Advertising and Public Relations at Hanyang University in South Korea and the 4th president of the Korean Health Communication Association. Prior to her current affiliation, she was an assistant professor at University of Georgia and then an associate professor at Michigan State University. Her research interests concern the ways social perception and norms influence, are influenced by, or interact with communication to promote people's health. So far, she has published about 100 peer-reviewed journal articles, two books, and 10 book chapters. Her research has been funded by Centers for Disease Control and Prevention (both United States and South Korea), National Institutes of Health, U.S. Department of Agriculture, Georgia Department of Human Sources, Blue Cross Blue Shield of Michigan, Michigan's Children Trust Fund, and Korean Health Promotion Foundation, among others.

Chapter 4

Christopher E. Beaudoin (PhD, University of Missouri-Columbia) is a professor in the Department of Communication at Texas A&M University. His program of research is on the social and health consequences of mediated communication. Conducted in domestic and international contexts, this research has commonly focused on the role of the media in promoting health behavior (e.g., cancer screening, smoking prevention, healthy diet, physical activity, family planning, and post-disaster safety) and in advancing social capital and civic participation.

Michael T. Stephenson (PhD, University of Kentucky) is associate vice provost for Institutional Effectiveness and professor in the Department of Communication at Texas A&M University. His research focuses on the media's role in changing or reinforcing health behavior and the moderating and mediating variables that affect health behavior. Most recently, he examined the role of parenting styles on the processing of anti-drug ads directed at parents of adolescents.

Chapter 5

Z. Janet Yang (PhD, Cornell University) is an associate professor of health and risk communication at the University at Buffalo. Her research centers on the communication of risk information related to science, health, and environmental issues. She is particularly interested in how cognitive and affective evaluations of risk influence individuals' decision-making processes. Much of her research is focused on social cognitive variables that influence information seeking, information processing, decision-making, and public perceptions of environmental and health risks. Some of her recent research projects involve climate change, energy, the H1N1 pandemic, and cancer clinical trial. Her research has been funded by the National Science Foundation and the Leukemia & Lymphoma Society.

Susan LaValley is a doctoral student in the Department of Community Health and Health Behavior in the University at Buffalo's School of Public Health and Health Professions. Her current research interests are health literacy, health information seeking, and patient-provider communication. As a former medical librarian, she has extensive experience helping clinical and consumer populations navigate online health information.

Chapter 6

Shoou-Yih Daniel Lee (PhD, University of Michigan) is Chairperson of the Department of Health Policy and Management at the University of North

Carolina at Chapel Hill. His current research addresses issues of health literacy, health care utilization and quality, patient-centered care, and HIT adoption and outcomes in health care organizations. His work has appeared in major health services research and management journals such as *Health Services Research, Medical Care, Medical Care Research and Review, Health Affairs, Health Care Management Review, Social Science & Medicine,* and *Journal of the American Medical Informatics Association.*

Tzu-I Tsai (Ph.D., University of California, Los Angeles, 2005) is a professor in the School of Nursing at National Yang-Ming University in Taiwan. Her research interests focus on health literacy, health education and promotion, maternal and child health, and immigrant health. Her work has appeared in health communication and nursing journals, such as *Journal of Health Communication, Health Education & Behavior, Health Promotion International, International Journal of Nursing Studies,* and *Journal of Clinical Nursing.*

Chapter 7

Bruce E. Pinkleton (Ph.D., Michigan State University, 1992) is Associate Dean of the Edward R. Murrow College of Communication at Washington State University. His research focuses on the role of individual motivations and information source use in individuals' decision-making processes in health and political contexts, including evaluating communication campaign effectiveness. His research has been funded by a variety of organizations including the National Center for Complementary and Integrative Health. His research has appeared in a number of communication and health-related journals including *Pediatrics, Communication Research,* the *Journal of Communication, Health Communication,* and the *Journal of Health Communication.*

Erica Weintraub Austin (Ph.D. Stanford University) is interim Co-Provost for Academic Affairs at Washington State University. Her research and outreach efforts focus on how media literacy and parent-child communication about media contribute to decision making about health and civic affairs among children, adolescents and young adults. Her research has been funded by a variety of organizations including the National Cancer Institute and the U.S. Department of Agriculture. Her research has appeared a number of communication and health-related journals including *Pediatrics, Communication Research,* the *Journal of Communication, Health Communication,* and the *Journal of Health Communication.*

Chapter 8

See Editors' Bio Sketch Above

Chapter 9

Seth M. Noar (PhD, University of Rhode Island) is a professor in The School of Media and Journalism at the University of North Carolina, Chapel Hill (UNC), and a member of UNC's Lineberger Comprehensive Cancer Center. His work addresses health behavior theories, message design and mass media campaigns, and eHealth applications. Dr. Noar has published more than 100 articles and chapters in a wide range of outlets in the social, behavioral, health, and communication sciences, and he serves on the editorial boards of several leading journals including *Health Communication*, *Communication Yearbook*, and *Journal of Communication*. Dr. Noar has been an investigator on several NIH-funded studies testing health communication strategies for health promotion and disease prevention. He is the co-editor of two books, most recently *eHealth Applications: Promising Strategies for Behavior Change*, published by Routledge. In 2014, Dr. Noar was recognized by Thomson Reuters as among the top 1% most cited researchers in the social sciences.

Jessica Gall Myrick (PhD, University of North Carolina at Chapel Hill) is an assistant professor in the Media School at Indiana University. Her primary research interests pertain to the intersection of health communication, media effects, and communication technology. Specifically, she is interested in the role of discrete emotions and affect in shaping risk perceptions, attitudes, and behaviors related to health and science messages. Her work has appeared in multiple journals, including *Health Communication, Journal of Health Communication, Science Communication,* and *Computers in Human Behavior.* She received her PhD. and a graduate certificate in Interdisciplinary Health Communication from the University of North Carolina at Chapel Hill in 2013. She also holds a BA. (Political Science) and an MA. (Journalism) from Indiana University.

Chapter 10

Claude H. Miller (PhD, University of Arizona) is an associate professor in the Department of Communication at the University of Oklahoma. He was awarded the Gerald R. Miller Outstanding Dissertation Award from NCA in 2001 for his dissertation *Indignation, Defensive Attribution, and Implicit Theories of Moral Character.* His current work investigates human affective responses to influences messages in various contexts by applying emotion, motivation, and social influence theories to a range of communication settings, particularly to mass mediated message designs targeting adolescent, elderly, and minority populations. Principle research areas include the effects of psychological reactance and the restoration of freedom on the inoculation process, and on health promotion and risk prevention messages; the effects of regulatory focus and subliminally induced mortality salience on social influence processes; the study, measurement, and mitigation of confirmation bias through the use of serious games; and the application of vested interest theory to health, crisis, and disaster-related communication.

Chapter 11

Melissa Wanzer (EdD., West Virginia University) is professor in the Communication Studies Department at Canisius College in Buffalo, New York, where she teaches graduate seminars in health communication, interpersonal communication and persuasion and undergraduate courses in health communication, family communication, interpersonal communication, gender, and humor. Her research focuses on the intrapersonal and interpersonal benefits of humor in health, instructional, and organizational contexts. She also studies health care provider-patient communication and the effectiveness of different types of health messages on audiences. Dr. Wanzer's research appears in *Communication Education, Communication Teacher, Communication Studies, Communication Quarterly, Health Communication, Journal of Health Communication, Western Journal of Communication, Qualitative Research Reports,* and *Communication Research Reports.* Dr. Wanzer, along with students enrolled in her health campaigns class, partnered with Roswell Park Cancer Institute (RPCI) to design and implement a comprehensive testicular cancer campaign at Canisius College. This campaign received two PRSA Silver Excalibur Awards.

Melanie Booth-Butterfield (PhD, University of Missouri) is a professor in the Department of Communication Studies at West Virginia. Her research focuses on humor, emotion, and interpersonal/relational interactions, emphasizing how communication patterns and traits affect message reception, encoding, and behavior. Dr. Booth-Butterfield's research has been published in *Communication Monographs, Human Communication Research, Communication Education, Journal of Applied Communication, Communication Quarterly, Southern Journal of Communication, Western Journal of Communication, Communication Studies, Communication Reports,* and *Communication Research Reports,* as well as numerous book chapters. She has been editor of *Communication Education, Communication Quarterly,* and *Communication Research Reports,* is past president of ECA, and author of the textbooks *Interpersonal Essentials* and *Influential Health Communication.*

Chapter 12

Xiaoquan Zhao (PhD, University of Pennsylvania) is associate professor in the Department of Communication at George Mason University. His research focuses on health message design and effects, evaluation of public communication campaigns, health information seeking, news effects on health and risk perceptions, and the role of the self in health behavior and persuasive communication. He has published widely in journals such as the *Journal of Communication, Human Communication Research, Communication Research, Communication Monographs, Health Communication*, and *Nature Climate Change*. His work has received support from both public and private funding sources, such as the FDA, NSF, and Merck Co. In 2013–2014, he was awarded the IOM/FDA Tobacco Regulatory Science Fellowship and conducted research at the FDA's Center for Tobacco Products.

Joseph N. Cappella (PhD, Michigan State University) is the Gerald R. Miller Professor of Communication at the Annenberg School for Communication at the University of Pennsylvania. His research has resulted in more than 150 articles and book chapters and four books. The articles have appeared in journals in psychology, communication, health, and politics. His research has been supported by grants from NIMH, NIDA, NSF, NCI, NHGRI, the FDA, The Twentieth Century Fund, and from the Markel, Ford, Carnegie, Pew, and Robert Wood Johnson foundations. His book with Kathleen Hall Jamieson on the spiral of cynicism has won prizes from the American Political Science Association and the ICA. He is a fellow of the International Communication Association and its past president, a distinguished scholar of the National Communication Association, and recipient of the B. Aubrey Fisher Mentorship Award.

Chapter 13

See Editors' Bio Sketch Above

Chapter 14

Jounghwa Choi (PhD, Michigan State University) is an associate professor in the Department of Advertising at Hallym University. Her current research interests focus on the effect of mass media and communication technologies on health behaviors and health-related beliefs, and health/risk message strategies for public communication campaigns. Her recent research has been published in related communication journals, such as *Health Communication, Journal* *of Health Communication, Korean Journal of Public Relations Research,* and *Korean Journal of Advertising & Public Relations.* Dr. Choi has served on the board of directors for Korean Health Communication Association and Korean Academic Society for Public Relations and is a member of the International Communication Association.

Hyunyi Cho (PhD, Michigan State University) is a professor in the Brian Lamb School of Communication at Purdue University. Current research investigates effects of communication on judgments and actions relevant to environmental risk and health risk and the role of messages and the media in social change and behavior change processes. While the immediate goal of this research program is to inform communicative approaches to risk prevention and health promotion efforts, the long term goal of this work is to contribute to advances in communication theory and research. She has edited two volumes, *Health Communication Message Design: Theory and Practice* (Sage, 2012) and the *Sage Handbook of Risk Communication* (2015). Cho is currently the principal investigator of a National Cancer Institute's R01 grant funded research project.

Chapter 15

Nick Carcioppolo (PhD, Purdue University) is an assistant professor of Communication Studies and director of the Cancer Communication Lab at the University of Miami. His research focuses on persuasion and health communication largely in the context of cancer prevention and screening. His research has been published in refereed outlets such as *Health Communication, Public Understanding of Science,* and *Journal of Communication.*

Chapter 16

Lee Ann Kahlor (PhD, University of Wisconsin—Madison) is an associate professor in the Stan Richards School of Advertising and Public Relations at the University of Texas at Austin. She researches risk information seeking in health, environmental, and science contexts. In that work she focuses on psychosocial predictors of seeking, avoiding, and sharing information. She also studies expert communication, with a focus on perceived norms and barriers related to the communication of science-focused information with lay audiences and the media. Her work has appeared in *Health Communication, Journal of Health Communication, Communication Research, Human Communication Research, Science Communication,* and other journals, and she co-edited the 2010 book *Communicating Science: New Agendas in Communication.*

Ming-Ching Liang (PhD, University of Texas at Austin) is an assistant professor from the Department of Communication, Writing, and the Arts at Metropolitan State University. His research mainly focuses on strategic communication about health, science, and environmental issues. His areas of interest include risk information behaviors, health campaigns, media coverage on health and environmental risks, and unintended consequences of risk communication. Liang's research can be found in *Health Communication, Journal of Health Communication, American Journal of Infection Control, American Journal of Health Behavior, Nature Nanotechnology,* and *Human Communication Research.*

Chapter 17

Brian L. Quick (PhD, Texas A&M University), is a pro¬fessor in the Department of Communication and the College of Medicine at the University of Illinois at Urbana-Champaign. His research interests involve health communication campaigns, media portrayals of health, and an examination of how individuals cognitively and emotionally process per¬suasive health messages. His research has resulted in more than 50 article and book chapter publications. The majority of his funded research on organ donation campaigns has been supported by NIH. Quick has received several teaching awards as well notoriety for his public outreach. He currently serves as a senior editor of *Health Communication* as well as serving on several editorial boards including *Communication Research, Communication Yearbook, Journal of Communication, Journal of Applied Communication Research,* and the *Journal of Health Communication.*

Tobias Reynolds-Tylus (M.A, University at Buffalo, The State University of New York, 2013), is a doctoral student in the Department of Communication at the University of Illinois at Urbana-Champaign. His research focuses on persuasion and health communication, largely in the contexts of organ donation and sexual decision making. His work has been presented at national and international conferences, and in refereed journals including *Journal of Health Communication* and *Progress in Transplantation.*

Chapter 18

Craig Trumbo (PhD, University of Wisconsin–Madison) is a professor in the Department of Journalism and Technical Communication at Colorado State University. His research addresses a range of interests involving health, risk, and the environment. Past and current projects include risk perception from suspected environmental cancer hazards, the effect of hazard proximity on risk perception, optimistic bias in risk perception, decision-making processes concerning hurricane evacuation, and social normative factors affecting use of electronic cigarettes. His areas of university teaching experience have included mass media effects, mass and interpersonal communication theory, research methods and applied statistics, communication of science and technology, and risk communication.

Se-Jin Kim is a doctoral student in the Department of Journalism and Technical Communication at Colorado State University. His current research interests pertain to science/risk and health/environmental communication. His dissertation project "Need for Affect and Cognition as Precursors to Risk Perception, Information Processing, and Behavioral Intent" proposes a hybrid theoretical model of risk-based behavioral attitude and intention that is based on the theory of reasoned action, dual processing risk perception, the heuristic systematic model, need for cognition, and need for affect. This work is aimed toward contributing to the creation of more effective messages as well as identifying appropriate channels for current and future science/risk and health/environmental communication. He has published several book chapters and journal articles, and also presented papers at numerous conferences.

Chapter 19

Erin L. Mead (PhD, 2014, Johns Hopkins University) is a post-doctoral fellow in the Tobacco Center of Regulatory Science at the University of Maryland, School of Public Health. Dr. Mead uses mixed methods to understand the multilevel factors that contribute to disparities in cancer prevention and tobacco use among high risk, priority populations, including low-income, minority, and young adult populations. Her work aims to inform tobacco control policy as well as the development and evaluation of theory-based, health communication and social and behavioral programs to promote tobacco cessation and cancer prevention.

Rajiv N. Rimal (PhD, Stanford University) is professor and chair of the Department of Prevention and Community Health at the Milken Institute School of Public Health at George Washington University. His scholarship focuses on developing and testing theory-based approaches for behavior change. Much of his work in the last 10 years in sub-Saharan Africa has focused on conducting and evaluating various interventions to prevent HIV/AIDS. He is particularly interested in understanding how risk perceptions and community norms affect behaviors.

Chapter 20

Nichole Egbert (PhD, University of Georgia) holds the rank of professor in the School of Communication Studies at Kent State University. Her research centers predominantly on social support in health contexts with a specific focus on family caregiving. Other research interests include spirituality/religiosity and health behavior and health literacy. She actively collaborates with a wide range of researchers, including those in the fields of nursing, public health, medicine, and communication. Her work can be found in outlets such as *Health Communication, Journal of Health Communication, Journal of Communication and Religion, Communication Yearbook,* and the 2011 *Routledge Handbook of Health Communication.*

Phillip R. Reed is a doctoral candidate in Communication and Information at Kent State University. His research focuses on ethical concerns in interpersonal conflict and persuasion. He situates himself at the intersection of social science and ethical philosophy, investigating each through the other's lens.

Chapter 21

See the Author's Bio Sketch for Chapter 10

Chapter 22

Stephen A. Rains (PhD, University of Texas at Austin) is associate professor of Communication at the University of Arizona. His research is situated in the general areas of communication and technology, health communication, and social influence. Much of his scholarship intersects these domains and explores the implications of new communication technologies for health communication. His research examining the use and consequences of new communication technologies for social support among adults coping with illness can be found in journals such as *Human Communication Research, Communication Monographs, Communication Research, Health Communication,* and *Journal of Computer-Mediated Communication.*

Chapter 23

Mary J. Bresnahan (PhD, University of Michigan) is a professor in the Department of Communication at Michigan State University. She is interested in obesity stigma and nutritional stigma experienced by people living in the inner city.

Jie Zhuang (PhD, Michigan State University) is a post-doctoral scholar in the Department of Communication at Michigan State University where she works as a grant manager. She has collaborated with Professor Bresnahan on several stigma studies.

Chapter 24

Kerk F. Kee (PhD, The University of Texas at Austin) is an assistant professor in the Department of Communication Studies, and a core faculty member in the interdisciplinary MS in Health & Strategic Communication program, at Chapman University. His research centers on the diffusion of innovations theory. He studies the flow of health information through social clusters in online communities, the spread of big data technologies through cross-disciplinary collaborations in scientific organizations, and more recently, the dissemination of pro-environmental behaviors through persuasive messages in modern societies. The interest in numeracy stems from observing the quantitative nature of health, scientific, and environmental information across his projects. Kerk's diffusion research has been funded by the National Science Foundation and the Bill & Melinda Gates Foundation. His work has appeared in journals such as *Health Communication*; *CyberPsychology, Behavior, & Social Networking*; *Journal of Computer-Mediated Communication*; *Computer Supported Cooperative Work*; *IEEE Computer*, etc.

Yuhua (Jake) Liang (PhD, Michigan State University) is an assistant professor in the Department of Communication Studies at Chapman University. His research focuses on persuasion in communication contexts enabled by technology. One area of focus examines how readers evaluate multiple sources of information they encounter on social media or participatory platforms (e.g., multiple product reviews and ratings on systems such as Amazon.com). Another area of focus involves how computer agents (e.g., autonomous programs) and robots may persuade and gain trust from humans in order to work collaboratively. As a rule, Jake aims to utilize the theoretical contributions from his work by applying them to real-life problems. For example, he has worked on a HRSA-funded health campaign promoting organ donation by managing advertisements on Facebook.com that drives inter-campus competition. He currently teaches in the BA in Strategic and Corporate Communication and the MS in Health and Strategic Communication programs.

Chapter 25

Roxanne Parrott (PhD, University of Arizona) is Distinguished Professor of Communication Arts & Sciences, and Health Policy & Administration at Penn State. She also serves as faculty for both the dual title graduate degree program in Bioethics & Humanities and the Homeland Security & Public Health Preparedness program. Her research focuses on efforts to derive theoretical insights to guide health message design, with her 2009 award-winning book, *Talking about Health: Why Communication Matters*, emphasizing the importance of clinical and public health communication about genomics to guide informed health decisions. Dr. Parrott's funded research has derived insights regarding the management of uncertainty related to genetic diagnoses, and the dualistic nature of genetic determinism, including both threat and essentialist components. She has developed a model to explain the effects of metaphor use on essentialist beliefs and involvement with genomic health messages.

Rachel A. Smith (PhD, Michigan State University) is an associate professor in the Department of Communication Arts and Sciences at Pennsylvania State University. Smith is a quantitative, social scientist who studies social influences in health. Her research centers on identifying message features and relational dynamics associated with the adoption and diffusion of positive and negative health beliefs and behaviors. For example, she has developed and tested theories focusing on the relationships and dynamics among communication, health, and stigmas. She uses a variety of quantitative methods, including dyadic analysis and social network analysis, to investigate these issues. She has expertise in health message design and evaluation, and extensive experience with the evaluation of funded programs nationally and internationally. She has made numerous presentations in scientific, technical, policy, and advocacy fora, and authored over 60 scientific, technical, and public health articles and chapters, the majority in peer-reviewed journals.

Amy E. Chadwick (PhD, Pennsylvania State University) is an assistant professor in the School of Communication Studies, Scripps College of Communication at the Ohio University. Her research is in the areas of persuasion, message design, health communication, and environmental communication. Much of her research examines how communication messages can affect attitudes, beliefs, and behaviors related to health and environmental issues, such as climate change, vaccination, advance care planning, and obesity. Dr. Chadwick is particularly interested in identifying intrinsic message features that create the discrete emotion hope and exploring how these messages and feelings of hope can promote pro-social change. She has developed and is continuously refining a theory of persuasive hope that identifies the causes and persuasive consequences of hope. In addition, she is examining the effects of hope on psychophysiological markers of stress. Dr. Chadwick also studies environmental and health disparities in rural Appalachia.

Chapter 26

Claude H. Miller
See the Author's Bio Sketch for Chapter 10

Bradley J. Adame (PhD, University of Oklahoma) is an assistant professor in the Hugh Downs School of Human Communication at Arizona State University. His research focuses on social influence, strategic message design, and behavioral outcomes in risk perception and crisis communication contexts. For example, he has studied how people respond to communication campaigns designed to promote disaster preparedness in areas of the country suffering high rates for weather disasters. His current work uses experimental techniques to understand the role of communication in preventing, creating, and mitigating organizational and community-based crises and disasters. Additional research areas include the roles of cognitive and affective processing of health campaign messages, the role of vested interest in predicting self-protective behavior, and the effects of fear in pro-social campaign messages.

Chapter 27

Kevin Wright (PhD, University of Oklahoma) is a professor of Communication at George Mason University. He has focused much of his research on social support processes and health outcomes in both face-to-face and computer-mediated contexts. He is the author of five books, including *Health Communication in the 21ˢᵗ Century* and *Computer-Mediated Communication in Personal Relationships*. He has published over 70 articles and book chapters, and his research appears in numerous journals such as *Communication Monographs, Journal of Computer-Mediated Communication, Journal of Communication, Health Communication, Journal of Health Communication, Journal of Applied Communication Research, Journal of Personal and Social Relationships, Communication Quarterly, Communication Studies,* and several other publications. Dr. Wright served from 2007 to 2010 as editor of the *Journal of Computer-Mediated Communication* published by the International Communication Association. He also serves on numerous editorial boards of various communication journals and is a frequent presenter at regional, national, and international communication conferences.

Index

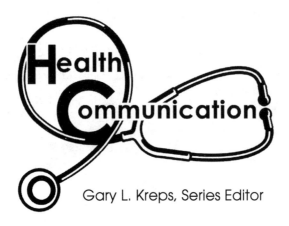

Gary L. Kreps, Series Editor

This series examines the powerful influences of human and mediated communication in delivering care and promoting health.

Books analyze the ways that strategic communication humanizes and increases access to quality care as well as examining the use of communication to encourage proactive health promotion. The books describe strategies for addressing major health issues, such as reducing health disparities, minimizing health risks, responding to health crises, encouraging early detection and care, facilitating informed health decisionmaking, promoting coordination within and across health teams, overcoming health literacy challenges, designing responsive health information technologies, and delivering sensitive end-of-life care.

All books in the series are grounded in broad evidence-based scholarship and are vivid, compelling, and accessible to broad audiences of scholars, students, professionals, and laypersons.

For additional information about this series or for the submission of manuscripts, please contact:

Gary L. Kreps
University Distinguished Professor and Chair, Department of Communication
Director, Center for Health and Risk Communication
George Mason University Science & Technology 2, Suite 230, MS 3D6
Fairfax, VA 22030-4444
gkreps@gmu.edu

To order other books in this series, please contact our Customer Service Department:

(800) 770-LANG (within the U.S.)
(212) 647-7706 (outside the U.S.)
(212) 647-7707 FAX

Or browse online by series:
www.peterlang.com